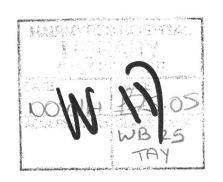

Qualitative Research in the Health Sciences

Methodologies, methods and processes

Bev Taylor and Karen Francis

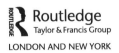

Routledge
Taylor & Francis Group

LONDON AND NEW YORK

First published 2013
by Routledge
2 Park Square, Milton Park, Abingdon, Oxon, OX14 4RN

Simultaneously published in the USA and Canada
by Routledge
711 Third Avenue, New York, NY 10017

Routledge is an imprint of the Taylor & Francis Group, an informa business

British Library Cataloguing in Publication Data
A catalogue record for this book is available from the British Library

Library of Congress Cataloging-in-Publication Data
Taylor, Beverley J. (Beverley Joan), 1951– author.
    Qualitative research in the health sciences : methodologies,
    methods, and processes / Beverley Taylor and Karen Francis.
        p. ; cm.
    Includes bibliographical references.
    I. Francis, Karen, 1959– author. II. Title.
    [DNLM: 1. Biomedical Research--methods. 2. Qualitative Research.
    W 20.5]
    610.72′4--dc23   2012049532

ISBN13: 978-0-415-68260-2 (hbk)
ISBN13: 978-0-415-68261-9 (pbk)
ISBN13: 978-0-203-77717-6 (ebk)

Typeset in Palatino by
HWA Text and Data Management, London

This book is dedicated by Bev Taylor to Carmen Zammit and Estelle Myers, two previous PhD students, now deceased, who lived life to the fullest and researched their lived experiences.

The book is dedicated by Karen Francis to her husband Peter and her family for their ongoing support. She is indebted to the staff with whom she works for their support, in particular, her assistant Juliearnah Kaandorp. The people in the background enable us to achieve our goals.

Contents

Contents

List of figures and tables

Figures

Tables

Preface

Bev Taylor and Karen Francis welcome readers to this book. Bev Taylor is an expert in qualitative research and reflective practice, who has published 11 research books. Karen Francis is recognized nationally and internationally for her contribution to the development of the discipline of rural nursing. Her highly successful research and publication agendas have focused on exploring the realities of nursing in rural environments, health workforce, preparation for practice, emergent contexts of practice, and rural populations' health issues.

This book covers a comprehensive range of qualitative research methodologies, methods and processes for health science teachers, clinicians and researchers, who have moved beyond basic research preparation to postgraduate levels. Therefore, the book has been written in a scholarly way to extend readers' knowledge, but it will also use accessible, practical language to extend readers' practical research skills.

The need for this book arose from a growing interest and acceptance in the health science disciplines of qualitative research approaches, as "stand alone" methodologies and/or integrated with quantitative designs in mixed methods approaches. The needs were sufficiently important to support a new book, because many existing research books are discipline-specific (i.e., written only for nurses or social workers), they are written for beginning researchers, they concentrate on a method, e.g., interviewing, focus groups, and/or they offer too little qualitative research information, and feature too much quantitative research. Therefore, this book responds to the need for an advanced, comprehensive research text with predominantly qualitative content, because of postgraduate teachers', clinicians' and researchers' needs for one book, which will provide deeper knowledge and application of qualitative methodologies, and congruent methods and processes.

The original impulse for writing the book came from a qualitative research module for the health sciences, written by Professor Desley Hegney, and taught by Professor Taylor for the first time in Semester One, 2010, at the National University of Singapore. The postgraduate students in this module enjoyed the content to such an extent, and texts that covered a broad range of content in a single book were so difficult to locate, that it became evident that a comprehensive research text was needed as soon as possible, giving a full, advanced level explication of the main qualitative research methodologies, methods and processes.

This book provides:

- A comprehensive collection of fully described qualitative research methodologies, methods and processes;

- High level theoretical content of the philosophies subsumed within the methodologies;

- Easy to follow practical advice for using research methods and processes congruent with the theoretical assumptions of the methodologies;

- A review of the main aspects of the process for developing a research project;

- A review of essential quantitative research designs to integrate with qualitative research in mixed methods approaches; and

- A full description of the uptake of qualitative research in the health sciences, in relation to evidence-based practice, practice development and research translation.

We hope you enjoy reading this book and that it becomes a practical resource for assisting you in undertaking high quality research using qualitative research methodologies, methods and processes.

Part I

Methodologies

In the first chapter of Part I of this book, our initial task as authors is to refresh your memory of some fundamental ideas relating to qualitative research, by clarifying what we mean by methodologies, methods and processes. We imagine you are most probably reading this book to assist you in undertaking research in the health sciences after basic research and practice preparation, so you already know about research in general, and you will have an interest in generating research evidence for your practice. By way of introduction, this book begins with some statements about each of the aforementioned foundational areas, before discussing world views guiding approaches to research, including quantitative and qualitative approaches, and the integration of both in mixed methods research. Lastly, we review some ideas about postmodern influences on paradigmatic shifts in research, before flagging the methodologies from Chapter 2 onwards.

1

Introduction

Bev Taylor

Differentiating methodologies, methods and processes

Qualitative research invites you to inquire about the human condition, because it explores the meaning of human experiences and creates the possibilities of change through raised awareness and purposeful action. People communicate their meanings through language, so words and language are fundamental tools for creating and validating knowledge in qualitative research. As it is with any other focus of human interest, specific words denote the fundamental ideas, and in qualitative research you must be conversant with these words and what they mean, in order to communicate meaningfully with other researchers and the research participants. In order to discuss qualitative research and 'do' it well, it is important to be clear about the definitions of key terms, and at the outset of reading this book, it is very important for you to differentiate between qualitative methodologies, methods and processes and understand their interrelationships.

In qualitative research, methodologies are particular sets of theoretical assumptions, which underlie the choice of data collection and analysis methods and processes (Taylor, Kermode and Roberts, 2006). This means that qualitative interpretive methodologies, such as grounded theory, historical research, ethnography and phenomenology, and qualitative critical methodologies, such as action research, critical ethnography, discourse analysis and feminism, all have deep, broad theoretical bases on which they base their search for new or amended, valid knowledge.

The methods and processes you use in collecting and analysing data depend on your choice of methodology. Methods are *what* you do to collect and analyse data, and processes are *how* you go about doing them. For example, in the methodology of grounded theory there are some well validated step-by-step methods for collecting and analysing data (Glaser and Strauss, 1967; Strauss and Corbin, 1998). The processes of how you undertake grounded theory will fit with the methodological assumptions of grounded theory and the nature of your researcher/participant relationship, so your inductive approach may include inviting participants to share their experiences of an area in which

3

little is known, through an exploratory data collection method, such as an interview, and of being aware constantly of how to undertake the grounded theory project authentically from the start to the finish.

The research methods and processes merge into a meshwork of what you are doing and how you are doing it, for example, in the grounded theory method of analysis of the first transcribed interview you will search for codes and when you are clear about the contributions of the first participant's account of the research area, you may need to extend the questions in the subsequent interview, and so on, to increase theoretical sampling until data are saturated, the codes fit into categories, and the integrated constructs lead to a grounded theory of the research area of inquiry. Therefore, the integrated grounded theory methods and processes involve having a sense of being on a mission of discovery, continually enacting the agreed ethical safeguards for and with participants, while following a systematic inductive approach, being open to what emerges, using memoing, conceptual diagrams and literature to extend your thinking, recognizing when no further codes are emerging in the data, and integrating the categories into meaningful theoretical statements. The methods and processes for other methodologies will vary according to the methodological assumptions of the specific approach and be in accord with your research aims, objectives and questions.

Differentiating the meaning of words is important, because basic problems arise by being unclear about terminology, which grow into major epistemological misunderstandings and debates, simply because words are used without due care, resulting in a lack of shared meaning. For example, the claims for the balanced, integrated innovation and benefits of mixed methods research are based to some extent on the complementarity of quantitative and qualitative methodologies (Tashakkori and Teddlie, 2010), when what is actually done is an adoption of an implicit postpositivistic orientation about mixed methods (Giddings and Williams, 2006; Hesse-Biber and Leavy, 2010).

Research after basic preparation

Increasingly, health sciences professionals are embracing qualitative research methodologies, methods and processes (Bhavnani and Fisher, 2010; Bower and Scambler, 2007; Égalité, Özdemir, and Godard, 2007; McKeown, Clarke, Ingleton, and Repper, 2010; Miller et al., 2008; Shaw, 2003; Skeat and Perry, 2008; Stein and Mankowski, 2004; Swift and Tischler, 2010). This book is geared towards people engaged in the health sciences and healthcare professionals, who have moved beyond their undergraduate research training, to postgraduate levels, although this book can be of help to anyone who takes the time and makes the effort to grapple with its ideas. As the book's authors, our intention is to engage you in epistemological conversations, which will help you to review your ideas about the 'big stories' that make up the pedagogy of qualitative methodologies, methods and processes. Our conversations will be facilitated through the tone and content of our writing and your willingness to engage in critical thinking about the ideas we put forward in exercises as 'food for thought'.

Qualitative research has moved into and beyond postmodernism, so as this book's authors we acknowledge that our writing puts us firmly into the role of agents of authority, but in the role of a reader, you have the freedom to mediate on our writing and decide for yourself the extent to which you take on the ideas. We are aware that multiple interpretations can be made about each and every methodology, method and process, so our intention as authors is to provide a practical way through the conceptual maze of qualitative research, so you can build your own ideas and make adaptations as you see fit. Therefore, two principles with which we align and apply throughout this book to qualitative research, are the need for epistemological congruency, and the need for some relatively stable conceptual structures.

The need for epistemological congruency

Congruency connotes links, connections, continuities, consistencies, coherence, cohesiveness and comprehensibility. In relation to qualitative research, congruency means linking and connecting ideas, so that there is a discernible flow and fit between the ideas arising from the entire research inquiry, from the questions, aims and objectives, right through to the data collection and analysis methods and processes, and the eventual research insights and implications, that show the application and progression of ideas 'faithful' to the foundational ideas of a respective methodology.

The faithfulness in congruency is akin to 'being true to the spirit or nature' of a particular methodology's basic ideas. For example, congruency is discernible in an ethnographic research project when the chosen methods and processes of data collection and analysis reflect knowledge about the habits, rituals, patterns, symbols and shared understandings of a particular culture or subculture, so you would expect to see the people who comprise the culture being described in their context. An ethnographic researcher looks closely as an interested and focused observer, at a group of people in their context, to generate, validate and report rich descriptions of their ways of being, which tell us more than we knew or understood previously about that group of people. The ethnographic research report becomes more comprehensible and 'believable' when it is found to be in tune with the basic assumptions of the anchoring ethnographic ideas.

In this postmodern era of extremely relative representations of knowledge, it may seem strange for us as authors to appeal to readers to be mindful of the need for congruency in qualitative research, but we recognize, and hold to the need to fulfil, some criteria for a project's trustworthiness. If there is no sign of congruency in a qualitative project, how can a reader discern if a study can be 'trusted'? If there is no flow, fit or match between a qualitative project's aims, objectives, methodological assumptions, methods and processes, and the new or amended insights it generates, what is it but a jumble of incoherent ideas with no purpose, direction or useful end point? Without congruency, a qualitative project's transitions and multiple end points may be interesting and poetic reading, but how can we know that the research is worthwhile for advancing the human-focused interests of the health sciences, and indeed, that it is not a hoax or 'fashionable nonsense' (Sokal, Bricmont, and Dawkins, 1998)?

Postmodern theorists have been criticized for creating an absurd philosophy through 'a pistache of Left-wing cant, fawning references, grandiose quotations, and outright nonsense' (Sokal, 1996, p. 217). In a well-publicized publication hoax, a New York University physics professor tricked the editors of *Social Text*, an influential academic journal of cultural studies, into publishing an article pretending to compare the similarities between quantum gravitational theory and postmodern philosophy. Sokal (1996) used the most fashionable postmodern terms and the 'silliest quotations' by postmodern academics that he could locate about mathematics and physics, to invent a position on '*Transgressing the boundaries: Towards a transformative hermeneutics of quantum gravity*'. Based on Sokal's reputation in physics and his ability to write obscure pseudo-postmodern arguments with academic authority, the journal's editor published the article without peer review. The exposure of the hoax by Sokal soon after, resulted in highly publicized academic and public quarrels internationally, about the scholarly merit of the journal, the right of authors to publish cross-disciplinary critiques, and the academic ethics of the matter.

To further advance his concerns about postmodern theorists' tendencies to misrepresent the science of mathematics and physics, Sokal teamed with Bricmont and Dawkins (1998), to 'thoughtfully and thoroughly dismantle the pseudo scientific writings of some of the most fashionable French and American intellectuals' (Sokal et al., 1998, book cover). In the book, entitled *Fashionable nonsense: Postmodern intellectuals' abuse of science*, the authors defended the foundations of the scientific method and its successful outcomes and discredited the postmodern idea that scientific theories are 'narrations' or social constructions. Interestingly, the original 'Sokal hoax' and the subsequent book (Sokal et al., 1998) have assisted in ushering in a reactionary turn against postmodernists, even to the point of ridiculing them, for example, in the form of a dictionary of fashionable nonsense, to be used if you are 'ever trapped at a party with a crowd of trendy academics' (Benson and Stangroom, 2004).

Even with wariness to watch out for postmodern hoaxes and safeguards for congruency in qualitative research, there are no guarantees of generating permanent, unshakeable 'truth', nor is there any intention to do so. Somewhere between the certainty of the absolute positivist research tradition and the extreme tentativeness of the ultra relativistic postmodern research tradition, there are multiple shifting points, which allow qualitative researchers to propose credible projects and follow them through with due care, so that the end points offer insights and suggestions can be 'trusted' and possibly transferable after careful scrutiny, debate, discussion and negotiation by the readers and research audience.

> **Food for thought**
> If we cannot create and validate knowledge that demonstrates congruency, have we done qualitative research, or have we engaged in some other form of literary expression or inquiry? What is your position on this epistemological issue?

The need for some relatively stable conceptual structures

In the postmodern era and beyond, knowledge loses its permanency and ideas are 'up for grabs' in highly relativistic epistemologies. However, the terrain of epistemology is perilous if you do not know where you are going, or how you hope to get there. While maintaining a degree of tentativeness about the nature of truth, given the relativistic, context-dependent and subjective forms of qualitative knowledge, as authors we hold on to the idea that some relatively stable conceptual structures are available, where you can rely on some depth and breadth of new understanding and rest a while on ultimately temporary, yet stable ideas. This epistemological positioning makes our grand narratives in qualitative methodologies a little less grand and a lot less arrogant, because we acknowledge the uncertain and unknowable aspects of inquiry into human experiences and constraints, while avoiding the epistemological emptiness in having no faith whatsoever in any kind of knowledge, as asserted in a sceptical postmodern view (Rosenau, 1992).

The need for relatively stable conceptual structures, even if they are by definition ultimately temporary, comes about because your health science research needs to be focused, manageable and useful, if it is to be judged well by examiners and readers and taken up as evidence in practice and academic settings. The need for focus, manageability and usefulness are inescapable in the health sciences, because all fields within health sciences have as their direct or indirect focus, the 'good of the patient' and the progression of their specific disciplinary knowledge and skills directed towards healthcare.

Relative stability in conceptual structures is an impermanent concept, because we realize that hope and faith in the stability of 'truth' keeps on changing over time. Kvale (1995, p. 23) provided a straightforward explanation of how the 'truthfulness' of knowledge has been construed over the ages, from the 'philosophy of the Enlightenment (which) was a reaction against the religious dogma of the medieval ages', to the modern era of positivism, when 'the belief in one true and objective reality, stable and universal' replaced the belief in one God. Kvale (1995) explained

> In a postmodern era the belief in foundations of true knowledge in an absolute God or an objective reality has dissolved. The conception of knowledge as a true mirror of reality is preplaced by knowledge as a linguistic and social construction of reality. There is a focus upon interpretation and negotiation of the meaning of the lived world … A move from knowledge as correspondence with an objective reality to

knowledge as a communal construction of reality involves a change in emphasis from observation to conversation and interaction. Truth is constituted though dialogue; valid knowledge claims emerge as conflicting interpretations and action possibilities are discussed and negotiated among the members of a community (p. 23).

While we do not subscribe to the existence of 'one true and objective reality, stable and universal', as this book's authors, we are aware of the need for some relatively stable conceptual structures as ideas which you can discuss and negotiate with members of your health science community, to clarify interpretations and decide on the possibilities for pragmatic action in your discipline. Therefore, even though our form of stable conceptual structures have no more permanency than for a frog landing on a lily pad, they do give you somewhere to sit for a while, while you decide on where to jump next in your ever-constant search for coherent knowledge, which is relevant and useful to your field of health science.

Research in the health sciences

As a postgraduate reader, the days are long behind you of grappling with questions, such as: What is health? What is disease? Of more importance to you now, we imagine, are the big health science issues and how to make sense of huge collections of data about health establishment, maintenance and restoration, from various sources, such as the World Wide Web, peer reviewed publications, books, professional conference presentations and the popular press. As a beginning point for considering the contribution of qualitative research in the health sciences globally, we need to return to some basic organizing ideas about health, health systems and the composition of the health sciences and take a fresh look at conceptualizing these areas.

Focusing on health

Health is a mainstream concern within and across nations and it is often a matter of public interest, with health issues featuring on radio and TV news broadcasts, alerting us to the personal dangers of risky lifestyle choices, such as smoking, high fat diets and alcohol, and galvanizing us into action when community threats occur, for example, the H1N1 influenza pandemic in 2009 and the radioactive contamination issues in Japan, during the tsunami aftermath in 2011. As a global issue, health is also a mainstream topic, the professional and public interest in which is maintained by recognized health-related organizations, such as the World Health Organization (WHO) and the Organisation for Economic Cooperation and Development (OECD). The WHO (www.who.int) and OECD (www.oecd.org) (Health Policies, Data and Policy Division) provide data on health statistics that are readily available in downloads of articles, reports and fact sheets.

Go to Google, type in www.who.int and follow the links to the WHO Statistical Information System (WHOSIS) and you will find the option to download the full report of World Health Statistics (WHO, 2010) in Arabic, Chinese, English or French. The WHO Health Statistics 2010 report is a prime example of how global health data are readily accessible for anyone with access to a computer and an interest in their country's health statistics and global comparisons.

Alternatively, go to www.oecd.org to the Directorate for Employment, Labour and Social Affairs, and you will locate key OECD health publications, analytical health projects, health data projects and health working papers to read online or download. Health is firmly in the public domain via online links, with easily accessible, up-to-date information, which can be used to educate people through public and professional agencies, as well as to be available as data sources for literature reviews and research projects. The wide availability of online health information from reputable sources, such as the WHO and OECD, helps to make health more of matter of informed personal knowledge and choices, taking the 'ownership' of health away from the exclusive possession of health science professionals and organizations, placing it into the hands of the health-seeking public.

Global differences in health systems

Detailed research reports on global differences in health systems are available online (e.g., www.who.int, www.oecd.org, www.commonwealthfund.org, www.kff.org). The relative success of global health systems is measured by the WHO by using the indicators of life expectancy and mortality rates. 'The indicators include overall life expectancy at birth, as well as infant and under-five mortality (the probability of dying between birth and 1 and 5 years of age, respectively), and adult mortality (the probability of dying between 15 and 60 years of age). Levels and trends for child mortality … are particularly relevant in understanding public health because globally almost 20% of all deaths are of children less than 5 years old' (WHO, 2010, p. 45).

Healthcare systems globally vary and they tend to show differences in health outcomes related directly to the wealthiness of a country (WHO, 2010). For example, 'neonatal mortality (death during the first 28 days of life per 1000 live births) accounts for a large proportion of child deaths in many countries, especially in low-income settings' (WHO, 2010, p. 45).

The global health report (WHO, 2010) was cautiously optimistic in its summation of the success of global health systems.

> With only five years remaining to 2015, there are signs of progress in many countries in achieving the health-related Millennium Development Goals (MDGs). In other countries, progress has been limited because of conflict, poor governance, economic or humanitarian crises, and lack of resources. The effects of the global food, energy, financial and economic crises on health are still unfolding, and action is needed to protect the health spending of governments and donors alike.
>
> (WHO, 2010, p. 12)

The inequities in global health systems are still evident, as shown in the WHO (2010) key points. (The emphasis in bold font is as in the original report.)

- **Undernutrition** is an underlying cause in about one third of all child deaths (p. 12).

- **Child mortality** continues to fall. The greatest reductions in child mortality have been recorded among the wealthiest households and in urban areas (p. 12).

- There have been increases in the coverage of relatively new **child health interventions**, such as the use of insecticide-treated nets to prevent malaria; efforts to prevent the mother-to-child transmission of HIV; and vaccination against hepatitis B and *Haemophilus influenzae* type B pneumonia (p. 13).

- The coverage of critical interventions such as oral rehydration therapy (ORT) for diarrhoea and case management with antibiotics for acute respiratory infections (ARIs) remains inadequate. As a result, diarrhoea and pneumonia still kill almost 3 million children under 5 years old each year, especially in low-income countries (p. 14).

- For the year 2005, half a million women – most of them in developing countries – die each year of complications during pregnancy or childbirth (p. 14).

- **Contraceptive prevalence** in developing countries increased from 50 per cent in 1990 to 62 per cent in 2005. Despite this, there remains a continuing unmet need for family planning (p. 15).

- In 2008, there were an estimated 243 million cases of **malaria** causing 863,000 deaths; mostly of children under 5 years old. Despite increases in the supply of insecticide-treated nets, their availability in that year was far below the level of need almost everywhere. The procurement of antimalarial medicines through public health services increased, but access to treatment (especially artemisinin-based combination therapy) was inadequate in all countries surveyed in 2007 and 2008. There are, however, indications that 9 African countries and 29 countries outside Africa are on course to meet the MDG target for reducing the malaria burden (p. 16).

- Latest estimates indicate that the incidence rate of **tuberculosis** continued to slowly decline (p. 16).

- New **HIV** infections have been reduced by 16 per cent globally between 2000 and 2008, due, at least in part, to successful HIV-prevention efforts. In 2008, it was estimated that 2.7 million people were newly infected with HIV … and there were 2 million **HIV/AIDS**-related deaths (p. 16).

- More than 1,000 million people are affected by **neglected tropical diseases** (p. 18).

- The percentage of the world's population using 'improved' **drinking-water** sources increased from 77 per cent to 87 per cent between 1990 and 2008 (p. 18).

- In 2008, 2,600 million people were not using 'improved' **sanitation** facilities, and of these 1,100 million were defecating in the open, resulting in high levels of environmental contamination and exposure to the risks of worm infestations (such as schistosomiasis) and microbial infections (such as trachoma, hepatitis and cholera) (p. 19).

- **Noncommunicable diseases and injuries** caused an estimated 33 million deaths in developing countries in 2004 and will account for a growing proportion of total deaths in the future. The health of individuals will also be undermined in the longer term by chronic conditions, sensory and mental disorders and violence. Tackling risk factors such as tobacco use, unhealthy diets, physical inactivity and the harmful use of alcohol (while also dealing with the socioeconomic impact of cardiovascular diseases, cancers, chronic respiratory diseases and diabetes) will depend not only upon effective healthcare services but also upon actions taken in a variety of policy domains (p. 20).

Socioeconomic inequities in global health systems cause some poorer countries to struggle to provide fundamental needs, such as adequate food and clean water, while affluent systems are trying to prevent and manage diseases brought about by lifestyle excesses. The WHO (2010) Health Statistics are inclusive of developed and under-developed countries and clearly show that wealthier countries have the resources and systems in place to produce good outcomes on population health indicators. Even so, a survey by the Commonwealth Fund (a private foundation working toward a high-performance health system) produced some interesting findings.

Schoen, Osborn, Doty, Squires, Peugh, and Applebaum (2009) undertook a survey study of more than 10,000 primary care physicians in 11 countries (Netherlands, New Zealand, United Kingdom, France, Italy, Germany, Sweden, Australia, Canada, Norway and the United States of America). Data were collected by mail, telephone, and the Internet, from February to July 2009. 'The bottom line' was that 'despite spending more on healthcare than other countries ... the United States lags behind on important measures of access, quality, and use of health information technology' (p. 2).

Health is fundamental to living well. Global health systems are geared towards assisting people to live as well as they can within the particular economic, social, cultural and political constraints operating of a specific country. While statistical information is needed to ascertain the overall patterns and trends of health and disease within countries and globally, this information does not capture descriptions of the human experiences in relation to their health needs, not does it involve collaborative methods and processes to empower people at local levels to make changes in their health systems. Qualitative research approaches, either as 'stand alone' methodologies with their concomitant methods and processes, or used in combination with quantitative methods, are necessary in the health sciences to get to the core of human experiences of health and illness and to facilitate change at personal and governmental levels.

The health sciences

The title of this book boldly promises a comprehensive compilation of qualitative methodologies, methods and processes for people engaged in all types of work in the health sciences. In its broadest sense, we are assuming that 'health scientists' are engaged directly or indirectly in some form of healthcare and that they are preparing or practising professionals from a broad range of healthcare knowledge and practice bases. As medical practitioners are 'health scientists' in managing, teaching, researching and practising medicine, doctors of all kinds are included in this book within the categorization of the health sciences, even though it is customary to see lists specifying 'medical *and* health sciences' in university website listings and research classifications globally.

Given the lack of an internationally agreed, comprehensive list of occupations and professions, which might be rightly placed under the banner of health sciences, and given our nationality, in Table 1.1 we have adapted the Australian and New Zealand Standard Research Classification (ANZRC, 2008), Division 11: Medical and Health Sciences, to try to be as inclusive as we possibly can, of any person in any health science area, who might benefit from reading this book.

Generating evidence for practice

From the 1990s to the present day, we have witnessed a movement in health sciences research and practice (Chiappelli, Brant, Oluwadara, Neagos, and Ramchandani, 2010; French et al., 2009; Gioia and Dziadosz, 2008; Isett et al., 2008; Kitson et al., 2008; Knox and Aspy, 2011; Ritchie, 2001; Tilburt, Mangrulkar, Goold, Siddiqui, and Carrese, 2008; Turner, Misso, Harris, and Green, 2008), which is firmly grounded in positivism and postpositivism and the medical profession's preference for the scientific method of empirico-analytical inquiry. Evidence based practice (EBP) was established by medical researchers in Canada, who wanted to ensure that medical practice was based on research evidence. Since that time EBP has become established in research and practice in other health sciences in the USA, UK, Europe and southern hemisphere countries.

EBP is 'the conscientious, explicit and judicious use of current best evidence in making decisions about the healthcare of patients' (Sackett, Rosenberg, Gray, Haynes, and Richardson, 1996, p. 2), which involves patients' values (Bennett and Bennett, 2000). Dawes et al. (2005, p. 4) suggests that EBP 'aims to provide the best possible evidence at the point of clinical (or management) contact'. Regardless of who defines it, the common feature of EBP is that the best evidence is used to direct effective medical and health sciences practice.

The evidence for EBP is gained by systematically searching for and analysing research articles and reports accessed though databases and libraries (Pearson and Wiechula, 2005). Pearson and Field (in Courtney, 2005, p. 74) claim that the systematic review process for accessing and analysing research projects is a form of research; indeed, it is frequently referred to as 'secondary research', because it includes undertaking a background literature review, formulating objectives and questions, and describing inclusion criteria, a search strategy for the literature, assessment criteria, data extraction and data synthesis.

Much has been done in the EBP movement, to be more inclusive of qualitative research findings as evidence of practice, but there are still some issues in recognizing the relative merits of qualitative research within a positivistic/postpositivistic framework. For example, I (BT) was keen to see the progress in peak health bodies' levels of evidence, so I went to Google, and found a pro-quantitative methods trend. In Australia, the peak health body, the National Health and Medical Research Council (NHMRC), upgraded its webpage (www.nhmrc.gov.au) on 26 October 2010 for levels of evidence gradings, to:

- I Evidence obtained from a systematic review of all relevant randomized controlled trials

- II Evidence obtained from at least one properly-designed randomized controlled trial

- III-1 Evidence obtained from well-designed control trials without randomization

- III-2 Evidence obtained from well-designed cohort or case-controlled analytic studies preferably from more than one centre or research group

- III-3 Evidence obtained from multiple time-series with or without the intervention. Dramatic results in uncontrolled experiments (such as the introduction of the penicillin treatment in the 1940s) could also be regarded as this type of evidence

- IV-1 Evidence from descriptive studies including case series, case reports and cross-sectional studies

- IV-2 Published policies, recommendations or opinions of recognized experts, organizations or learned colleges including endorsement of

- IV-3 evidence by recognized Australian bodies (such as RACGP, Urological Society of Australia etc.)

- IV-4 Consensus opinion of the working party not endorsed formally by recognized bodies

- N/A Not applicable – not possible to apply a level of evidence.

In the UK, the Oxford Centre for Evidence-based Medicine (CEBM) posted its levels of evidence for 2009 (www.cebm.net) in a more detailed form, but

Table 1.1 Medicine and health sciences – Australian and New Zealand classifications

Classification	Description	Professional areas of coverage
Medical biochemistry and metabolomics.	Human biochemistry or the chemistry of human living organisms and the human life process	Medical Biochemistry: Amino Acids and Metabolites; Carbohydrates; Inorganic Elements and Compounds; Lipids; Nucleic Acids; Proteins and Peptides (incl. Medical Proteomics); Metabolic Medicine
Cardiovascular medicine and haematology		Cardiology (incl. Cardiovascular Diseases); Haematology; Respiratory Diseases
Clinical sciences	Specific clinical aspects of medicine, including causes, diagnosis, treatment and management of specific diseases and conditions	Anaesthesiology; Clinical Chemistry (diagnostics); Clinical Microbiology; Dermatology; Emergency Medicine; Endocrinology; Gastroenterology and Hepatology; Geriatrics and Gerontology; Infectious Diseases; Intensive Care; Medical Genetics (excl. Cancer Genetics); Nephrology and Urology; Nuclear Medicine; Orthopaedics; Otorhinolaryngology; Pathology (excl. Oral Pathology); Physiotherapy; Podiatry; Psychiatry (incl. Psychotherapy); Radiology and Organ Imaging; Rehabilitation and Therapy (excl. Physiotherapy); Rheumatology and Arthritis; Surgery; Venereology
Complementary and alternative medicine		Chiropractic; Naturopathy; Traditional Aboriginal and Torres Strait Islander Medicine and Treatments; Traditional Chinese Medicine and Treatments; Traditional Maori Medicine and Treatments
Dentistry		Dental Materials and Equipment; Dental Therapeutics, Pharmacology and Toxicology; Endodontics; Oral and Maxillofacial Surgery; Oral Medicine and Pathology; Orthodontics and Dentofacial Orthopaedics; Paedodontics; Periodontics; Special Needs Dentistry
Human movement and sports science		Biomechanics; Exercise Physiology; Motor Control; Sports Medicine
Immunology	Processes and reactions of the human immune system	Allergy; Applied Immunology (incl. Antibody Engineering, Xenotransplantation and T-cell Therapies); Autoimmunity; Cellular Immunology; Humoural Immunology and Immunochemistry; Immunogenetics (incl. Genetic Immunology); Innate Immunity; Transplantation Immunology; Tumour Immunology

Medical microbiology	Microbiology associated with human health and disease, other than clinical microbiology	Medical Bacteriology; Medical Infection Agents (incl. Prions); Medical Parasitology; Medical Virology
Neurosciences	Processes and reactions of the human nervous system, including neurology and neuromuscular disease	Autonomic Nervous System; Cellular Nervous System; Central Nervous System; Neurology and Neuromuscular Diseases; Peripheral Nervous System; Sensory Systems
Nursing		Aged Care Nursing; Clinical Nursing; Primary (Preventative); Clinical Nursing; Secondary (Acute Care); Clinical Nursing: Tertiary (Rehabilitative); Mental Health Nursing; Midwifery
Nutrition and dietetics		Clinical and Sports Nutrition; Dietetics and Nutrigenomics; Nutritional Physiology; Public Nutrition Intervention
Oncology and carcinogenesis	Cancer cell biology; cancer diagnosis; and cancer therapy	Cancer Cell Biology; Cancer Diagnosis; Cancer Genetics; Cancer Therapy (excl. Chemotherapy and Radiation Therapy); Chemotherapy; Haematological Tumours; Molecular Targets; Radiation Therapy; Solid Tumours
Ophthalmology and optometry		Ophthalmology; Optical Technology; Vision Science

the CEBM criteria basically reflect the thinking in the NHMRC levels, giving preference to randomized controlled trials and other controlled, objective methods and measures. The same pattern for levels of evidence is replicated in the USA (e.g. www.cochrane.org, www.ahrq.gov/clinic/epc/).

Most levels of evidence feature quantitative methods as the best sources of information, because of their fit with the generation and validation of biomedical science. The almost total absence of qualitative research data as evidence has been a source of critique of EBP and researchers have attempted to address this deficit (Greenhalgh and Taylor, 1997; Horsburgh, 2003; Morse, 2003; Whittemore, Chase, and Mandle, 2001). The Joanna Briggs Institute in Australia has compiled a hierarchy of four levels of evidence, which is inclusive of qualitative research (Pearson, 2002), and judges the merit of research according to feasibility, appropriateness, meaningfulness and effectiveness (FAME). You can view these criteria online at: www.joannabriggs.edu.au/pubs/approach.php#B. In this book, Chapter 10 describes mixed methods research in detail and deals with some of the pragmatic issues of EBP in integrated quantitative/qualitative projects.

World views guiding approaches to research

A paradigmatic or world view of traditions of research allows us to 'see the big picture' and appreciate some of the epistemological differences and track changes in theoretical positioning over time. For simplicity's sake, and for the benefit of taking a macro view of major epistemological differences and changes, we will review the generally accepted classifications of quantitative and qualitative research and some key postmodern influences (Table 1.2).

The quantitative research tradition

The original quantitative research tradition, aka positivism and logical positivism, came about as a rejection of hope and faith in one true God as the source of absolute knowledge, in favour of scientism's quest for the *only* true, scientific knowledge, in the form of verifiable statements, such as those generated by mathematics and deductive logic. Other key positivistic assumptions of quantitative research included 'taking a pro-observation stance, taking an anti-cause stance (preferring lawful relationships), downplaying explanations, and taking an antitheoretical stance towards entities' (Johnson and Gray, in Tashakkori and Teddlie, 2010, p. 82).

Postpositivism developed in response to debunking the logic of verification (Popper, 1959) and from multiple challenges from researchers and scholars within the qualitative interpretive and critical traditions (Fay, 1987; Foucault, 1980; Habermas, 1972; Heidegger, 1962; Lather, 1988). Although the criticisms of positivism were broadly based from a variety of perspectives, 'collectively they destabilized the positivist notions of absolute truth, provable hypotheses, and unbiased, value-free researchers'. Even so, positivistic quantitative researchers do not unanimously accept the amended conceptualizations of

Table 1.2 Generally accepted research traditions

	Quantitative	Qualitative interpretive	Qualitative critical	Beyond postmodernism
		Postmodern influences		
Also known as:	positivism, positivistic, Cartesian, reductionism, reductionist, empirico-analytical, hypothetico-deductive, postpositivism, postpositivistic	interpretative, interpretivism, interpretivist, constructivism, constructivist	radical, poststructuralism, poststructuralist	post post postmodernism
Knowledge is:	absolute, about finding cause and effect links, deductive	relative, context-dependent, subjective, richly descriptive	relative, context-dependent, intersubjective, critiqued as power	ultra relativistic, localized to personal narratives, highly subjective, all research traditions critiqued as grand narratives
Research areas and questions are:	reduced to their smallest parts, hypothesized, tested empirico-analytically, analyzed using numbers, interpreted as mathematical relations	part of the whole, left open as tentative ideas, explored through a variety of means, analyzed through language, interpreted according to methodological assumptions	part of the whole, left open as tentative ideas, explored through a variety of means, analyzed through language, interpreted according to methodological assumptions	open, allow room for difference, work with people's narratives to emphasize relative self-understandings
Research conditions require:	validity through control of variables, reliability through test-retest, objectivity without human distortion and bias	participants' validation, attention to context, acknowledgement of human subjectivity without human distortion and bias	participants' validation, attention to context, acknowledgement of human subjectivity without human distortion and bias	openness to multiple, tentative, contradictory interpretations by readers of the research
Findings and outcomes:	are quantified in numbers, need to be statistically significant, claim to be predictive and generalizable	are qualified in words, make relativistic statements about human experiences, provide meaningful insights into experiential possibilities, are specific to local phenomena	are qualified in words, make relativistic statements about power relationships and institutions, provide critique of the status quo and possibilities for social-political change, are specific to identified constraints	make no universal truth claims or prescriptions, offer options for public debate, are left open to constant questioning as possibilities for local and personal solutions

the postpositivists and the 'underpinning assumptions of postpositivism are continuous with positivism' in many ways (Giddings and Grant, 2007, p. 54). As Giddings and Grant (2007) point out

> Postpositivists maintain (determinism) in a modified form: rather than assuming a linear process of cause and effect, they perceive outcomes as the result of a complex array of causative factors that are in interaction with their outcomes ... and the assumption of reductionism ... that experience can be reduced to a discrete set of ideas or concepts that be described and tested ... (is modified by postpositivists to) factor in the unpredictable and contradictory nature of human experience ... Postpositivists diverge from positivists significantly (on objectivism) ... to argue that reality is socially and culturally constructed and researcher objectivity is impossible ... and (postpositivists) ... tend to talk about 'supporting' rather than 'proving' hypotheses ... Postpositivists also maintain ... that the scientific method is best; however, they believe that choice of method is guided by the research question and that research can incorporate multiple methods, including non-traditional ones, especially for triangulation (p. 55).

Quantitative research designs reflect positivistic and postpositivistic assumptions about the creation and validation of knowledge as truth, while 'rarely acknowledging the philosophical and theoretical underpinnings of their research' (Giddings and Grant, 2007, p. 55). As seen in levels of evidence for EBP globally, the gold standard of quantitative research designs is the randomized controlled trial, followed by: other well-designed control trials without randomization; well-designed cohort or case controlled analytic studies, preferably from more than one centre or research group; multiple time-series with or without the intervention; and descriptive studies including case series, case reports and cross-sectional studies.

Rigour is ensured in quantitative research through reliability and validity measures, which reflect the underlying epistemological assumptions of the positivist and postpositivist perspectives in the quantitative research tradition. These measures can be studied and applied in detail in sources dedicated to the quantitative research tradition (e.g., Campbell, Machin, and Walters, 2007; Harris and Taylor, 2009; Rao and Murthy, 2008).

The qualitative research tradition

The qualitative research tradition grew out of the critiques of the epistemological positions of positivism and postpositivism by philosophers in phenomenology (Edmund Husserl, 1859–1938); anthropology (Franz Boas, 1858–1942); symbolic interactionism (Herbert Mead, 1863–1931); critical theory (Karl Marx, 1818–1883); poststructuralism (Michel Foucault, 1926–1884); and postmodernism (Jean Baudrillard, 1929–2007). Although the epistemological concepts vary between the various interpretive and critical methodologies represented by these great thinkers, qualitative research essentially attempts to explore the relative nature of knowledge, which is subjective, unique and context dependent. Qualitative research may use inductive thinking that starts from a specific instance and moves to the general pattern of combined instances, to grow from 'the ground up' to make larger statements about the nature of the thing being investigated (Glaser and Strauss, 1967), but it may also use radical critiques of existing knowledge and agencies of power within organizations (Foucault and Sheridan, 1991). People are acknowledged as sources of information and their subjective expressions of their personal awareness are valued as being integral to the meaning that comes out of the research.

Qualitative research acknowledges that people and phenomena may change according to their circumstances, so it is inappropriate to generalize research findings to the wider group of people or things being studied, rather transferability may be possible, if findings resonate with the readers of research. The measures for ensuring validity in qualitative research involve asking the participants to confirm that the interpretations represent, faithfully and clearly, what the experience was/is like for the people acting as sources of information in the research. Reliability is often not an issue in qualitative research, as it is based on the idea that knowledge is relative and dependent on all of the contextual features of the people, place, time and other circumstances.

There are many ways of categorizing qualitative research, however, in this book we adopt qualitative interpretive and critical classifications (Taylor, Kermode and Roberts, 2006) and take account of postmodern influences, such as in mobilizing some qualitative methodologies. Essentially, the major difference between interpretive and critical qualitative research is the main intention of what they hope to achieve through the research process. Interpretive research aims mainly to generate meaning through rich description, to make sense out of phenomena of interest. Critical research aims to bring about changes in the status quo, by working systematically through research problems to find answers and to cause change activity in light of those answers.

Interpretive and critical qualitative research methodologies generate meaning and they can bring about change, but they differ in the intensity of their change intentions. Qualitative interpretive research methodologies bring about change through raised awareness of phenomena and critical methodologies tend to have explicit change agendas for people and organizations.

Mixed methodologies

In concert with the EBP movement, there has been a push towards integrating qualitative and quantitative methodologies in what has been mostly called mixed methods research (MMR). MMR has been heralded as the 'third paradigm' in research (Plano Clark and Wang, 2010; Ploeg et al., 2010; Tashakkori and Teddlie, 2010; Thogersen-Ntoumani, Fox, and Ntoumanis, 2005). However, as the support for MMR grows, some cautionary notes have been sounded and some qualitative researchers are calling for a closer inspection of the claims for epistemological integration and balance, by pointing out methodological differences between qualitative data collection and analysis (QUAL) and quantitative data collection and analysis (QUAN) (Giddings, 2006; Giddings and Grant, 2007) and the risk of the qualitative research tradition being subsumed by the persistently dominant quantitative research tradition.

Tashakkori and Teddlie (2010) describe the benefits of MMR, as inferred in the characteristics of MMR as:

- methodological eclecticism (freedom to combine the best methods for answering the research questions) (p. 8);
- paradigmatic pluralism (a variety of paradigms can serve as underlying philosophies) (p. 9);
- an emphasis on diversity at all levels of the research enterprise (p. 9);
- an emphasis on continua rather than a set of dichotomies (p. 10);
- an iterative, cyclical approach to research (p. 10);
- a focus on the research question (or research problem) in determining the methods employed within any given study (p. 10);
- a set of basic 'signature' research designs and analytical processes (p. 10);
- a tendency towards balance and compromise that is implicit within the 'third methodological community' (p. 11); and
- a reliance on visual representations (e.g., figures, diagrams) and a common notational system (p. 11).

The limitations of MMR are addressed well by Giddings and Grant (2007), who argue that MMR

has been captured by a pragmatic postpositivism ... which secures mixed methods within the broader positivist project to know the world in particular ways. The effect of this capture is to reinstall the marginalization of other forms of knowing. Moreover, the resultant narrowing of focus means more circumscribed fields of values at play, questions being asked, forms of data being collected, modes of analysis being undertaken, and possible outcomes being generated (p. 52).

Food for thought

What is your position on the integrative claims of MMR and the counter claims by qualitative researchers, who are concerned that qualitative research is at risk of being subsumed into the epistemological initiatives and methods of the quantitative research tradition?

The challenge of integrating quantitative ideas about rigour and qualitative ideas about a project's trustworthiness has been addressed through various means. For example, traditionally the approach has been to discuss validity from a QUAL and QUAN perspective, but to not mix them (Tashakkori and Teddlie, 1998), to extend the idea of construct validity to cover all phases of the MMR (Leech, 2010), to link inferences in evaluation standards with validity (Teddlie and Tashakkori, 2009), to develop nine forms of legitimation (Onwuegbuzie and Johnson, 2006) and to review validity concerns as related to types of designs (D.T. Campbell, 1986; Creswell, Plano Clark, and Garrett, 2008). MMR will be discussed in detail in Chapter 10.

Postmodern influences on paradigmatic shifts in research

Postmodernism evolved in response to the epistemological assumptions of positivism and postpositivism, and also as critique of interpretive and critical qualitative research methodologies (Derrida, Allison, and Garver, 1996; Lyotard, 1984). Rosenau (1992) differentiated between a range of overlapping extreme to moderate forms of sceptical and affirmative postmodernism.

Rosenau (1992, p. 15) explains that the sceptical postmodernists offer 'a pessimistic, negative, gloomy assessment (and) argue that the post-modern age is one of fragmentation, disintegration, malaise, meaninglessness, a vagueness or even absence of moral parameters and societal chaos'. Contrastingly, affirmative postmodernists, while agreeing with the critique of modernity, nevertheless have a 'more hopeful, optimistic view of the post-modern age' (p. 15).

Sceptical postmodernism

Extreme forms of sceptical postmodernism abandon modernity, leaving no reasons for, or ways of, doing research, because they claim authors use their authority as writers to control and censure readers. The human as subject is rejected because s/he is a humanist product of modernity representing a subject–object dichotomy, and s/he is criticized 'for seizing power, for attributing meaning, for dominating and oppressing' (Rosenau, 1992, p. 42). Effectively, these criticisms prevent the human subject from asking or pursuing research questions.

Truth 'claims are a form of terrorism', that threaten and provoke, silencing those who disagree (Rosenau, 1992, p. 78), thereby making research tantamount to a terrorist activity. Words, images, meanings and symbols constitute a 'fixed system of meaning', and, as representations, they are rejected by sceptical postmodernists, because they do not allow for diversity (p. 96). The inability to place (even tentatively) some faith in language renders researchers incapable of transmitting ideas gleaned by any research means. In summary, sceptical postmodernism leaves no reasons for, or ways of, doing research, making research endeavours unnecessary and impossible.

Affirmative postmodernism

Affirmative postmodernists allow room for different, less pessimistic interpretations, while still holding on to some central ideas. Affirmative postmodernists do not abandon the author completely, but they reduce the author's authority, so that s/he 'makes no universal truth claims, has no prescriptions to offer' (Rosenau, 1992, p. 31), and offers only options for public debate. This position allows researchers, as the authors of projects, to offer tentative insights for readers' interpretations and discussion. The human as subject returns 'not as the same subject banished' by sceptical postmodernists, but as a 'post-modern subject with a new non-identity', who 'will reject total explanations and the logocentric view that implies a unified frame of reference' (Rosenau, 1992, p. 57). This allows researchers to focus on humans as subjects, but in ways that do not make bold, broad theory claims.

History is a source of criticism, but it is revised radically 'to focus on the daily life experience of ordinary people', in narrations of small events on the margins of human existence, left open to constant questioning as possibilities, rather than statements of fact and truth. Time is not linear or bounded, and truth is rejected as universal in favour of 'specific, local, personal and community forms of truth' (Rosenau, 1992, p. 80). This allows researchers to work with people's narratives to emphasize the relative nature of their self-understandings. Representation is permissible, but in improved political forms that assist oppressed minorities and women to find voice, leaving room for participatory and emancipatory research that focuses on the specific circumstances of participants and finds multiple and contradictory personal and local solutions. In summary, affirmative postmodernism does not sever ties with organized research, rather it can influence projects by the application of redefined ideas about people and the sense they make out of their knowledge and existence.

Postmodernism and qualitative research methodologies

By virtue of their underlying theoretical assumptions, qualitative methodologies fit into the postmodern categorization of 'grand narratives' (Lyotard, 1984), because they hold as foundational, large series of interrelated concepts and theories, presented as 'big stories' about the nature of certain kinds of knowledge. For example, historical research bases its quest to generate historical knowledge on the assumption that knowledge of the past is valuable, indeed historical researchers may assert that history 'is probably stronger than language in the moulding of human consciousness' (Yuginovich, 2000, p. 70). Similarly, all the other qualitative methodologies assert certain epistemological ideas about the nature of knowledge generation and validation, according to the basic interests and principles of their respective approaches. The broad range of methodologies described in detail in Part One of this book, are here to assist you in making informed choices about congruent research methods and processes for your projects.

Interestingly, naming qualitative methodologies as grand narratives, positions them as dominant discourses, with the self-appointed authority to influence epistemological inquiry. As dominant discourses, they fall into the same discourse category as the quantitative research paradigm, from which qualitative methodologies have long since distanced themselves, because of well-debated epistemological differences (Derrida et al., 1996; Foucault, 1980; Lyotard, 1984; Rosenau, 1992). Being branded with the quantitative research tradition as dominant discourses, is a paradox for qualitative methodologies, because many of their theoretical assumptions relate to increasing human awareness through deep and rich description (Lincoln and Guba, 1985), and to deliberately questioning the status quo to unseat political agendas (Heron and Reason, 1997). Even with their interpretive and critical intentions, qualitative research methodologies do not escape postmodern critique, because they are indeed grand narratives, by virtue of their well-held, specific, foundational epistemological assumptions.

However, the postmodern naming of qualitative methodologies as grand narratives does not necessarily condemn them to being arrogant and overbearing ultimate authorities, nor render them ineffective as knowledge sources, simply because they lack the extreme relativism of postmodern views of knowledge, especially of the sceptical postmodern type (Rosenau, 1992). To the contrary, researchers using qualitative methodologies have responded to postmodern critiques along cherished methodological lines, for example, feminists do not want to abandon their emancipatory intentions for women to give them voice and free them from patriarchal oppression (Lather, 1993). Some critical feminists have taken on the relativity and creativity of postmodern ideas, while holding true to the central assumptions of feminism and critical social science (Glass, 2000; Glass and Davis, 1998; Hardin, 2003), demonstrating that epistemology in the postmodern era does not have to be about an either/or option.

Although they have been criticized for advocating and creating unreliable and disconnected 'truths' (Sokal, 1996) the ultra relativistic, postmodernist proponents of knowledge have actually created the potential for qualitative researchers to redefine themselves more clearly and to free themselves from their epistemological confines, by engaging in deeper levels of introspection and epistemological debate.

Even though it may not be received well nor be applied by some healthcare professionals and researchers, postmodern thought has caused us to think about, argue, debate, and in some cases, ridicule the ideas, but in our reactionary phases, it has caused a shakeup of rigid ideas of what and how a qualitative research project *should* be, making broader views of epistemology possible, while unseating claims that one qualitative methodology is superior to another. The influences of postmodern thought are also that qualitative researchers have become more open to epistemological critique, becoming more transparent about their fundamental ideas, more flexible in adapting and shifting their paradigmatic positions by creating mobile methodologies, and more tentative in making 'truth' claims at a project's completion.

Chapter summary

Definitions of methodologies, methods and processes must be clear, as you embark on extending your knowledge and undertaking research in the health sciences after your basic research preparation. Even though you already have some knowledge about research in general, to make our epistemological assumptions clear to you, we described our position on the need for epistemological congruency and some relatively stable conceptual structures, on which you can build your own ideas and make adaptations as you see fit. In the first section of this chapter, we also presented a comprehensive list of health sciences and reviewed some fundamental ideas relating to evidence-based practice, world views guiding approaches to research, and postmodern influences on paradigmatic shifts in qualitative research.

The first part of this book, Chapters 2 to 10, is about a range of qualitative methodologies, including grounded theory, historical research, ethnography, phenomenology, narrative inquiry, case study research, critical ethnography, feminisms, action research and mixed methodologies. As methodologies are composed of sets of interrelated theoretical concepts, for each methodology showcased, we describe its definitions, theoretical assumptions, epistemological origins, common concepts and methods, plus examples of how the methodologies have been interpreted by qualitative researchers in healthcare professions.

Key points

- Qualitative research invites researchers to inquire about the human condition, because it explores the meaning of human experiences and creates the possibilities of change through raised awareness and purposeful action.

- In qualitative research, methodologies are particular sets of theoretical assumptions, which underlie the choice of data collection and analysis methods and processes.

- Qualitative interpretive methodologies, such as grounded theory, historical research, ethnography and phenomenology, and qualitative critical methodologies, such as action research, critical ethnography, discourse analysis and feminism, all have deep, broad theoretical bases on which they base their search for new or amended, valid knowledge.

- The methods and processes qualitative researchers use in collecting and analysing data depend on their choice of methodology.

- Methods are *what* you do to collect and analyse data, and processes are *how* you go about doing them.

- Multiple interpretations can be made about methodologies, methods and processes, so our intention as authors is to provide a practical way through the conceptual maze of qualitative research, so you can build your own ideas and make adaptations as you see fit.

- In relation to qualitative research, congruency means linking and connecting ideas, so that there is a discernible flow and fit between the ideas arising from the entire research inquiry, from the questions, aims and objectives, right through to the data collection and analysis methods and processes, and the eventual research insights and implications, that show the application and progression of ideas 'faithful' to the foundational ideas of a respective methodology.

- While maintaining a degree of tentativeness about the nature of truth, given the relativistic, context-dependent and subjective forms of qualitative knowledge, some relatively stable conceptual structures are available.

- The epistemological positioning of congruency and relatively stable conceptual structures makes grand narratives in qualitative methodologies a little less grand and a lot less arrogant, because we acknowledge the uncertain and unknowable aspects of inquiry into human experiences and constraints, while avoiding the epistemological emptiness in having no faith whatsoever in any kind of knowledge, as asserted in a sceptical postmodern view.

- The original quantitative research tradition, aka positivism and logical positivism, came about as a rejection of hope and faith in one true God as the source of absolute knowledge, in favour of scientism's quest for the *only* true, scientific knowledge, in the form of verifiable statements, such as those generated by mathematics and deductive logic.

- The qualitative research tradition grew out of the critiques of the epistemological positions of positivism and postpositivism.

- Much has been done in the EBP movement, to be more inclusive of qualitative research findings as evidence of practice, but there are still some issues in recognizing the relative merits of qualitative research within a positivistic/postpositivistic framework.

- In concert with the EBP movement, there has been a push towards integrating qualitative and quantitative methodologies in what has been mostly called mixed methods research (MMR).

- As the support for MMR grows, some cautionary notes have been sounded and some qualitative researchers are calling for a closer inspection of the claims for epistemological integration and balance, by pointing out methodological differences between QUAL and QUAN and the risk of the qualitative research tradition being subsumed by the persistently dominant quantitative research tradition.

- By virtue of their underlying theoretical assumptions, qualitative methodologies fit into the postmodern categorization of 'grand narratives', because they hold as foundational, large series of interrelated concepts and theories, presented as 'big stories' about the nature of certain kinds of knowledge.

- The ultra relativistic, postmodernist proponents of knowledge have created the potential for qualitative researchers to redefine themselves more clearly and to free themselves from their epistemological confines, by engaging in deeper levels of introspection and epistemological debate.

Critical review questions

1 In what ways are the EBP and mixed methods research movements complementary?

2 To what extent is congruency possible in qualitative research in an era of postmodernism and mixed methods research?

References

ANZRC. (2008). Australian and New Zealand Standard Research Classification (ANZSRC) Retrieved 9 June 2011, http://www.abs.gov.au/ausstats/abs.

Bennett, S., & Bennett, J.W. (2000). The process of evidence based practice in occupational therapy: informing clinical decisions. *Australian Occupational Therapy Journal, 47*(4), 171–180.

Benson, O., & Stangroom, J. (2004). *The Dictionary of Fashionable Nonsense: A Guide for Edgy People.* London: Souvenir Press.

Bhavnani, V., & Fisher, B. (2010). Patient factors in the implementation of decision aids in general practice: a qualitative study. *Health Expectations, 13*(1), 45–54.

Bower, E., & Scambler, S. (2007). The contributions of qualitative research towards dental public health practice. *Community dentistry and oral epidemiology, 35*(3), 161–169.

Campbell, D.T. (1986). Relabeling internal and external validity for applied social scientists. *New Directions for Program Evaluation, 1986*(31), 67–77.

Campbell, M.J., Machin, D., & Walters, S.J. (2007). *Medical statistics: A textbook for the health sciences.* West Sussex: Wiley-Interscience.

Chiappelli, F., Brant, X., Oluwadara, O., Neagos, N., & Ramchandani, M. (Eds.). (2010). *Evidence-based practice: Toward optimizing clinical outcomes.* Berlin: Springer.

Courtney, M.D. (2005). *Evidence for nursing practice.* Sydney: Churchill Livingstone.

Creswell, J.W., Plano Clark, V., & Garrett, A.L. (2008). Methodological issues in conducting mixed methods research designs. *Advances in mixed methods research: Theories and applications.* Los Angeles: Sage, 66–84.

Dawes, M., Summerskill, W., Glasziou, P., Cartabellotta, A., Martin, J., Hopayian, K., & Osborne, J. (2005). Sicily statement on evidence-based practice. *BMC Medical Education, 5*(1), 1.

Derrida, J., Allison, D.B., & Garver, N. (1996). *Speech and phenomena: And other essays on Husserl's theory of signs.* Evanston, IL: Northwestern University Press.

Égalité, N., Özdemir, V., & Godard, B. (2007). Pharmacogenomics research involving racial classification: qualitative research findings on researchers' views, perceptions and attitudes towards socioethical responsibilities. *Pharmacogenomics, 8*(9), 1115–1126.

Fay, B. (1987). *Critical social science: Liberation and its limits.* Ithaca, NY: Cornell University Press.

Foucault, M. (1980). *The History of Sexuality, Vol. 1* (1976). Trans. R. Hurley. New York: Vintage.

Foucault, M., & Sheridan, A. (1991). *Discipline and punish: The birth of the prison.* Penguin Books: New York.

French, B., Thomas, L.H., Baker, P., Burton, C.R., Pennington, L., & Roddam, H. (2009). What can management theories offer evidence-based practice? A comparative analysis of measurement tools for organisational context. *Implementation Science, 4*(1), 28 (15 pages).

Giddings, L. (2006). Mixed-methods research. *Journal of Research in Nursing, 11*(3), 195–203.

Giddings, L., & Grant, B. (2007). A trojan horse for positivism?: a critique of mixed methods research. *Advances in Nursing Science, 30*(1), 52–60.

Giddings, L., & Williams, L.A. (2006). *A challenge to the postpositivist domination of mixed methods research: A review of nursing journals 1998–2005.* Paper presented at the Mixed Methods Conference 2006, Cambridge, UK.

Gioia, D., & Dziadosz, G. (2008). Adoption of evidence-based practices in community mental health: a mixed-method study of practitioner experience. *Community mental health journal, 44*(5), 347–357.

Glaser, B.G., & Strauss, A.L. (1967). *The discovery of grounded theory: Strategies for qualitative research.* New Jersey: AldineTransaction.

Glass, N. (2000). Speaking feminisms in nursing. In Greenwood, J. (Ed.), *Nursing theory in Australia: Development and application.* Frenchs Forest: Pearson Education Australia.

Glass, N., & Davis, K. (1998). An emancipatory impulse: a feminist postmodern integrated turning point in nursing research. *Advances in Nursing Science, 21*(1), 43–52.

Greenhalgh, T., & Taylor, R. (1997). How to read a paper: papers that go beyond numbers (qualitative research). *BMJ, 315*(7110), 740–743.

Habermas, J. (1972). *Knowledge and human interests,* Beacon Press, USA.

Hardin, P.K. (2003). Shape shifting discourses of anorexia nervosa: reconstituting psychopathology. *Nursing Inquiry, 10*(4), 209–217.

Harris, M., & Taylor, G. (2009). *Medical and health sciences statistics made easy* (2nd edn). Sudbury: Jones and Bartlett.

Heidegger, M. (1962). Being and time (trans. J. Macquarrie & E. Robinson). New York: Harper & Row.

Heron, J., & Reason, P. (1997). A participatory inquiry paradigm. *Qualitative Inquiry, 3*(3), 274–294.

Hesse-Biber, S.N., & Leavy, P. (2010). *The practice of qualitative research.* Thousand Oaks: Sage.

Horsburgh, D. (2003). Evaluation of qualitative research. *Journal of Clinical Nursing, 12*(2), 307–312.

Isett, K., Burnam, M., Coleman-Beattie, B., Hyde, P., Morrissey, J., Magnabosco, J., & Goldman, H. (2008). The role of the state mental health authorities in managing change for the implementation of evidence-based practices. *Community Mental Health Journal, 44,* 195–211.

Kitson, A.L., Rycroft-Malone, J., Harvey, G., McCormack, B., Seers, K., & Titchen, A. (2008). Evaluating the successful implementation of evidence into practice using the PARiHS framework: theoretical and practical challenges. *Implementation Science, 3*(1), doi.10.1186/1748-5908-3-1.

Knox, L.M., & Aspy, C.B. (2011). Quality improvement as a tool for translating evidence based interventions into practice: what the youth violence prevention community can learn from healthcare. *American Journal of Community Psychology,* 1–9.

Kvale, S. (1995). The social construction of validity. *Qualitative Inquiry, 1*(1), 19.

Lather, P. (1988). *Feminist perspectives on empowering research methodologies.* Paper presented at the annual meeting of the American Educational Research Association, Washington DC. (ERIC Document Reproduction Service. No. 283 858).

Lather, P. (1993). Fertile obsession: Validity after poststructuralism. *Sociological quarterly, 34*(4), 673–693.

Leech, N. (2010). Interviews with the early developers of mixed methods research. In Tashakkori A. & Teddlie, C. (Eds.), *SAGE handbook of mixed methods in social and behavioral research* (2nd edn). Thousand Oaks: Sage.

Lincoln, Y.S., & Guba, E.G. (1985). *Naturalistic inquiry.* Thousand Oaks: Sage.

Lyotard, J.F. (1984). *The postmodern condition: A report on knowledge.* Minnesota: University of Minnesota Press.

McKeown, J., Clarke, A., Ingleton, C., & Repper, J. (2010). Actively involving people with dementia in qualitative research. *Journal of Clinical Nursing, 19*(13/14), 1935–1943.

Miller, K.L., Reeves, S., Zwarenstein, M., Beales, J.D., Kenaszchuk, C., & Conn, L.G. (2008). Nursing emotion work and interprofessional collaboration in general internal medicine wards: a qualitative study. *Journal of advanced nursing, 64*(4), 332–343.

Morse, J.M. (2003). Principles of mixed methods and multimethod research design. *Handbook of mixed methods in social and behavioral research,* 189–208.

Onwuegbuzie, A.J., & Johnson, R.B. (2006). The validity issue in mixed research. *Research in the Schools, 13*(1), 48–63.

Pearson, A. (2002). Nursing takes the lead: redefining what counts as evidence in Australian healthcare *Reflections on Nursing Leadership,*(4th quarter), 18–21.

Pearson, A., & Wiechula, R. (2005). The JBI model of evidence based healthcare. *International Journal of Evidence Based Healthcare, 3*(8), 207–215.

Plano Clark, V., & Wang, S. (2010). Adapting mixed methods research to multicultural counseling. *Handbook of multicultural counseling,* 427–438.

Ploeg, J., Skelly, J., Rowan, M., Edwards, N., Davies, B., Grinspun, D., & Downey, A. (2010). The role of nursing best practice champions in diffusing practice guidelines: a mixed methods study. *Worldviews on Evidence Based Nursing. 7*(4): 238–251.

Popper, K. (1959). *The logic of scientific discovery.* London: Hutchinson.

Rao, N., & Murthy, N. (2008). *Applied statistics in health sciences.* New Dehli: Jaypee Brothers.

Ritchie, J. (2001). Case series research: a case for qualitative method in assembling evidence. *Physiotherapy theory and practice, 17,* 127–135.

Rosenau, P.M. (1992). *Post-modernism and the social sciences: Insights, inroads, and intrusions.* New Jersey: Princeton University Press.

Sackett, D.L., Rosenberg, W., Gray, J., Haynes, R.B., & Richardson, W.S. (1996). Evidence based medicine: what it is and what it isn't. *BMJ, 312*(7023), 71–72.

Schoen, C., Osborn, R., Doty, M.M., Squires, D., Peugh, J., & Applebaum, S. (2009). A survey of primary care physicians in eleven countries, 2009: perspectives on care, costs, and experiences. *Primary care, 28,* w1171.

Shaw, I. (2003). Qualitative research and outcomes in health, social work and education. *Qualitative research, 3*(1), 57–77.

Skeat, J., & Perry, A. (2008). Exploring the implementation and use of outcome measurement in practice: a qualitative study. *International Journal of Language & Communication Disorders, 43*(2), 110–125.

Sokal, A. (1996). Transgressing the boundaries: Toward a transformative hermeneutics of quantum gravity. *Social Text* (46/47), 217–252.

Sokal, A., Bricmont, J., & Dawkins, R. (1998). Intellectual impostures. *Nature, 394*(6689), 141–142.

Stein, C.H., & Mankowski, E.S. (2004). Asking, witnessing, interpreting, knowing: Conducting qualitative research in community psychology. *American Journal of Community Psychology, 33*(1), 21–35.

Strauss, A.L., & Corbin, J.M. (1998). *Basics of qualitative research: Techniques and procedures for developing grounded theory.* Thousand Oaks: Sage.

Swift, J., & Tischler, V. (2010). Qualitative research in nutrition and dietetics: getting started. *Journal of Human Nutrition and Dietetics, 23*(6), 559–566.

Tashakkori, A., & Teddlie, C. (1998). *Mixed methodology: combining qualitative and quantitative approaches.* Thousand Oaks: Sage.

Tashakkori, A., & Teddlie, C. (2010). *Sage Handbook of Mixed Methods in Social & Behavioral Research.* Thousand Oaks: Sage.

Taylor, B., Kermode, S. & Roberts C. (2006). *Research in nursing and healthcare: Evidence for practice.* Melbourne: Thomson.

Teddlie, C., & Tashakkori, A. (2009). *Foundations of mixed methods research: Integrating quantitative and qualitative approaches in the social and behavioral sciences.* Thousand Oaks: Sage.

Thogersen-Ntoumani, C., Fox, K.R., & Ntoumanis, N. (2005). Relationships between exercise and three components of mental well-being in corporate employees. *Psychology of sport and exercise, 6*(6), 609–627.

Tilburt, J.C., Mangrulkar, R.S., Goold, S.D., Siddiqui, N.Y., & Carrese, J.A. (2008). Do we practice what we preach? A qualitative assessment of resident–preceptor interactions for adherence to evidence based practice. *Journal of evaluation in clinical practice, 14*(5), 780–784.

Turner, T., Misso, M., Harris, C., & Green, S. (2008). Development of evidence-based clinical practice guidelines (CPGs): comparing approaches. *Implementation Science, 3*(1), 45.

Whittemore, R., Chase, S.K., & Mandle, C.L. (2001). Validity in qualitative research. *Qualitative health research, 11*(4), 522.

WHO. (2010). World Health Statistics 2010 Retrieved 9 June 2011, from http://www.who.int/whosis/whostat/2010/en/index.html.

Yuginovich, T. (2000). A potted history of 19th century remote area nursing in Australia and, in particular, Queensland. *Australian Journal of Rural Health, 8*(2), 63–67.

2

Grounded theory

Bev Taylor

Grounded theory (GT) is the first methodology in Part One of this book, because it is positioned on the quantitative/qualitative methodological interface. In this chapter I introduce you to various foundational GT definitions and theoretical assumptions, before reverting to the origins of GT. My reasons for moving directly to definitions and assumptions are to 'cut to the chase', to get some grounding in what is meant by GT, and why it qualifies as a methodology, before making a temporal shift back to where it all began (Glaser and Strauss, 1967).

We then take the well-worn track traversed by many other GT information seekers, by looking at Strauss and Corbin's (1990b) adaptation of the original GT method, to draw comparisons between their approaches from reading their work and by reviewing other peoples' summations of the differences (Boychuk Duchscher and Morgan, 2004; Charmaz, 2006; Heath and Cowley, 2004; Kendall, 1999). Crucial to this journey of discovery of GT are Barney Glaser's replies to researchers, who have made adaptations to the original GT, plus his own extensions of thought on GT over the years. Barney Glaser has responded vigorously to adaptations that have strayed from his original and subsequent interpretations of GT.

Notwithstanding the fundamental differences in the GT objectivist approaches of Glaser and Strauss, and Strauss and Corbin, and constructivist versions of GT, we then negotiate a 'middle road' to locate and describe some common GT concepts. As an interface qualitative methodology, GT offers researchers a way beyond a focus on quantitative verification methods solely, to the processes of generating theory, and as such, it has been embraced widely by researchers from the social and health sciences. In the last part of this chapter we look at some examples of research claiming to inductively generate theory from the data from various GT approaches.

Defining grounded theory

Definitions of GT vary according to the originators' essential views of the methodology and other authors' successive adaptations. Glaser and Strauss (1967) did not come to a direct definition of GT quickly in their book. However, Strauss and Corbin (1998) 'cut to the chase' when defining GT, because they were keen to identify their adaptations to the original GT ideas.

Glaser and Strauss's GT definition

Although every chapter in their book built up their emerging views on GT, in the first few chapters Glaser and Strauss (1967) set a context for their writing and provided some basic epistemological GT ideas that inferred a definition. Glaser and Strauss were writing mainly for sociologists, whose work at that time was based firmly in positivistic research, so they clarified at the outset that their development of GT was in part due to an attempt 'to close the gap between theory and research' (Glaser and Strauss, 1967, p. 4). They wanted to remedy what they saw as an overemphasis in quantitative research to verify, rather than to generate theories, and to register their dismay at reading poorly constructed explanations of research findings. For example, they disapproved of any 'highly empirical study which at its conclusion has a tacked-on explanation taken from a logically deduced theory' (Glaser and Strauss, 1967, p. 4). After omitting all of the non-inclusive (male) pronouns in the original quote, Glaser and Strauss's (1967) meaning is still very clear on their concerns about opportunistic (ungrounded) theories, in which

> The author tries to give … data a more general sociological meaning, as well as to account for or interpret what (was) found … because (of training) to research and verify … facts, not (to) research and generate (an) explanation of them. The explanation is added afterward … as a tacked-on explanation …
>
> (Glaser and Strauss, 1967, pp. 4–5)

Although Glaser and Strauss (1967) described their initial thoughts about GT fully in their book, it is up to the reader to locate and construct a clear and succinct definition. They flagged that their 'basic position (was) that generating grounded theory is a way of arriving at theory suited to its supposed uses' (Glaser and Strauss, 1967, p. 3). Hints are given as to the precise identity of GT in the quotes:

> Our approach, allowing substantive concepts and hypotheses to emerge first, on their own, enables the analyst to ascertain which, if any, existing formal theory may help him [sic] generate his [sic] substantive theories … (to) be more faithful to … data, rather than forcing it to fit a theory … (to) be more objective and less theoretically based … Substantive theory in turn helps to generate new grounded formal theories and to reformulate previously established ones. Thus it becomes a strategic link in the formulation and development of formal theory based on data … Suffice it to say that we use the word *grounded* here to underlie the point that the formal theory we are talking about must be contrasted with the 'grand' theory that is generated from logical assumptions and speculations about the 'oughts' of social life. Within these relations existing among social research, substantive and formal theory is a design for the cumulative nature of knowledge and theory. The design involves a progressive building up of facts, through substantive to grounded

formal theory … (the comparative analysis of) many ethnographic studies and *multiple theories* are needed so that various substantive and formal areas of inquiry can continue to build up to more inclusive formal theories.

(Glaser and Strauss, 1967, pp. 34–35)

Also, at the end of Chapter 2, Glaser and Strauss (1967, p. 43) wrote

… we wish to emphasize one highly important aspect of generating theory that pervades this and other chapters of our book. Joint collection, coding, and analysis of data is [*sic*] the underlying operation. The generation of theory, coupled with the notion of theory as process, requires all three operations be done together as much as possible. They should blur and intertwine continually, from the beginning of an investigation to its end.

Based on these quotes and the general tenor of the book, my attempt at defining the originators' approach to GT is that grounded theory is an objective process of discovery and theory generation using theoretical sampling and constant comparative data analysis to collect, code, and analyse data continually until substantive and formal areas of inquiry emerge and build up to more inclusive formal grounded theories that fit and are relevant to the areas they claim to explain.

Strauss and Corbin's GT definition

Strauss and Corbin's (1998) definition of GT is easier to locate in the second edition of their text, which was in the publication process when Anselm Strauss died. Strauss and Corbin (1998) approached the question of a definition for GT directly.

What do Strauss and Corbin mean when they use the term 'grounded theory'? They mean theory that is derived from data, systematically gathered and analysed through the research process. In this method, data collection, analysis, and eventual theory stand in close relationship to one another. A researcher does not begin a project with a preconceived theory in mind (unless his or her purpose is to elaborate and extend existing theory). Rather, the researcher begins with an area of study and allows the theory to emerge from the data. Theory derived from data is more likely to resemble the 'reality' than is theory derived by putting together a series of concepts based on experience or solely through speculation (how one thinks things ought to work). Grounded theories, because they are drawn from data, are likely to offer insight, enhance understanding, and provide a meaningful guide to action.

(Strauss and Corbin, 1998, p. 12)

Charmaz's GT definition

Variations on the foundational definitions of GT continue to be published, often reflecting authors' adherence to the originators' ideas, or adapting their ideas to suit a refashioning of some of the key ideas. For example, Charmaz (2006, 2008) took up the postmodern challenge to reconstruct GT using constructivist epistemological assumptions, which 'have sought to loosen key grounded theory strategies from their positivistic foundations evident in both Glaser's and Strauss and Corbin's versions of the method' (Charmaz, 2008, p. 469). She described the properties of GT as 'an inductive, comparative, emergent, and interactive method' and added that these 'properties take full form in its constructivists versions and shape how researchers invoke its strategies' (Charmaz, 2008, p. 470). The full meanings of each of these words within Charmaz's constructivist GT definition are elaborated in her well-argued publication (Charmaz, 2008), which is described later in this chapter.

Theoretical assumptions of grounded theory

Grounded theory qualifies as a qualitative interpretive methodology moving between objectivist and constructivist standpoints. Positioned originally on the interface of quantitative/qualitative epistemologies, GT's assumptions are derived from a reactionary turn against an overemphasis on data verification in positivism and postpositivism, and from a paradigmatic shift brought about by postmodern and narrative turns towards constructivism.

The theoretical assumptions of GT vary to some extent, from an objectivist to a constructivist standpoint (Charmaz, 2000). In Table 2.1 three groups of key GT authors are outlined, in relation to their respective key publications, epistemological influences, concepts and their paradigmatic positioning.

Many of the terms introduced in this first section may be fairly familiar to you, as they have framed the broad structure of GT since 1967. We now return to Barney Glaser and Anselm Strauss's foundational work, to get a better understanding of their discovery of GT, so you can see how the adaptations to GT over time have become adjusted to later epistemological trends, such as constructivism.

Origins of grounded theory

Grounded Theory (GT) originated with the work of Glaser and Strauss (1967) in their book: *The Discovery of Grounded Theory: Strategies for Qualitative Research*. The copy of the book I borrowed from a large Asian university in May 2011 indicated to me that successive readers had grappled with the book's content, as it was strewn with pencil marks, underlining, ticks and asterisks and the pages had yellowed from shelving for more than four decades. In writing this chapter, I enjoyed collating many sources, including peer reviewed journal articles, books, book chapters and editorials. Having Barney and Anselm's little black book beside me as I typed gave me the greatest joy, however, as I

Table 2.1 GT theoretical assumptions

	Glaser and Strauss/ Glaser	Strauss/ Strauss and Corbin	Other GT authors
Key publications	(Glaser and Strauss 1967; Glaser 1978, 1992; Strauss and Glaser 1970)	(Strauss and Corbin 1990a, 1994; Strauss and Glaser 1967; Glaser and Strauss 1970)	(Bryant 2002, 2003; Charmaz 2000, 2005, 2006, 2008; Henwood and Pidgeon 2003; Seale 1999)
Philosophical influences	Glaser: Structural functionalism Quantitative methods	Strauss: Pragmatism Symbolic interactionism Ethnographic field research Corbin: Strauss's version of GT	In general: Postmodern and narrative turns Constructivism
Key theoretical assumptions			
Reality is:	External, discoverable	External, discoverable	Multiple, constructed
Data are:	Discovered	Discovered	Mutually constructed
Researchers' views are:	Prioritized	Prioritized	Prioritized
The observer is:	Neutral, passive, authoritative	Neutral, passive, authoritative	Participant-informed
Data analysis is:	An objective process	An objective process	Intersubjective, interactive Co-constructive, reflexive
Representation of data is:	Unproblematic	Unproblematic	Problematic, due to knowledge relativity, situatedness and partiality
Concepts:	Emerge from data	Emerge from data	Are researcher-constructed categories
Generalizations are:	Context-free	Context-free	Partial and context-dependent
Aims:	To develop abstractions, To offer parsimonious explanations	To develop abstractions, To offer parsimonious explanations	To construct possible interpretations, To understand interpretively
Paradigmatic positioning	Objectivist GT	Objectivist GT	Constructivist GT

Food for thought

As the writer of this chapter, I am assuming a certain entry level in readers. I assume that as a postgraduate researcher you are conversant with various terms, which are, in fact, dense with meaning. Please take some time to 'unpack' the message in the sentence above, which reads:

Grounded theory qualifies as a qualitative interpretive methodology moving between objectivist and constructivist standpoints. Positioned on the interface of quantitative/qualitative research approaches GT's epistemological assumptions are derived from a reactionary turn against an overemphasis on data verification in positivism and postpositivism, and from a paradigmatic shift brought about by postmodern and narrative turns towards constructivism.

What do all these words mean and how do they relate to one another? Try speaking out aloud, or write your own paraphrased version of these sentences. It may help to highlight and define the main words and track them throughout this chapter and various parts of the book.

was aware that this book started GT and contributed to researchers breaking away from positivistic and post-positivistic research methods, to embrace other ways of researching and knowing about human experiences.

Barney Glaser and Anselm Strauss have been cited so often that they appear in the free, public domain dictionary, Wikipedia, and even though it may not enjoy much credibility as an academic source, a segment in Wikipedia shows that they are both public figures. Go to Google, type in their names, and it will take you to Wikipedia to read Barney and Anselm's reviews.

Glaser and Strauss's GT approach

Glaser and Strauss (1967, pp. vi–vii) were clear in the preface to their book, that it

was directed toward improving social scientists' capacities for generating theory that *will* be relevant to their research. Not everyone can be equally skilled at discovering theory, but neither do they need to be a genius to generate useful theory. What is required, we believe, is a different perspective on the canons derived from vigorous quantitative verification on issues such as sampling, coding, reliability, validity, indicators, frequency distributions, conceptual formulation, construction of hypotheses, and presentation of evidence. We need to develop canons more suited to the discovery of theory. These guides, along with associated rules of procedure, can help release energies for theorizing that are frozen by the undue emphasis on verification.

Even though they had clear intentions in mind to loosen up sociologists' imaginations and abilities to generate theory, Glaser and Strauss began tentatively in their approach to GT in sociology, aware of the need to keep 'the discussion open-minded, to stimulate rather than freeze thinking about the topic' (Glaser and Strauss, 1967, p. 9). Another point seemingly lost in the ensuing developmental years, is that Glaser and Strauss made it very clear that the book was written *for sociologists specifically*, for their theorizing. They emphasized that their book intended

> to underscore the basic sociological activity that only sociologists can do: generating sociological theory. Description, ethnography, fact-finding, verification (call them what you will) are all done well by professionals in other fields and by layman [sic] in various investigative agencies. But these people cannot generate sociological theory from their work. Only sociologists are trained to want it, to look for it, and to generate it.
>
> (Glaser and Strauss, 1967, pp. 6–7)

So, very clearly at the outset, the originators of GT emphasized the point that sociological theorizing is the sole domain of sociologists. Even so, Glaser and Strauss were aware that their GT had applications in other disciplines, because they worked originally with nurses and the writing of their book 'was made possible by the Public Health Service Research Grant ... from the Division of Nursing ...' (Glaser and Strauss, 1967, p. ix). However, given that their book on discovering GT was directed mainly to sociological theorizing and they placed the ownership of that activity in the domain of sociologists, one wonders whether some of the confusion and debates that ensued since may have been in part due to the authors' directly worded conviction that sociologists are the only people who can theorize legitimately on sociological phenomena.

The definition of Glaser and Strauss's original GT that I offer in this chapter is that it is an objective process of discovery and theory generation using theoretical sampling and constant comparative data analysis to collect, code, and analyse data continually until substantive and formal areas of inquiry emerge and build up to more inclusive formal grounded theories that fit and are relevant to the areas they claim to explain. This being basically so, we need to unpack the key words and ideas in the definition to review the originators' thoughts on what became known later as classic (Glaserian) GT.

An objective process

The process of discovery for Glaser and Strauss's (1967) GT was anchored firmly in the roots of positivism and postpositivism, which would be later referred to by Charmaz (2000) as objectivist GT. Glaser and Strauss clarified that their quest was to discover theory, which emerged from data, and this process involved thoroughly meticulous and systematic observations, comparisons and analyses of like groups and data sources. Their original intention in assisting sociologists to discover and generate GT was to 'forestall the opportunistic use of theories that have dubious fit and working capacity' (Glaser and Strauss, 1967, p. 4), which amounted to 'tacked-on' explanations by sociologists to account for their quantitative findings. Glaser and Strauss's (1967) intention was, by association, to emphasize and actually refine scientific inquiry through an objective process for generating theory, which reflected the rigour of quantitative coding methods in generating qualitative summaries (grounded theories) for explaining the association between variables (codes and categories).

Their foundational quantitative training was so enmeshed in their thinking, that Glaser and Strauss (1967) did not even tackle the question of the researcher's orientation to the research, as to whether it is objective, subjective or intersubjective, because they took for granted the basic requirement of all scientific inquiry, that the researcher is objective and that the inquiry process is objective. Therefore, no other stance but objectivity was imaginable to them in generating scientific research and theorizing, so nothing but objectivity was required in their original GT process.

Their epistemological position and objectivist assumptions were made even clearer, when Glaser and Strauss made an early stand for mixed methods research, in writing

> … there is no fundamental clash between the purposes and capacities of qualitative and quantitative methods or data. What clash there is concerns the primacy of emphasis on verification or generation of theory – to which heated discussions on qualitative versus quantitative data have been linked historically … We believe that each form of data is useful for both verification and generation of theory, whatever the primacy of the emphasis … In many instances, both forms of data are necessary – not quantitative to test qualitative, but both used as supplements, as mutual verification and, most important for us, as different forms of data on the same subject, which, when compared, will each generate theory.
>
> (Glaser and Strauss, 1967, pp. 17–18)

Glaser and Strauss (1967) did not question the inherent differences in the epistemological assumptions of qualitative and quantitative research, given the postpositivistic (pragmatic) influences in their philosophical training, nor did they restrict the use of their GT to qualitative data, as can be seen in Part Two of their book, in which they described new sources for qualitative data and their theoretical elaboration of quantitative data. Their call to quantitative researchers was to free up and make more flexible 'at strategic points, the rigorous rules for accuracy of evidence and verification', 'so as to facilitate the generation of theory' (Glaser and Strauss, 1967, p. 186), through a process of secondary analysis of quantitative data.

In effect, for Glaser and Strauss (1967), the GT process could be nothing else *but* an objective process. Objectivity in the GT discovery process was such an obvious choice to them that it needed no mention nor defence, as it was taken for granted as a given. Even though they were moving to a more creative position than on the quantitative/qualitative divide existing at that time, Glaser and Strauss were still very much in tune with the basic positivist and postpositivist epistemological assumptions of their philosophical training. Glaser and Strauss held true to their stated intention, to make more scientific sociologists' explanations for their quantitative research findings, so that they became legitimate grounded theories rather than 'tacked-on' explanations.

Discovery and theory generation

Discovery and theory generation are linked inextricably in Glaser and Strauss's (1967) GT, because the generation of grounded theories must always be through discovery as they emerge, after an intensive period of systematic and constant comparative analysis. Throughout their book, they refer often to discovery, as a process of finding knowledge, which exists, and can be located through constant, systematic searching, comparisons and analyses. For example, in 'discovering theory, one generates conceptual categories or their properties from evidence' (Glaser and Strauss, 1967, p. 23), and 'verifying as much as possible with as accurate evidence as possible is requisite while one discovers and generates (the) theory – but *not* to the point where verification becomes so paramount as to curb generation' (Glaser and Strauss, 1967, p. 28). Hence, the constant comparison process used to discover and generate theory had to be as rigorous and scientifically thorough as possible, but they were nevertheless keen to encourage sociologists to free up some of their verification criteria in the process of theory generation.

Theoretical sampling

'Theoretical sampling is the process of data collection for generating theory whereby the analyst jointly collects, codes and analyses (the) data and decides what data to collect next and where to find them, in order to develop (the) theory as it emerges' (Glaser and Strauss, 1967, p. 45). Glaser and Strauss (1967) devoted 32 pages of their book to theoretical sampling (pp. 45–77), but their essential ideas are that theoretical sampling:

- Begins with 'local' concepts as what is known broadly about the research features, e.g., people within the research context (p. 45);

- Involves the researcher continually developing 'theoretical sensitivity' to build up 'an armamentarium of categories and hypotheses on substantive and formal levels' (p. 46);

- Asks the questions: 'What groups or subgroups does one turn to *next* in data collection? And for *what* theoretical purpose? … How does (one) select multiple comparison groups?' (p. 47);

- Involves selecting comparison groups based on 'their *theoretical relevance* for furthering the development of emerging categories' (p. 49);

- Continues until *theoretical saturation* is reached, which means 'that no additional data are being found' and similar instances are being 'seen over and over again' (p. 61);

- Is in 'a variety of slices of data' (p. 66) at a depth appropriate to the category, especially *core* theoretical categories (p. 70); and

- Involves collecting, coding and analysing data at the same time; in 'continual intermeshing' (p. 73) for as long as it takes to saturate all the groups of data to form a substantive theory.

From substantive to formal grounded theory

Having reached data saturation, the GT process is ready to advance the 'substantive theory grounded in one particular substantive area' (Glaser and Strauss, 1967, p. 79), to a formal theory, by continuing the intensive constant comparative analysis of the core categories giving rise to properties and hypotheses from which an 'exceedingly complex and well-grounded formal theory can be developed' (Glaser and Strauss, 1967, p. 85), which fits and works with the area being explained.

In summary, originally, Glaser and Strauss (1967) viewed GT as an objective process of discovery and theory generation using theoretical sampling and constant comparative data analysis to collect, code, and analyse data continually until substantive and formal areas of inquiry emerge and build up to more inclusive formal grounded theories that fit and are relevant to the areas they claim to explain.

Strauss and Corbin's GT approach

In the second edition of their co-authored book, Strauss and Corbin's (1998) approach to GT had evolved into some key assumptions about GT and how it is undertaken. For Strauss and Corbin (1998), GT:

- Is about discovery (p. 1);

- Involves *description* ('depicting, telling a story, sometimes a very graphic and detailed one, without stepping back to interpret events or explain why certain events occurred and not others'), *conceptual ordering* ('classifying events and objects along various explicitly stated dimensions, without necessarily relating the classifications to each other to form an overarching explanatory scheme') and *theorizing* ('the act of constructing … from data an explanatory scheme that systematically integrates various concepts through statements of relationship') (p. 25);

- Can include 'a true interplay' between 'qualitative and quantitative methods in supplementary or complementary forms', 'to carry out the most parsimonious and advantageous means for arriving at theory', which requires 'sensitivity to the nuances in data, tolerance for ambiguity, flexibility in design, and a large dose of creativity' (p. 34);

- Involves choosing a problem and stating the research question;

- Requires the researcher to maintain a balance between objectivity ('to arrive at an impartial and accurate interpretation of events') and sensitivity ('to perceive the subtle nuances and meanings in data and recognize the connections between concepts') (pp. 42–43);

- Advocates using literature, but not to stifle creativity if 'it is allowed to stand between the researcher and the data'. Rather, it is 'used as an analytic tool … (to) foster conceptualisation' (p. 53);

- Analyses data through microscopic examination, which is the 'detailed line-by-line analysis necessary at the beginning of a study to generate initial categories (with their properties and dimensions) and to suggest relationships among properties; a combination of open and axial coding' (p. 57);

- Comprises the 'basic operations' of asking questions ('an analytic device to open up the line of inquiry and direct theoretical sampling') and making comparisons ('an analytic tool used to stimulate thinking about properties and dimensions of categories') (p. 73);

- Uses open coding, which is 'the analytic process through which concepts are identified and their properties and dimensions are discovered in the data' (p. 101);

- Develops and names the discovered concepts as categories and subcategories, 'in terms of their properties and dimensions' (p. 116);

- Uses axial coding, which is the conceptual 'process of relating categories to their subcategories, termed 'axial' because coding occurs around the axis of a category, linking categories at the level of properties and dimensions' (p. 123);

- Involves selective coding, in which 'the major categories are finally integrated to form a larger theoretical scheme' (p. 143) as a grounded theory; and

- Uses memos ('written records of analysis that may vary in type and form'), code notes ('memos containing the actual products of the three types of coding: open, axial and selective'), theoretical notes ('that contain an analyst's thoughts and ideas about theoretical sampling and other issues'), operational notes ('memos containing procedural directions and reminders') and diagrams ('visual devices that depict the relationships among the concepts') (p. 217).

In summary, Strauss and Corbin's (1998) approach to GT is that it is an objective discovery process, involving description, conceptual ordering and theorizing, to make microscopic analyses of data, aided by memos and diagrams and by asking questions and making comparisons in open, axial and selective coding, to form a grounded theory. The actual method for undertaking the three types of coding is best assimilated by reading their book and by practising their method, as you build up your expertise as a GT researcher.

Epistemological debates

Exploring GT leads inevitably to understanding adaptations of the original version of GT put forward by Glaser and Strauss. Information seekers need to look at Strauss and Corbin's (1990b) adaptation of the original GT method. Thereafter, multiple, inevitable comparisons emerge between Glaser and Strauss's original GT, and Strauss and Corbin's GT, as described by the authors, and by other people's summations of the differences (Boychuk Duchscher and Morgan, 2004; Charmaz, 2006; Heath and Cowley, 2004; Kendall, 1999). Crucial to this journey of exploration of GT are Barney Glaser's replies to adaptors of the original GT, plus his own extensions of thought on GT over the years.

If you choose to use GT in your postgraduate research, it will be most likely that you will need to deal in depth with the primary GT authors' methodological differences, to decide on and justify your choice of a GT approach to inform your research. As the differentiation of the two main versions of GT is somewhat inevitable, there are many published explanations of how they differ, making the task quite complex for researchers attempting to track the precise twists and turns of epistemological claims and counter claims since the original GT publication by Glaser and Strauss (1967).

The precise methods for generating grounded theories vary and they have been debated in detail for decades. For example, Kendall (1999) reflected very frankly on the problems she encountered when she tried to use Strauss and Corbin's axial coding, and how she eventually reverted to Glaser's GT approach. Kendall (1999, p. 746) explained that

> Both Glaser (1978, 1992) and Strauss and Corbin (1990b) described coding as an essential aspect of transforming raw data into theoretical constructions of social processes. Glaser distinguished two types of coding processes, substantive (open) and theoretical, and Strauss and Corbin described three: open, axial, and selective ... Glaser (1978) described substantive (open) coding as a way to 'generate an emergent set of categories and their properties which fit, work and are relevant for integrating into a theory' (p. 56). Strauss and Corbin (1990b) define open coding as 'the process of breaking down, examining, comparing, conceptualizing, and categorizing data' (p. 61). The approaches to open coding are similar although Glaser places more emphasis on the importance of allowing codes and theoretical understandings of the data to emerge than do Strauss and Corbin.

Other differences in the application of GT definitions of coding are also apparent. Selective coding (Strauss and Corbin, 1990b) and theoretical coding (Glaser, 1978, 1992) involve the selection of a central, core category, around which all the other categories are integrated and find their main messages. Even though Strauss and Corbin (1990a) and Glaser (1978, 1992) define these coding processes similarly, they apply them differently, thereby creating different end products in grounded theory generation.

Herein lies the central epistemological dilemma of applying GT coding to the eventual interpretation of human experiences. Codes and categories are foundational to GT, because they are formed from the raw data of accounts of human experience. The problem arises in divergent approaches to GT when the codes and categories are subject to interpretation through the process of *emergence*.

Kendall (1999, p. 746) revisited Glaser's foundational GT concept that emergence 'is the process by which codes and categories of the theory fit the data, not the process of fitting the data to predetermined codes and categories'. Glaser (1978) made it very clear that meaning is derived from generating codes and categories directly from the data. When Strauss and Corbin introduced axial coding, they intended to find a process for reconstructing fragmented data, which are separated by open coding. Axial coding uses a coding paradigm involving conditions, phenomena, context, action/interactional strategies, and consequences (Strauss and Corbin, 1990b, p. 96), by 'making connections between the categories and subcategories'. The idea behind Strauss and Corbin's paradigm model for axial coding is to question the findings systematically and thoroughly for a more comprehensive elaboration of the resulting grounded theory.

However, Glaser (1978) warned against 'forcing' the data into a framework, such as Strauss and Corbin's paradigm model, because the data should speak for themselves. Glaser's main complaint with Strauss and Corbin's GT coding method is that it places more emphasis on operational steps than on theory development and emergence. Strauss and Corbin (1990b) defended the paradigm model as complex, systematic, 'real world' thinking to construct complex and meaningful theory.

It seems to me that Strauss and Corbin's paradigm model for axial coding is actually an attempt to address issues of rigour, by producing an intricate measure of reliability and validity. The complex meshwork of coding reflects a modified deterministic view of 'outcomes as the result of a complex array of causative factors that are in interaction with their outcomes' (Giddings and Grant, 2007, p. 54). However, in adding another layer of complexity in axial coding, for all their good intentions for establishing rigour, Strauss and Corbin may have moved away from the GT basic principles, which value data emerging directly from the analysis of the research participants' accounts of their experiences.

Returning to Kendall (1999), the researcher admitted in her article that not only did she have difficulty in applying Strauss and Corbin's GT method due to the complexity of axial coding, she also came to a point of agreement with Glaser that the best way to use GT was by his original intention of discovering a core category in a GT, which has emerged from a substantive (open) and theoretical coding process.

Glaser has had a great deal to say to researchers and scholars about their various interpretations and applications of his classic (Glaserian) version of GT. Sounding like a disgruntled teacher (Glaser and Holton, 2004, paras 7–8), frustrated by *yet again* having to clarify certain fundamental ideas about GT to less than attentive audiences, he writes:

> I wish to remind people, yet again, that classic GT is simply a set of integrated conceptual hypotheses systematically generated to produce an inductive theory about a substantive area. Classic GT is a highly structured but eminently flexible methodology. Its data collection and analysis procedures are explicit and the pacing of these procedures is, at once, simultaneous, sequential, subsequent, scheduled and serendipitous, forming an integrated methodological 'whole' that enables the emergence of conceptual theory as distinct from the thematic analysis characteristic of QDA research. I have detailed these matters in my books 'Theoretical Sensitivity' (Glaser, 1978), 'Basics of Grounded Theory Analysis' (Glaser, 1992), 'Doing Grounded Theory' (Glaser, 1998), and 'The Grounded Theory Perspective' (Glaser, 2001). Over the years since the initial publication of 'Discovery of Grounded Theory' (Glaser and Strauss, 1967), the transcendent nature of GT as a general research methodology has been subsumed by the fervent adoption of GT terminology and selective application of discrete aspects of GT methodology into the realm of QDA research methodology. This multi-method cherry picking approach, while obviously acceptable to QDA, is not compatible with the requirements of GT methodology.

Throughout the article, Glaser and Holton (2004, para 6) addressed 'the myriad of remodeling blocks to classic GT analysis brought on by lacing it with qualitative data analysis [QDA] descriptive methodological requirements'. Authors' works came in for criticism for misinterpreting Glaserian GT, including Creswell (1998), May (1994), and Morse (1994). In all cases, Glaser unpicked and criticized each methodological point, before he delivered a tutorial on GT procedures, including theoretical sensitivity, getting started, 'all is data', use of literature, theoretical coding, open coding, theoretical sampling, constant comparative method, core variable, selective coding, delimiting, interchangeability of indicators, pacing, memoing, sorting and writing up and analytic rules developed during sorting. My response to all of this is: '*Why is it then, if GT is so straightforward and simple, as Barney would have us believe, that so many of us get it wrong?*'

At the risk of being seen as an inattentive reader, my interpretation of Glaser's response to qualitative data analysis (QDA) is that while he is at pains to point out that GT is scientific (systematic, objective, exhaustively detailed in tracking codes and so on), he seems to be missing the point that various qualitative research approaches differ on their epistemological assumptions about researcher objectivity. For Glaser, the tendency is abhorrent to subsume GT into the category of descriptive qualitative research and to use it for QDA.

Glaser does not want to place GT into a research grouping seemingly beset with methodological issues.

Glaser does not appreciate that what he is calling QDA is actually a much broader field of qualitative inquiry extending to extreme postmodernist viewpoints, in which methodological issues are openly acknowledged and debated as being intrinsic to subjective, relativistic epistemologies. The honest debate of epistemological issues by qualitative researchers, for example, of their vexed questions relating to the nature of truth and how knowledge is generated and validated, are seen as fundamental core issues by qualitative researchers. Discussions of the nature of, and measures for 'rigour' in qualitative research, the inherent problems of 'generalizability' of research findings, and the subjective positioning of the researcher within the research, are taken by Glaser as failings and weaknesses of QDA. Rather than seeing methodological disclosures as signs of the epistemologically mature debate, which one might reasonably expect to find in a strong and critically aware research paradigm, Glaser sees these frank discussions as signs of methodological flaws.

It seems to me that Glaser has missed the main points that differentiate the various forms of qualitative research from the epistemological assumptions of positivism and postpositivism. Most importantly, he does not seem to take into account the relativistic and subjective nature of knowledge, which assumes that there are no certain, absolute truths and that human research and the interpretation of knowledge through human agency cannot help but be influenced to some extent by aspects of human agency and subjectivity. Glaser makes some epistemological concessions about the effects of context on knowledge, but he basically hangs on to treasured postpositivistic notions of 'scientific' inquiry, as defined and determined by determinism, objectivity, tireless checking and cross-checking of information, and the ultimate sense of faith in generating absolute knowledge, when all the parts of the conceptual puzzle have been located, labelled, put in place and explained objectively.

As assessed by Glaser, the score card is also low for most readers of classic GT on conceptualization (Glaser, 2002). Glaser reiterates his contention that conceptualization has been misinterpreted and misused as description, by 'many immensely funded description-producing agencies such as newspapers, police, FBI and so forth, as well as an immense qualitative data analysis (QDA) research movement'. In this statement Glaser makes it clear that he relegates QDA to everyday descriptive levels and that 'it is sociologists, psychologists, social psychologists, and other social researchers who are mandated to conceptualize in the social science' (Glaser, 2002, p. 3).

Here again, Glaser's tone is of a disappointed and somewhat irritated teacher, admonishing errant students, reminding would-be researchers not to claim they are undertaking GT if they are unwilling to adhere to specific epistemological requirements that raise the inquiry above description to scientific conceptualization.

> All that GT is, is the generation of emergent conceptualizations into integrated patterns, which are denoted by categories and their properties.

This is accomplished by the many rigorous steps of GT woven together by the constant comparison process, which is designed to generate concepts from all data. Most frequently, qualitative data incidents are used. Through conceptualization, GT is a general method that cuts across research methods (experiment, survey, content analysis, and all qualitative methods) and uses all data resulting therefrom. Because of conceptualization, GT transcends all descriptive methods and their associated problems, especially what is an accurate fact, what is an interpretation, and how is the data constructed. It transcends by its conceptual level and its 3rd and 4th level perceptions. By transcending, I do not say implicitly that description is 'bad', 'wrong', or 'unfavourable'. Description is just different with different properties than conceptualization, yet these different properties are confused in the qualitative research literature. Actually, descriptions run the world, however vague or precise (and mostly the former). Precious little conceptualization affects the way the world is run.

(Glaser, 2002, p. 3)

In this section I described some of the comparisons between Glaser and Strauss's original GT, and Strauss and Corbin's GT, as described by the authors, and by other people's summations of the differences. I offered as an example Kendall's (1999) comparison of Glaser's and Strauss and Corbin's definitions and uses of coding, with particular emphasis on the problem of axial coding. Barney Glaser's replies to authors of GT, correcting their erroneous interpretations, were also described. In the next section, we turn our attention to another major adaptive interpretation of GT and to Glaser's responses to it.

Charmaz's constructivist approach to GT

Charmaz (2008) wrote an informative book chapter about reconstructing grounded theory. I recommend this chapter to you, as it will give you a firm grounding on the origins and various iterations of GT, plus a sound appreciation of a constructivist interpretation of GT. Essentially, constructivist GT calls for 'flexible, open-ended strategies … to conduct systematic, directed inquiry and to engage in imaginative theorizing from empirical data' (Charmaz, 2008, p. 436). Charmaz (2008, p. 469) identified with the growing number of scholars, who 'have sought to loosen key grounded theory strategies from their positivistic foundations'.

Charmaz (2008, p. 469) is of the view that researchers 'can use grounded theory strategies without endorsing mid-century assumptions of an objective, external reality, a passive neutral observer, or a detached narrow empiricism'. While acknowledging the overall contributions of Glaser and Strauss to the development of GT specifically, and qualitative research in general, Charmaz critiques their various original, adapted and sustained views of GT, as essentially reductionist and mechanistic. Instead, Charmaz takes a constructivist view, that 'social reality is multiple, processual, and constructed', so a 'researcher's position, privileges, perspective, and interactions' are also part of constructed reality (Charmaz, 2008, p. 469).

Charmaz (2008) tracked the evolution of GT in key debates between the original version and subsequent iterations. Following on from the original text (Glaser and Strauss, 1967), Charmaz noted the progression of thought in Strauss's (1987) publication of *Qualitative Analysis for Social Scientists*, to Strauss and Corbin's (1990b, 1998) books, which revised GT towards increased verification through technical procedures. Glaser's (1992) response to increased verification in GT was to claim that Strauss and Corbin's axial coding 'forced the data' with unnecessary analytical complexity. Even so, Glaser's justification of the original GT and his insistence on emergence, rested on an adherence to comparative approaches including 'avoidance of extant theories, a delayed literature review, and on a direct and, often, narrow empiricism' (Charmaz, 2008, p. 466).

While Glaser was stringent in his criticism of Strauss and Corbin's pragmatic tendencies towards microscopic detailed analysis in procedural methods, such as the conditional/consequential matrix, Glaser's epistemological arguments, nonetheless, rested on similar positivistic assumptions. As Charmaz (2008, p. 467) asserted, 'Strauss and Corbin's and Glaser's versions of grounded theory assume an external reality independent of the observer, a neutral observer, and the discovery of data. Notions of what researchers see, define, and describe as data, do not permeate their texts'.

Objectivist GT requires a researcher to be detached, unbiased and value free, as an essential attitude for ensuring the proper functioning of the scientific method. Contrastingly, constructivist GT calls for relativistic views of epistemology, and the idea that human phenomena are socially constructed. Constructivist GT, therefore, holds to the idea of socially constructed realities, and it acknowledges the relative 'messiness' that is integral to co-constructing a project's methods and processes, while the researcher works actively and reflexively through multiple, complex, contextual issues in selecting, collecting and analysing data.

It would seem that Glaser does not agree with changing GT to anything other than his view of it. Responding to Charmaz's (2000) publication, Glaser (2002) refuted constructivist GT soundly, on all counts. His response is peppered with criticism of Charmaz's (2000) article specifically, for example, in relation to 'forcing type interview guides', being simplistic about the potential knowledge outcomes of interviews, and of avoiding researcher bias issues. Using capital letters to emphasize key words and ideas, Glaser delivered more GT clarification. For example, Glaser claimed constructivist GT is a misnomer, because 'all is data'. He clarified that '"All is Data" is a GT statement, NOT applicable to Qualitative Data Analysis (QDA)' (Glaser, 2002, para. 2). Glaser's (2002) responses to Charmaz (2000) are direct, unflinching and 'forensic'. For example, Glaser (2000, para 16) wrote: Charmaz claims

the 'grounded theorist's analysis tells a story about people, social processes, and situations. The researcher composes the story; it does not simply unfold before the eyes of an objective viewer. The story reflects the viewer as well as the viewed.' … Again, absolutely NO, the GT researcher does not 'compose' the 'story.' GT is not description, and the unfolding is emergent from the careful tedium of the constant comparative method and theoretical sampling – fundamental GT procedures. These are not story making, they are generating a theory by careful application of all the GT procedures. The human biasing whatever is minimized to the point of irrelevancy in what I have seen in hundreds of studies. The GT reflections of the researcher are his/her skill at doing GT. This remodeling by CHARMAZ [*sic*] of GT is clearly just not correct and is implicitly supporting the QDA requirements for accuracy. CHARMAZ [*sic*] has not considered the properties of conceptualization in her offer of a constructivist GT.

In defence of Charmaz's constructivist GT, Antony Bryant (2003) wrote 'A Constructive/ist Response to Glaser'. Bryant had also written an article on epistemological issues in GT (Bryant 2002), so when he realized Glaser had replied to Charmaz's publication on constructivist GT, he was keen to read Glaser's response. However, his 'pleasure turned to dismay' (Bryant, 2003, para 1), when instead of a coherent, well-argued response, Bryant perceived Glaser's article to be 'an incoherent and inconsistent article formatted like a poor piece of tabloid journalism' (Bryant, 2003, para 2). As has been the case with other authors who have interpreted GT, Glaser subjected Charmaz to criticism on each and every substantive aspect of her writing, by pulling them apart and refuting them mercilessly.

Charmaz's (2000, 2006, 2008) writing distinguishes between objectivist and constructivist GT. As Bryant (2003, para 3) explains, objectivist GT 'assumes the reality of an external world, takes for granted a neutral observer, and views categories as derived from data'. Contrastingly, constructivist GT 'recognizes that the viewer creates the data and ensuing analysis through interaction with the viewed' (Charmaz, 2000, p. 523). Bryant argued that Charmaz 'is not prescribing the constructivist view as the only valid one, but she is making the case for a full and proper consideration of issues of constructivism as they impact upon some of the central – and oft-repeated – defining phrases of GTM (grounded theory method)' (Bryant, 2003, para 4).

Bryant (2003, para 5) quite rightly points out that all of Glaser's and Strauss and Corbin's epistemological assumptions about the role of the researcher are 'objectivist – i.e. positivist – in the sense that representation is seen as ultimately unproblematic once a neutral point of reference can be assured for the researcher'. In defence of a constructivist view of GT, Bryant (2003, para 7) suggests that

The essential issues are that the positivist stance of a neutral observer, gathering data about the world, from which theories somehow emerge is now so severely discredited that one of the few places in which one can find such unreconstructed positivism is in the work of some of those claiming adherence to GTM – including, but not restricted to, Barney Glaser.

In summary, the evolution of GT from objectivist to constructivist methodologies has been highlighted by adaptations to Glaser and Strauss's (1967) original version, to Glaser's various iterations of researcher-neutral GT, to one in which researchers own and value their own positioning and subjectivity within the research process. From my perspective as the author of this chapter, I venture to offer an opinion on Glaser and his summation of what he calls QDA. It seems to me that Glaser mistakes as a failing, the honesty qualitative researchers use, when they discuss the problems of rigour or trustworthiness they encounter in creating and validating relativistic knowledge. Having no faith in the discovery of absolute truth, qualitative researchers seek instead to explore the margins of possibilities, being content to offer tentative insights into human phenomena. Glaser has not grasped the idea that, beyond the structured promises of positivistic epistemology, knowledge is seen as partial, incomplete, subjective, and ever-changing, according to its unique contexts of time, place and person. Holding on to the knowledge assumption of the certainty of a discoverable, objective reality, Glaser assumes that the researcher must use tireless, value-free analytical measures to discover and validate that knowledge. In effect, Glaser's responses to all errant interpreters of his GT are along the lines that they have mistakenly taken a relativistic view of what, to him, is essentially an objective epistemological method and process. In Glaser's GT one cannot 'construct' a reality, because it already exists, out there, waiting for emergence, by being discovered, analysed and interpreted objectively.

Common grounded theory concepts

Even though there are fundamental differences in the objectivist GT approaches of Glaser and Strauss, Glaser individually, Strauss and Corbin, and the constructivist approach of Charmaz, it is possible to negotiate a 'middle road' to locate and describe some common GT concepts. Even with its adaptive differences, GT offers researchers a way beyond a focus on quantitative verification methods alone, to the comparative processes of generating middle range theory, and as such, it has value for researchers in the social and health sciences.

While various GT commonalities have been suggested (e.g., Creswell, 1998), Charmaz (2008, p. 472) suggests GT guidelines in accord with Glaser's comparative approach of:

- Comparing data with data
- Labeling data with active, specific codes
- Selecting focused codes
- Comparing and sorting data with focused codes
- Raising telling focused codes to tentative analytic categories
- Comparing data and codes with analytic categories

- Constructing theoretical concepts from abstract categories

- Comparing category with concept

- Comparing concept and concept.

Charmaz's comparative guidelines are helpful in finding commonalities in GT methods and processes, but they are, of necessity, broad so they mask the various differences in GT approaches. If you are intending to use a GT approach for your research project, you need to explore in depth the differences in GT, so you can make an informed choice as to which version suits your needs best. A microscopic, all-inclusive analysis of the GT differences will take some time and several PhDs, so the best you can do at this stage may be to get a sense of GT from this chapter, and then pursue in depth the type of GT that best approximates your epistemological assumptions and the nature of your project.

Food for thought
Imagine that you are interested in researching an area of interest in which little is known, as shown by gaps and silences in relevant literature and in your experience. Compare and contrast objectivist (Glaser and Strauss, Strauss and Corbin) and constructivist (e.g., Charmaz) approaches and decide by whose approach your project will be informed. Given the divergent GT views, you will need to justify your choice, so think about *why* you have chosen the GT approach in relation to the aims and objectives your project, and your own potential to undertake successfully that specific GT approach.

Grounded theory research projects in the health sciences

From my reading of GT projects, I have observed varying ways of undertaking GT research. Some examples of research claim to inductively generate theory from the data in the Glaser and Strauss, or Glaserian sense (Lindqvist and Hallberg, 2010; Wiese and Oster, 2010), or they claim to apply Strauss and Corbin's approach (Malm and Hallberg, 2006; Wagman, Björklund, Håkansson, Jacobsson and Falkmer, 2011). Other projects take on a constructivist approach (McCreaddie, Payne and Froggat, 2010), or they use a non-specific form of GT, by claiming to be informed broadly by a selection of common GT epistemological ideas (Kalischuk, 2010), while others seem to tack GT on to their project with the barest justification. GT has also been combined successfully with other methodologies, such as feminism (Plummer and Young, 2009), critical realism (Oliver, 2011), ethnomethodology (Lester and Hadden, 1980), extended case method (Tavory and Timmermans, 2009), narrative analysis (Floersch, Longhofer, Kranke and Townsend, 2010), and phenomenology (Skodol Wilson and Hutchinson, 1991).

For example, Lindqvist and Hallberg (2010, p. 456) used 'the constant comparative method of grounded theory (GT), developed by Glaser and Strauss (1967)' and Glaser (1992), to 'illuminate the main concern of people suffering from chronic obstructive pulmonary disease (COPD) and how they handle their everyday life'. Twenty-three people with COPD at different stages were interviewed and from the analysis of their transcribed accounts, Lindqvist and Hallberg (2010, p. 456) claimed:

> a substantive theory was generated showing that the main concern was *feelings of guilt due to self-inflicted disease* associated with smoking habits. This core category was related to five managing strategies termed *making sense of existence, adjusting to bodily restrictions, surrendering to fate, making excuses for the smoking-related cause* and *creating compliance with daily medication.*

If we take as a beginning point, that a project's 'worth' lies in two main components – its methodological justification and the congruency between the methodological assumptions and the project's outcomes (results, findings, insights, implications, recommendations) – then this article scores fairly well on both criteria.

In this article, Lindqvist and Hallberg (2010) give readers insights into the feelings of guilt related to self-inflicted disease and there is a reasonable (given the word limitation) description of GT. However, I wonder how Glaser would view their application of his GT, given that he has often strenuously insisted that these ideas have been misrepresented. Take the methodological justification, for instance. The researchers claimed they used Glaserian GT for their project, because theirs was an essentially inductive task, and GT offered them a constant comparison method and the ability to generate a core concept. However, the article shows no real evidence (as Barney might expect) of the meticulous method of constant comparison, leading to the formation of the core category. To claim the use of a GT method reflecting key GT concepts is one matter, to do that with the extreme precision and analytic accuracy demanded by Glaser is yet another matter. In effect, most projects claiming to use Glaser's GT (other than Barney's projects) would have shortfalls of some kind.

Read research texts to see how various authors present GT (e.g., Birks and Mills, 2011).

Also gather and read GT research articles, paying special attention to a project's 'worth' or trustworthiness. As you study the research articles, ask yourself two main questions:

- What is the author(s)' methodological justification of this type of GT?

- What is the degree of congruency between the stated GT assumptions and the project's reported outcomes (results, findings, insights, implications, recommendations)?

As you have seen from this chapter, the nature and application of GT is not as clear as the originators may have expected or reasonably hoped. While the blurriness of methodologies is philosophically acceptable as a 'mind field', especially in terms of the potential for spirited epistemological debates, it can turn out to be a 'mine field' for researchers, whose work is to be assessed by journal reviewers and thesis examiners.

Chapter summary

There are many key messages to be gleaned from this chapter, the first of which is that GT is positioned on the quantitative/qualitative methodological interface. GT began with Glaser and Strauss (1967), and it was then adapted (Strauss and Corbin, 1990b, 1998). In this chapter, we reviewed the original GT and its adaptations, and we also noted Barney Glaser's replies to researchers, who have made adaptations to Glaserian GT.

Definitions of GT vary. I subsumed the originators' approach to GT into a definition of an objective process of discovery and theory generation using theoretical sampling and constant comparative data analysis to collect, code, and analyse data continually until substantive and formal areas of inquiry emerge and build up to more inclusive formal grounded theories that fit and are relevant to the areas they claim to explain. Essentially, Strauss and Corbin's (1998) definition of GT is 'theory that is derived from data, systematically gathered and analysed through the research process'. For Charmaz (2008, p. 469), GT is 'an inductive, comparative, emergent, and interactive method' and these 'properties take full form in its constructivists versions and shape how researchers invoke its strategies' (Charmaz, 2008, p. 470). Therefore, we have seen that the definitions and theoretical assumptions of GT vary, from an objectivist to a constructivist standpoint.

Even though there are fundamental differences in the objectivist and constructivist GT approaches, it is possible to locate and describe some common GT concepts. Charmaz (2008, p. 472) suggests GT guidelines in accord with Glaser's comparative approach, which are helpful in finding commonalities in GT methods and processes, but they mask the various differences in GT approaches. If you are intending to use a GT approach for your research project, you need to explore the differences in GT in depth, so you can make an informed choice as to which version suits your needs best.

In the health sciences, GT projects have claimed to inductively generate theory from the data in the Glaser and Strauss, or Glaserian sense, or they claim to apply Strauss and Corbin's approach. Other projects have taken on a constructivist approach, or they used a non-specific form of GT, by claiming to be informed broadly by a selection of common GT epistemological ideas, while others seem to tack GT on to their project with the barest justification. GT has also been combined successfully with other methodologies, such as feminism, critical realism, ethnomethodology, extended case method, narrative analysis, and phenomenology.

As you gather and read GT research articles, pay special attention to a project's 'worth'. Ask yourself about the author(s)' methodological justification of their type of GT, and the degree of congruency between the stated GT assumptions and the project's reported outcomes. The nature and application of GT is not as clear as the originators may have expected or reasonably hoped. Be careful that you do not stumble unwittingly into a GT 'mine field'. If you choose GT for a research project, have a sound rationale for its use, and show clearly how you have applied it, with reference to the methodological assumptions and methods of that type of GT.

Key points

- Grounded theory is a qualitative interpretive methodology moving between objectivist and constructivist standpoints.

- Glaser and Strauss's original definition of GT was that it is an objective process of discovery and theory generation using theoretical sampling and constant comparative data analysis to collect, code, and analyse data continually until substantive and formal areas of inquiry emerge and build up to more inclusive formal grounded theories that fit and are relevant to the areas they claim to explain.

- Strauss and Corbin (1998) define GT as an objective discovery process, involving description, conceptual ordering and theorizing, to make microscopic analyses of data, aided by memos and diagrams and by asking questions and making comparisons in open, axial and selective coding, to form a grounded theory.

- For Charmaz (2008) GT is 'an inductive, comparative, emergent, and interactive method' whose 'properties take full form in its constructivists versions and shape how researchers invoke its strategies' (p. 470).

- Given that Glaser and Strauss's (1967) book on discovering GT was directed mainly to sociological theorizing and they placed the ownership of that activity in the domain of sociologists, some of the confusion and debates that ensued since may have been in part due to the authors' original convictions.

- Exploring GT leads inevitably to understanding adaptations of the original version of GT put forward by Glaser and Strauss.

- If you choose to use GT in your postgraduate research, it will be most likely that you will need to deal in depth with the primary GT authors' methodological differences, to decide on and justify your choice of a GT approach to inform your research.

Critical review questions

1 In what ways is it difficult to follow a grounded theory approach *exactly* to the steps in the method?

2 Is it possible to develop a grounded theory that will explain specific human experiences in *all* cases? Defend your answer with a reasoned rationale.

References

Birks, M., & Mills, J. (2011). *Grounded theory: A practical guide*. Thousand Oaks: Sage.

Boychuk Duchscher, J.E., & Morgan, D. (2004). Grounded theory: reflections on the emergence vs. forcing debate. *Journal of Advanced Nursing, 48*: 605–612.

Bryant, A. (2002). Re-grounding grounded theory. *Journal of Information Technology Theory and Application* 4(1): 25–42.

Bryant, A. (2003). A constructive/ist response to Glaser. *FQS: Forum for Qualitative Social Research,* 4. www.qualitative-research.net/fqs/-texte/1-03/1-03bryant-e. htm. Accessed September 2011.

Charmaz, K. (2000). Constructivist and objectivist grounded theory. In N.K. Denzin, & Y. Lincoln (Eds.) *Handbook of qualitative research,* 2nd edn. Thousand Oaks: Sage.

Charmaz, K., (2005). Grounded theory in the 21st Century. N.K. Denzin, & Y.S. Lincoln, (Eds.), *The Sage handbook of qualitative research*. Thousand Oaks: Sage.

Charmaz, K. (2006). *Constructing grounded theory: A practical guide through qualitative analysis*. Thousand Oaks: Sage.

Charmaz, K. (2008). Reconstructing grounded theory. In P. Alasuutari, L. Bickman & J. Brannen (Eds.) *The SAGE Handbook of social research methods*. London: Sage.

Creswell, John W. (1998). *Qualitative inquiry and research design*. Thousand Oaks: Sage.

Floersch, J., Longhofer, J.L., Kranke, D., & Townsend, L. (2010). Integrating thematic, grounded theory and narrative analysis: A case study of adolescent psychotropic treatment. *Qualitative Social Work, 9*(3), 407–425.

Giddings, L.S., & Grant, B.M. (2007). A trojan horse for positivism?: A critique of mixed methods research. *Advances in Nursing Science,* 30, 52.

Glaser, B.G. (1978). *Theoretical sensitivity: Advances in the methodology of grounded theory*. Mill Valley: Sociology Press.

Glaser, B.G. (1992). *Emergence vs forcing: Basics of grounded theory analysis*. Mill Valley: Sociology Press.

Glaser, B.G. (1998). *Doing grounded theory: issues and discussions*. Mill Valley, CA: Sociology Press.

Glaser, B.G. (2000). Constructivist grounded theory? *Forum Qualitative Sozialforschung / Forum: Qualitative Social Research* [On-line Journal], 3(3), Art. 12. Available at: http://www.qualitative-research.net/fqs-texte/3-02/3-02glaser-e.htm.

Glaser, B.G. (2002). Constructivist grounded theory? *Forum: Qualitative Social Research,* 3(3), [47 paragraphs].

Glaser, B.G., & Holton, J. (2004). Remodeling grounded theory. *Forum: Qualitative Social Research* 5(2), [80 paragraphs].

Glaser, B.G., & Strauss, A.L. (1967). *The discovery of grounded theory: Strategies for qualitative research*. Chicago: Aldine.

Heath, H., & Cowley, S. (2004). Developing a grounded theory approach: A comparison of Glaser and Strauss. *International Journal of Nursing Studies*, 41, 141–150.

Henwood, K. and Pidgeon, N. (2003) Grounded theory in psychological research. In P.M. Camic, J.E Rhodes & L. Yardley, Lucy (Eds.) *Qualitative research in psychology: Expanding perspectives in methodology and design*. Washington, DC: American Psychological Association.

Kalischuk, R.G. (2010). Cocreating life pathways: Problem gambling and its impact on families. *The Family Journal: Counselling and Therapy for Couples and Families, 18*(1): 7–17.

Kendall, J. (1999). Axial coding and the grounded theory controversy. *Western Journal of Nursing Research, 21*(6), 743–757.

Lester, M., & Hadden, S.C. (1980). Ethnomethodology and grounded theory methodology: An integration of perspective and method. *Journal of Contemporary Ethnography, 1980*(9), 3–33.

Lindqvist, G., & Hallberg, L.R. (2010). Feelings of guilt due to self-inflicted disease: A grounded theory of suffering from chronic obstructive pulmonary disease (COPD). *Journal Health Psychology, 15*(3): 456–466.

Malm, D. & Hallberg, L.R.-M. (2006). Patients' experiences of daily living with a pacemaker: A grounded theory study. *Journal of Health Psychology, 11*(5), 787–798.

May, K. (1994). The case for magic in method. In J. Morse (Ed.), *Critical Issues in Qualitative Research Methods*. Thousand Oaks: Sage, 10–22.

McCreaddie, M., Payne, S., & Froggat, K. (2010). Ensnared by positivity: A constructivist perspective on 'being positive' in cancer care. *European Journal of Oncological Nursing, 14*(4), 283–290.

Morse, J. (1994). Emerging from the data: Cognitive processes of analysis in qualitative research. In J. Morse (Ed.), *Critical issues in qualitative research methods*. Thousand Oaks: Sage, 23–41.

Oliver, C. (2011). Critical realist grounded theory: A new approach for social work research. *British Journal of Social Work, 42*(2): 1–17.

Plummer, M., & Young, L.E. (2009). Grounded theory and feminist inquiry: Revitalizing links to the past. *Western Journal of Nursing Research,* published online 29 December DOI: 10.1177/0193945909351298.

Seale, C. (1999) Quality in qualitative research. *Qualitative Inquiry* 5 (4): 465–478.

Skodol Wilson, H., & Hutchinson, S.A. (1991). Triangulation of qualitative methods: Heideggerian hermeneutics and grounded theory. *Qualitative Health Research, 1*(2), 263–276.

Strauss A.L. (1987) *Qualitative analysis for social scientists*. Cambridge: Cambridge University Press.

Strauss, A.L., & Corbin, J.M. (1990a) *Basics of qualitative research: Grounded theory procedures and techniques*. Thousand Oaks: Sage.

Strauss, A.L., & Corbin, J.M. (1990b) Open coding. *Basics of qualitative research: Grounded theory procedures and techniques*. Thousand Oaks: Sage, 101–121.

Strauss, A.L., & Corbin, J.M. (1994) 'Grounded theory methodology: an overview'. In N.K. Denzin, & Y.S. Lincoln, (Eds.), *Handbook of qualitative research*. Thousand Oaks: Sage.

Strauss, A.L., & Corbin, J.M. (1998). *Basics of qualitative research: Techniques and procedures for developing grounded theory*. Thousand Oaks: Sage.

Strauss, A.L. and Glaser B.G. (1970) *Anguish*. San Francisco: Sociology Press.

Tavory, I., & Timmermans, S. (2009). Two cases of ethnography: Grounded theory and the extended case method. *Ethnography, 10*(3), 243–263.

Wagman, P., Björklund, A., Håkansson, C., Jacobsson, C., & Falkmer, T. (2011). Perceptions of life balance among a working population in Sweden. *Qualitative Health Research, 21*(3), 410–418.

Wiese, M., & Oster, C. (2010). 'Becoming accepted': The complementary and alternative medicine practitioners' response to the uptake and practice of the traditional medicines therapies by the mainstream health sector. *Health, 14*(4), 415–433.

Historical research

Karen Francis

Understanding the past to inform the present and the future is a recognized field of qualitative research inquiry. Since the very dawn of time mankind has reflected on their lives and passed their experiences on to others through oral traditions, capturing illustrations of life experiences, written accounts and through fashioned artefacts. In this chapter historical research methodologies are described and the methods adopted to generate and analyse data are highlighted.

Origins of historical research

Looking at the past to inform the future is a common feature of research. Interest in how people lived in the past has and will continue to captivate future generations of people globally. Attempting to imagine what it must have been like to live without mobile phones will interest new generations of people who will communicate by different means that are as yet unimaginable. Warelow and Edward (2007, p. 57) affirmed that understanding of the present is made clearer when we are able to look to the past and the present, and examine how the present has been informed by the past, and acknowledge that both, the preceding and the present, are mutually important.

Future generations of researchers like those of today who are interested in history will need to be mindful not to judge yesterday on contemporary beliefs and understandings (Sweeney, 2005). Artefacts such as documents, art works, monuments, buildings and utensils left behind by past generations, are pieces of a puzzle that allow a single lens through which to look. Historical researchers have a duty to familiarize themselves with the societal norms of the day, recognize that cultural context is important and that persuasive influences that have shaped the lives of former generations are not always overt (McMurray, Pace, and Scott, 2004). It is appropriate to gather, collate and speculate on what the past may have been in order to generate an evidence-informed illustration of yesteryear, of specific events and of the daily lives of the people who once lived in the time and the context under investigation (Sweeney, 2005).

Defining historical research

There are many approaches that can be adopted to explore research questions that are historically situated (Brennan, 2011). Ashley (cited in Sweeney, 2005, p. 63) suggested that historical studies are '... an integrated written record of past events, based on the results of a search for truth'. This definition however does not accommodate the diversity of other records that can be accessed that reflect how people existed in preceding times, nor does it provide for the multiple realities, a tenet that underpins qualitative research epistemology. For our purposes historical research is defined as the study of the past. The simplicity of this definition is purposive as it accommodates the breath of philosophical traditions and captures the key intent of this type of research, investigations that are contextualized as occurring in former times. There are many types of historical research approaches such as oral histories, historiography, social and chronological historical accounts, all of which offer a window to glimpse what has occurred in times gone by.

Theoretical assumptions of historical research

Historical research like most other qualitative traditions has been informed by logical positivism, a tradition that accepts singular truths and uses verification of evidence as the method by which a truth is reached (Sweeney, 2005). Historical researchers are influenced by paradigmatic assumptions. Some historians favour a singular truth methodology reflective of the empiricist worldviews, while others prefer approaches that align with the interpretivists' tenets that value individuality, and accept that there are multiple realities and therefore multiple truths. Other researchers are influenced by the critical interpretivist paradigm and seek to uncover oppressive forces that have influenced individuals and societies (Brennan, 2011; Carr, 1990; Lewenson, 2011; Lusk, 1997).

Sweeney (2005, p. 65) cautioned that historical data, no matter what the orientation of the researcher, is subjected to a level of interpretation. He declared that researchers are removed in time and often place and their scholarship is therefore influenced by contemporary preconceptions that impact on their construction of the history they are re-creating (Sweeney, 2005). The warning proffered by Sweeney (2005) affirms that while historical studies are illuminating and provide a sense of what it was like, the studies present an informed hypothesis only. To ensure that the histories produced are as reliable an interpretation of the past as possible, the data generation methods adopted and the processes used to analyse and make sense of the data must be subjected to rigorous interrogation (McMurray et al., 2004). As suggested by Sweeney (2005) researchers should be true to the research tradition that they utilise, and the underpinning philosophical assumptions of the tradition should guide the research processes of data generation and analysis.

Undertaking a historical research study

The common feature of all historical research approaches is the intent to make sense of the past in order to inform the present and the future. Authors have commented that the process of undertaking historical research is like detective work (Schneider, Elliot, LoBiondo-Wood, and Haber, 2003; Sweeney, 2005). Historical research is always time specific and involves the interpretation of data generated from intensive rigorous investigation. The data is gathered from many sources that the researcher believes will provide insight into the period of time or foci of research interest. Piecing together a history, particularly when there are no people living to tell their story, is reliant on researcher interpretation of the evidence (data) collected. Historians begin their quest initially by posing a question that is historically contextualized, such as what were the experiences of Australian nurses in the Malayan Emergency (McLeod and Francis, 2007a) or what is the history of mental health nursing in Victoria, Australia (Sands, 2009; Sweeney, 2005). Other researchers identify a need for knowledge that requires a historical investigation. For example Guscott et al. (2007), in locating the development of new practices such as mental health trauma responses to disaster in Australia, tracked the impetus and subsequent evolution of this practice to the Bali bombings in 2002 (Guscott, Guscott, Mallingambi, and Parker, 2007).

Once a researchable phenomenon has been identified, a hypothesis is formed and research question/s delineated (Sweeney, 2005). The next phase in the process is to source data, categorize and analyse, formulating and testing conclusions, followed by a process of accepting or refuting conceptualized hypotheses (Sweeney, 2005). At each stage the researcher interrogates the data, seeking to verify authenticity.

A criticism of historical research is the contention that the demonstration of rigour in the research endeavour is reliant on development of theory to explain phenomenon that cannot be irrefutably proved. Keeping an open mind and letting the historical evidence speak for itself is a method of ensuring rigour in historical research investigations.

Data for historical studies is generated using techniques that include reviewing texts often located in libraries and other archival repositories (Lusk, 1997), collecting artefacts that provide insight into the lives of people in the past and through investigation of archival or documentary evidence. Data sources may include primary and secondary sources. Primary data sources are evidence left by those who have lived during the time or events being studied (Wood, 2011). This evidence includes artefacts such as architecture, maps, tools, personal and utilitarian items such as hair brushes, sewing kits, cooking pots, crockery, tools, clothing, quilts, tapestries and paintings or printed and hand-written records (Sweeney, 2005). Oral historians rely on conversations with people who have lived and experienced events that are of interest to them, such as war memories, being part of political or social movements or having lived through timeframes of interest. Collecting stories from people who have experienced a phenomenon that is time specified, such as nursing

Table 3.1 Understanding and evaluating historical sources (Wood, 2011, p. 27)

Criteria	Critique
Provenance	What kind of document is it? Who created the document? Why was the document created? What does the preservation suggest about its authenticity?
Purpose	What was the writer's purpose in creating the document? Who was the document written for? How did the writer's purpose influence the way the document was written?
Context	How does the document relate to its temporal, geographic, social, political, cultural and professional contexts? How representative is the document of other documents in the field? How representative is the writer of other people in the field?
Veracity	How credible is the writer? How might the writer's purpose in creating the document have introduced bias? What values and assumptions are evident in the document? How important is it that evidence in this document is accurate? How does the information differ from others?
Usefulness	How useful is the document for the research purpose? How does the document offer information not available from other sources?

in the Malayan Emergency, can challenge researchers to consider the ethical implications of the study. McLeod and Francis described the problem of protecting participants' identity when the numbers of people still living who could be involved in their study was minimal (McLeod and Francis, 2007b). They opted to use pseudonym names for each participant and to de-identify the names of places and people as a further safety net for ensuring compliance with the ethical approval of the study. Being familiar with ethical guidelines for human research is as important for historical studies as it is for other approaches.

Establishing the reliability of the data is an expected and necessary stage in all historical studies. Wood (2011) outlined four criteria for establishing the reliability of primary written data sources – see Table 3.1. Accessing archival materials is a negotiated process. Locating where information is and how it can be accessed is time consuming and can mean travelling to a repository to view information. Thankfully, many written documents have been digitalized, improving access (Lewenson, 2011). Computer programs such as NVivo, Ethnograph and websites that support searching family histories have enhanced the capacity of historical researchers to isolate and manage data.

Carbon dating of materials is another technique used to determine the age of carbon-based materials. This technique predicts the rate of carbon decay in order to estimate age. Carbon dating has been used extensively to date artefacts

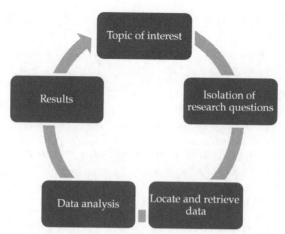

Figure 3.1 Steps in conducting a historical research investigation

such as building remains, plant and animal life including human remains (Anon, 2012). The age of cultures has been estimated using this method. Researchers drawing on non-written records such as illustrations, paintings, etchings, or utilitarian utensils may also need to establish the producer of such items as part of the evidence criterion. Depending on the item, processes such as comparing craftsmanship technique with known practices of the era is a commonly adopted practice (Ciceri, 2012; Matthaes, 2011).

Secondary sources of data are accounts of historical events and/or time provided by others who may or may not have used primary data sources to construct and theorize on the same foci as a new researcher to the field of study (Lewenson, 2011). These are valuable for researchers beginning a historical study. Reviewing the historical commentaries of others provides insight and often clues to data sources that may not have been considered. This approach may also provide a level of confirmation for researchers when the interpretations of others' investigations align with their own. Godden and Forsyth in Schneider et al. (2003) advocated this process, suggesting that ensuring familiarity with events of the day including the social, economic and political situations, provides background for understanding the period and the people. Wineberg suggested that historians must be tempered in their analysis and interpretation of data and report the findings of their investigations after thorough interrogation and cross-referencing of their information with other sources cited (Toman and Thifault, 2012). Sweeney (2005) supported this process, advocating that the data should be subjected to external criticism, that is, establishing the genuineness of the data source. Further, internal criticism is another method recommended by Sweeney (2005) to verify data authenticity. This process involves determining the intent of the data source and the meaning of that data. Holmes (2008) cautioned that historical information retrieved by researchers may have been produced as tools to manipulate. His warning to historical researchers is to be careful when constructing accounts of the past that the motivations of the authors are exposed, otherwise falsehoods can be perpetuated and accepted as truths (Holmes, 2008, p. 102). Holmes utilized the example of the dogma of Aryan supremacy purported by Hitler prior to, and during World War 2. He reasoned that Hitler and his supporters advanced their overt agenda to indiscriminately murder Jewish people (the Holocaust) by overtly advocating the superiority of the Aryan people. Many Germans and other cultural groups disaffected by the impact of the depression that occurred prior to the war accepted this propaganda, however following the war this doctrine was challenged internationally. Holmes argued that the intent of Hitler's propaganda was interrogated and the hidden agenda revealed. His message to researchers was that revealing the covert intent is as important as establishing the overt. Recognizing that secondary data sources are always another's interpretation is central to the process of critique and establishing an audit path for the study.

As discussed previously, there is no single approach to historical research. Researchers begin their quest with a problem and through a systematic process of uncovering information piece together a story that informs contemporary understanding. Interpreting the data that leads to the generation of the story/history is supported by an evidence trail and clear articulation of the assumptions the researcher has drawn to proffer an understanding of the historical phenomenon being investigated. Clarifying the intent of the research through enunciation of a research question or questions defines the parameters of the study and guides the data generation and analysis methods to be employed (Lewenson, 2011). Figure 3.1 provides direction for undertaking a historical investigation.

Case example of a nursing history

Many researchers are drawn to historical research when questions they ask of the present cannot be answered. My own doctoral study was a historical study of the beginnings of community health nursing in the colony of New South Wales. The impetus for this study was to uncover why community nurses in Britain were highly regarded yet community nursing in Australia had not been privileged to the same degree. I began the study with the hypothesis that community nursing in Australia should reflect the same development as had occurred in Britain. My study was guided by Michel Foucault, a French 20th-century historian who became interested in understanding the relationship between power, discourse and disciplinary knowledge. Foucault was a historian who challenged traditional chronological historical accounts by illuminating the covert powers that control societies, groups and individuals (McHoul and Grace, 1993). My investigation was informed by the philosophical assumptions of the critical interpretivist paradigm. This was appropriate theoretically as I was asking the data I collected critical questions that included who is speaking and why, who has allowed them to speak and why?

Preliminary readings of historical accounts were silent on the evolution of community nursing in Australia in the 19th century but these allowed me to construct a chronology of events that directed my investigation. As my interest was piqued I began to ask questions of the texts as described above that I was able to locate and then began a process of tracking primary source data generally isolated from reading potted historical accounts of nursing, social and military commentaries. I developed a very close relationship with a librarian who specialized in history at my university. As I identified primary source data that included policy documents, personal diaries, hospital reports, correspondence and secondary data namely, historical commentaries, biographies of significant persons and discussions with experts, my librarian associate tracked the texts. Throughout the study tracking data sources was a challenge but I am pleased to report, my librarian's tenacity and skill was such that we not only located digital copies, but were sent original reports dating back as far as the middle of the 19th century from repositories in Ireland, England and Australia. I was given permission to keep many of these, which were added to materials of my university library.

The period of time initially targeted that would define the study was from white colonization of Australia, 1788 to 1998. As the study progressed, it became apparent that understanding why the history of community nursing in the colony took an alternative path to that in Britain, could only be revealed by tracing back in time, and across continents. My study drew on data generated from Ireland, England and France and dated back to the 17th century.

My thesis was that community nursing in Australia is an artefact of the work of the Catholic religious women who arrived in Australia in 1832. The Sisters of Charity, an Irish order of religious women, established community nursing services to treat the poor of Sydney prior to establishing St Vincent's Hospital in 1857. The establishment of professional nursing practice in Australia has been attributed to Lucy Osburn, the first Matron appointed to the Sydney Hospital in 1868. The Catholic religious women who preceded Osburn were trained nurses, hospital administrators and one was an apothecary, yet their professional status and the contribution they made to nursing and healthcare was silenced. Using a Foucauldian lens to examine the chronological history I constructed, I hypothesized that while the religious women were well-educated women of their day their religiosity limited their capacity to write history. I concluded that their contribution was silenced and an alternative history of nursing and healthcare in the colony of New South Wales has been perpetuated and accepted (Francis, 1998). My study highlighted an alternative version of the development of nursing, specifically community nursing, and raised awareness of covert agendas that had shaped understanding of the past (Brennan, 2011).

Limitations of historical research

Describing the past is fraught with difficulty. The more removed the researcher is from the time and place that contextualize the study, the more likely it is that the interpretation constructed is limited. Historical studies, even those that draw on the lived accounts of people who have experienced the phenomenon of interest, are influenced by time and as some have argued their memories will have faded, impacting on their recall. Historical studies are useful and provide understanding but like other research approaches are not infallible.

Chapter summary

This chapter has provided an overview of historical research. A description of the research process was provided to guide understanding. Limitations of this methodology were highlighted and an example of a study provided.

Key points

- Understanding the present is made clearer when we are able to look to the past and the present, and examine how the present has been informed by the past, and acknowledge that both are mutually important.

- Historical researchers have a duty to familiarize themselves with the societal norms of the day, recognize that cultural context is important and that persuasive influences that have shaped the lives of former generations are not always overt.

- Stated simply, historical research is defined as the study of the past.

- Some historians favour a singular truth methodology reflective of the empiricist worldviews, while others prefer approaches that align with the interpretivists' tenets that value individuality, and accept that there are multiple realities and therefore multiple truths. Other researchers are influenced by the critical interpretivist paradigm and seek to uncover oppressive forces that have influenced individuals and societies.

- The common feature of all historical research approaches is the intent to make sense of the past in order to inform the present and the future.

- Researchers begin their quest with a problem and through a systematic process of uncovering information piece together a story that informs contemporary understanding.

- Interpreting the data that leads to the generation of the story/history is supported by an evidence trail and clear articulation of the assumptions the researcher has drawn to proffer an understanding of the historical phenomenon being investigated.

- Clarifying the intent of the research through enunciation of a research question or questions defines the parameters of the study and guides the data generation and analysis methods to be employed.

Critical review questions

1 Discuss the relevance of historical studies as a research enterprise.

2 Identify and describe the range of data generation research on methods and consider the strengths and weaknesses of each.

3 Discuss the statement 'Historical research informs the future'.

4 Describe how rigour can be maintained in historical research studies.

References

Anon. (2012). Carbon dating. Retrieved 19 November 2012, from http://hyperphysics.phy-astr.gsu.edu/hbase/nuclear/cardat.html.

Brennan, D. (2011). Telling stories about ourselves: historical methodology and the creation of mental nursing narratives. *Journal of Psychiatric and Mental Health Nursing*, 18, 657–663.

Carr, E. (1990). *What is history?* London: Penguin.

Ciceri, G. (2012). Ten steps to verify the authenticity of antique silverwares. Retrieved 19 November 2012, from http://www.ascasonline.org/articoloaa31ING.html.

Francis, K. (1998). Poverty, chastity and obedience: the foundations of community nursing in the colony of New South Wales. PhD thesis, University of Adelaide, Adelaide.

Guscott, W.M., Guscott, A.J., Mallingambi, G., & Parker, R. (2007). The Bali bombings and the evolving mental health response to disaster in Australia: Lessons from Darwin. *Journal of Psychiatric and Mental Health Nursing*, 14(3), 239–242.

Holmes, C.A. (2008). Historical inquiry and understanding our past. *Contemporary Nurse*, 30(2), 101–106.

Hung, P., & Popp, A. (2012). Learning to do historical research: a primer, how to frame a researchable question. Retrieved 10 September 2012, from http://www.williamcronon.net/researching/questions.htm.

Lewenson, S.B. (2011). Historical research method. In H.J. Streubert & D. Rinaldi Carpenter (Eds.), *Qualitative Research in Nursing* (pp. 225–248). Philadelphia: Wolters Kluwer, Lippincott, Williams & Wilkins.

Lusk, B. (1997). Historical methodology for nursing research. *Journal of Nursing Scholarship*, 29(4), 355–359.

Matthaes, G. (2011). Determining the authenticity of antique and modern paintings Retrieved 19 November 2012, from http://www.paintingsauthenticity.com/.

McHoul, A.W., & Grace, W. (1993). *A Foucault primer: Discourse, power and the subject.* Melbourne: Melbourne University Press.

McLeod, M., & Francis, K. (2007a). Invisible partners: the Royal Australian Army Nursing Corps pathway to the Malayan Emergency. *International Journal of Nursing Practice*, 13(6), 341–347.

McLeod, M., & Francis, K. (2007b). A safety net: use of pseudonyms in oral nursing history. *Contemporary Nurse*, 25(1–2), 104–113.

McMurray, A.J., Pace, R.W., & Scott, D. (2004). *Research: a common sense approach.* Southbank, Victoria: Thomson.

Sands, N.M. (2009). Round the bend: a brief history of mental health nursing in Victoria, Australia 1848–1950s. *Issues in Mental Health Nursing*, 30(6), 364–371.

Schneider, Z., Elliot, D., LoBiondo-Wood, G., & Haber, J. (2003). *Nursing research* (2nd edn). Sydney: Mosby.

Sweeney, J.F. (2005). Historical research: examining documentary sources. *Nurse Researcher*, 13(3), 61–73.

Toman, C., & Thifault, M.-C. (2012). Historical thinking and the shaping of nursing identity. *Nursing History Review*, 20, 184–204.

Warelow, P., & Edward, K.-L. (2007). Evidence-based mental health nursing in Australia: our history and our future. *International Journal of Mental Health Nursing.*, 16, 57–61. doi: 10.1111/j.1447-0349.2006.00445.x.

Wood, P. (2011). Understanding and evaluating historical sources in nursing history research. *Nursing Praxis in New Zealand*, 27(1), 25–33.

4

Ethnography

Karen Francis

This chapter provides an overview of ethnographic research. Like other qualitative research approaches there are many adaptations of ethnography, however all are concerned with the study of culture or cultural groups. The origins of this methodology are identified and the philosophical tenets that underpin the approach discussed. Data generation methods and a process to guide data analysis are featured.

Defining ethnography

Ethnography is the study of culture. This methodology is the oldest of the qualitative research approaches (Strauss et al., 1984; Hoare, 2012) developed from the traditions of anthropology and sociology (Polit and Beck, 2001; Genzuk, 2003; Giampietro, 2011; Lambert et al., 2011). Ethnography evolved to address researchers' desire to understand cultures and cultural knowledge (Giampietro, 2011). Muecke (1994 in Streubert and Rinaldi Carpenter, 2011) proffered that there is no single ethnographic approach; rather, the process adopted reflects the training and belief systems of the individual researcher. Nonetheless, Muecke (1994 in Streubert and Rinaldi Carpenter, 2011) categorized ethnographic research into four major schools of thought/approaches:

1 Classical

2 Systematic

3 Interpretative or hermeneutic

4 Critical.

Classical ethnography involves extensive time in 'the field' observing behaviours and explicating why and under what circumstances these occur. Systematic ethnography is interested in the organization of culture while interpretive or hermeneutic ethnography seeks to uncover the meanings of interactions and behaviours (Streubert and Rinaldi Carpenter, 2011). Critical ethnographies investigate culture adopting a critical lens to identify internal and external power relationships that influence how the group behaves (Foley and Valenzuela, 2008; Streubert and Rinaldi Carpenter, 2011). Critical ethnographies aim to empower the cultural group by raising individuals and the group's awareness. Critical ethnographies are characterized as having a political intent. A heightened awareness provides the group with opportunity to effect change if they decide it is necessary (Schneider et al., 2003; Baumbusch, 2010). Foley and Valenzuela (2008) make the point that some critical ethnographers are extremely politically motivated and use their research credentialing to assume positions of authority and become public spokespersons for the 'oppressed'. In recent years two new ethnographic approaches have emerged and are gaining popularity. Ethnonursing, conceptualized by Leininger (1985), provides a framework for ethnographic investigations of nursing specific phenomenon, and auto-ethnography is a study of personal experience that is culturally positioned.

Ethnography provides researchers with an approach to examine in depth and holistically, cultural groups. Spradley (1979) maintains that ethnography is a useful research methodology for health researchers and in particular nurse researchers as this approach provides a lens for seeing the whole, not just a glimpse of a part and enables insight into group beliefs and practices (Streubert and Rinaldi Carpenter, 2011).

Theoretical assumptions of ethnography

Ethnographic research, the study of cultures, evolved from anthropology, the investigation of people, their ways of living, what they believe and how they adapt to change (Burns and Grove, 2005). In the latter years of the 19th century and early 20th century social anthropology began to emerge as new methodology for examining cultures. Ethnographic studies of all types aim to interpret culture by explicating the nuances of what makes a culture or cultural group distinct, albeit from different perspectives. They are always conducted in naturalistic settings, involve the collection of data using multiple methods that include both emic and etic perspectives of data generation, case numbers are small and there are a myriad of ethical issues that need to be negotiated prior to, and during data collection (Lambert et al., 2011).

Understanding the world of cultures or cultural groups provides a rich tapestry for making sense of the knowledge that is integral to the culture of interests' collective identity. This knowledge underpins the dynamics of the group's interactions, behaviours and the way in which the group is structured and the sense that they have of their cultural group. Ethnographic researchers are interested in identifying the cultural norms, patterns of social interaction and the methods used to ensure cultural cohesiveness that are indicative of how the cultural group functions. The knowledge generated is socially constructed, that is, it is an outcome of the interaction between people and their world (Lambert et al., 2011). Spradley added to the discourse on this methodology arguing that ethnographic research involves learning from others (cited in Streubert and Rinaldi Carpenter, 2011).

Critical ethnographic studies seek to identify issues of inequality that may be related to race, gender and class in cultures and cultural groups in order to comprehend them (McMurray et al., 2004). A critical ethnographic study was undertaken in Western Australia to explore the experiences of eight women nurses working in public hospital middle management roles or the corporate sector. The researchers believed that women are disadvantaged because of their gender. The study found that the participants were oppressed because of the patriarchal nature of management structures and practices and of the dominance of the medical model that underpins health services and health service delivery (Pannowitz et al., 2009).

Common ethnography research characteristics and concepts

The centrality of the researcher as investigator, the cyclical nature of data generation and analysis and cultural immersion are fundamental characteristics that underpin ethnographic research. Cultural immersion is a central point of difference between ethnography and other qualitative research methodologies (Baumbusch, 2010). Spending time in the cultural setting, listening, observing and asking questions to gain insight into the cultural milieu and the day-to-day relationships that influence how individuals behave and why and under what conditions, is the fundamental data generation techniques utilized by proponents of ethnography.

Discerning how cultures see themselves and view the world is an intrinsic aspect of ethnographic research and can be achieved through cultural immersion. Being immersed in a culture amplifies the researcher's awareness and appreciation of what is being observed, thus facilitating data analysis (Allen et al., 2008). Malinowski proposed that investigations of cultures should bridge the gap between extrinsic and intrinsic knowing. Observing from an outsider (etic) perspective provides researchers with a single dimensional level of understanding (Polit and Beck, 2001; Hoare et al., 2012) that relies on the researchers' frames of reference to contextualize and make sense of the information they collect (observation, asking questions, reviewing texts) and process. Adding depth and legitimizing understanding of what is observed by the researcher is achieved through the adoption of emic data generation techniques; that is, through insider perspectives. Asking members of the culture to share their experiences and to seek clarification when needed adds clarity to the research, strengthens the trustworthiness of the data and analysis. As Polit and Beck (2001) offered, ethnographers seek to reveal tacit knowledge that they define as:

> … information about the culture that is so deeply embedded in cultural experiences that members do not talk about it or may not even be consciously aware of it. (p. 213)

By using etic and emic approaches for data generation, ethnographers can achieve this research goal as demonstrated in the following exemplar.

A study undertaken of Sri Lankan nurses' management of pain in cancer patients involved the researcher undertaking 3 months observation of nurses working in a specialist cancer hospital. This data was supplemented by interviews with 10 nurse participants. The researcher kept a diary throughout that was used to make notations of what was observed, and reflections and interpretation of what was happening and why. Findings from this study highlighted that nurses did not manage effectively cancer patients' pain. The nurses were task oriented, not well resourced and had limited knowledge of aetiology and symptomology of cancer, which impeded their capacity to pre-empt and respond to pain exacerbation (De Silva, 2008). This exemplar illustrates the strength of ethnographic research. The nurses in this study were unable to meet patient needs as the model of care, task orientation restricted their practice. The researcher argued that high workloads, nursing shortages and poor understanding of pain management were factors that contributed to their practice inertia.

Ethnographic research draws on symbolic interactionism to appreciate the meanings that the culture affords to objects, interactions, beliefs and the way in which members communicate (Anderson and Taylor, 2009). It is this insight that provides the depth of understanding required to make sense of, and understand, how a cultural group functions and the rules that guide behaviours.

Data collection methods

The collection of data for ethnographic studies aims to capture the social meanings and ordinary activities of members of the cultural group of interest (informants) in naturally occurring settings, or contexts (e.g. home, community, workplace, educational setting). The context is referred to as the 'field' (Genzuk, 2003; Lambert et al., 2011). Typically, ethnographers enter the world of the culture, the field of study they are investigating to generate data that will allow them to answer the research questions they have posed. Entering the field requires ethnographers to identify biases that may potentially limit their capacity to see and understand the world of the cultural group as they experience it (Baumbusch, 2010). If preconceived ideas and beliefs are not subjected to such interrogation, misunderstanding may occur and there is likelihood that data analysis will become ethnocentric, providing, at best, a stifled biased etic description (Omohundra, 2008; Vandenberg and Hall, 2011). Genzuk (2003) cautions that reporting factually what is observed is necessary to avoid researcher biases, while Baumbusch (2010) advocates researchers engage in an ongoing process of reflexivity. She describes this process as a self-critique of values and belief systems that incorporates identifying the researchers' social positioning and their relationship with the group.

Ethnographers traditionally generate data using a variety of techniques that include but are not limited to observation, interviews, focus groups, review of documentary evidence and keeping field notes. Prior to entering the field, ethics approval to undertake a study involving humans must be obtained (Nagy et al., 2010; Baumbusch, 2010; Allbutt, 2010). The intent of the research, the expectations of participants who agree to take part and their options for withdrawing consent must be clearly explicated. A signed consent is generally required prior to individuals being included in ethnographic studies. This process ensures that the research study meets the ethical guidelines for research conducted on humans and limits harm to those who agree to be involved (Genzuk, 2003; National Health and Medical Research Council, 2012). Ethnographic studies are labour intensive and time consuming as extensive periods of time are spent in the field collecting data.

Prior to entering the field, it is often the practice of ethnographic researchers to familiarize themselves with the cultural group and their context (workplace, community, school). This is achieved by reading the literature, visiting the context and introducing the researcher and providing a forum for members of the cultural group to ask questions (Genzuk, 2003; Eberle and Maeder, 2011; Allen et al., 2008). This process establishes researcher credibility and facilitates the development of relationships between the researcher and members of the culture (Allbutt, 2010). Some ethnographic researchers entering the field have intimate and/or expert knowledge of the culture that facilitates their research journey (Allen et al., 2008). Blogg and Hyde (2008) undertook a study of carers of people undergoing home haemodialysis. These researchers acknowledged that having a background in renal nursing and home support raised their awareness of the necessity to better understand the needs of carers who support these people and facilitated their access to the field for data generation. The authors advocated that health professionals including nurses recognize that carers require information, support and counselling when they become overwhelmed. They argued that while nurses are providing care to people on home dialysis they can also provide support to carers by engaging them in activities, inviting questions, assessing how they are managing and facilitating additional support when required (Blogg and Hyde, 2008).

Ethnographic data is generally of three types:

- Cultural behaviours (what members do)

- Cultural artefacts (what members make and use)

- Cultural speech (what people say) (Polit and Beck, 2001).

These data types are produced using a number of methods that include recording what the researcher sees and interpretation of this information through field notations. Field notations are written and/or recorded (audiotaping, digital voice recordings or video recordings) to capture initial ideas of what is being observed and reflections on the information generated. Pannowitz et al. (2009) suggested that the reflective musings of the researchers are largely internalized critical conversations that facilitate processing of the information generated, and initial theorizing about the data.

Observational data is perhaps the mainstay of an ethnographer's data collecting tool-box. Observation involves being immersed (Roberts, 2009) in the field, that is, being present and watching what happens in the context of the cultural group (Eberle and Maeder, 2011). Researchers may watch without participating in the activities of the group. This process is termed non-participant observation (Eberle and Maeder, 2011; Baumbusch, 2010). Observing and participating in the activities of the cultural group is termed participant observation (Baumbusch, 2010). Participant observation, argues Genzuk (2003):

> is an omnibus field strategy in that it simultaneously combines document analysis, interviewing of respondents and informants, direct participation and observation, and introspection.

Pannowitz et al. (2009) completed an ethnographic study. They supported the technique of being with participants in their practice world to gain insight of the culture as it is experienced by the participants, while Vandenberg and Hall (2011) promoted Carspeckens' (1996) approach to observational data collection that involved initial passive observation of the cultural group until little new information is captured. At this point they recommended closer scrutiny of the group and individuals' behaviour patterns should occur. To reduce researcher bias and focus their data collection, they also supported keeping field notations of identified issues that they felt required further clarification. These researchers offered that by speaking with participants about the issues and/or engaging in more observation the clarification required was achieved.

Asking questions to clarify observational data is a technique employed by ethnographers and it is also a way for validating tentative thoughts about the meaning of generated data (Bland, 2006; Allen et al., 2008). Approaching participants or key informants (people the ethnographer has recognized as being able to answer specific questions) to gain further insight or clarify issues is one strategy to authenticate initial theorizing. Referring to processes or practices that have been observed or gleaned from review of other data sources such as documents, records or organizational charts is another way of confirming beliefs about the data. Using tools such as interview schedules to direct conversations enabling the researcher to collect targeted information, is a method that can also be employed to generate information and to further clarify assumptions about the culture (Nawafleh et al., 2012). King et al. in their study of Aboriginal Health Workers used this approach to explore with participants the impact of a diabetes educational programme on their practice (King et al., 2007).

Making sense of the world of the cultural group requires understanding of how meaning is ascribed to the objects, behaviours and others. Ethnography is deeply influenced or indeed is informed by symbolic interactionism. Symbolic interactionism theory asserts that:

- people act toward things on the basis of the meanings they ascribe to those things;
- that the meanings ascribed to these things are derived from, or arise out of, the social interaction that one has with others and the society; and
- that these meanings are handled in, and modified through, an interpretative process used by the person in dealing with the things he/she encounters (Nelson, 1998, p. 1).

Ethnographic research aims to ask and answer questions about cultures that make visible this knowledge. Continually asking the data as it is generated the following questions is a useful strategy for refining the analysis process:

- what beliefs and practices inform how the group construct their world,
- what is it like for each person in this context,
- how do individuals shape their lives within the context, and
- what environmental factors influence coping and adaptation.

(Nawafleh et al., 2012, p. 66)

The generation of data generally involves more than one method (Allen et al., 2008; Lambert et al., 2011). Participant observation, field notes, interviews, and surveys are examples of commonly adopted methods of collection. Interviews may be conducted with individuals or groups (focus groups) to explore issues and/or to clarify observed behaviours or documentation. These data are generally audio recorded and subsequently transcribed for data analysis. Field notes are used to capture observations, initial thoughts or reflections, and may include initial analyses and conceptualizations. Secondary data sources such as document retrieval and analysis are often accessed to uncover 'rules' or 'codes of behaviour' that direct interactions and the manner in which groups function. Historical information may be accessed to inform understanding of the past, which can inform understanding of where patterns of thoughts, behaviours and practices observed evolved from (Nawafleh et al., 2012).

In order to make the data collection and interpretation transparent, researchers creating ethnographies often attempt to be 'reflexive'. Reflexivity refers to a method adopted by researchers to critically reflect on the ways in which their involvement in a study influences, acts upon and informs the research (Barton, 2008). Despite engaging in this process, no researcher can be totally unbiased, which has provided the basis for critique of this methodology.

Data analysis

Ethnographic studies typically use multiple data generation techniques as described previously. Each individual data set (transcriptions of interviews, field notations, documentary analysis) is reviewed for overall content. Content refers to the key themes or ideas that are overtly identifiable, with reference to the research questions that underpin the study. These initial themes generally direct the next stage of analysis that involves rereading the text, interrogating the data for covert information (surreptitious or hidden meaning) and allocating data segments of text to named codes that explain elements of the culture under investigation.

Next, all the generated coded data segments (themes) are again reviewed and like codes grouped as a category code. The created category code/s are given a new name that captures the common meanings inherent in each smaller code (subcode). The process follows a hierarchical method of synthesizing

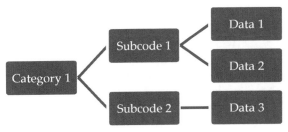

Figure 4.1 Conceptualization of the steps in data analysis for each data set

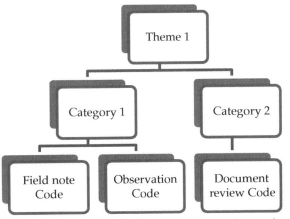

Figure 4.2 Conceptualization of individual data set code synthesis

and reducing as the analysis moves from the initial to the finalized stage of analysis. As each level of analysis occurs the level of abstraction of the data also increases (Figure 4.1).

Individual analysed data sets (those from the field notes, observations, interviews/focus groups and document reviews) are compared and commonalities and differences identified (Genzuk, 2003). Figure 4.2 illustrates the process of examining data codes from each data set and synthesizing the information to create themes that reflect the final level of analysis. It is at this stage that the researcher is able to describe the culture under investigation and answer the research questions that underpin the study.

Describing in detail the theorizing that has guided the research provides an audit trail that is a useful strategy for limiting researcher bias (Roberts, 2009). This strategy, combined with the reflexive process discussed previously strengthen claims that the research has followed a rigorous, analytical, sequenced investigation consistent with the methodology of ethnography (Roberts, 2009).

Interpretation involves attaching meaning and significance to the analysis. Identified patterns of activity and other social processes must be explained. This procedure can involve revealing relationships and linkages that direct and/or influence these that the group may or may not be conscious of

(Lambert, 2011). Once these steps have been completed the researcher reports on their interpretations, providing a rationale for how data were managed and a justification for the conclusions offered. Contexualized examples are included as evidence of the intellectualizing process. It is usual for ethnographers to provide a detailed description or ethnography of the culture in which the typical activities, relationships and rules that guide the group's actions are explicated. Recommendations proffered arising from the research should reflect the findings and correspond with the research questions initially posed.

Limitations

The flexibility of ethnographic methodologies has raised questions about the rigour of this type of research. The reliance on researcher interpretation and on cultural immersion as a data collection approach are cited as key limitations of this methodology. However these features are also the strengths of this research approach that is concerned with the study of culture.

Chapter summary

Ethnographic research is a widely used methodology in health research. Studying culture and cultural groups allows insight into social actions and how groups of people construct and live in their worlds. For health researchers, ethnographic studies are a mechanism or window for viewing and making sense of the life worlds, and the rules that inform understanding and behaviours of people they encounter in therapeutic interactions and through professional encounters.

Key points

- Ethnography is the study of culture.
- Classical ethnography involves extensive time in 'the field' observing behaviours and explicating why and under what circumstances these occur.
- Systematic ethnography is interested in the organization of culture while interpretive or hermeneutic ethnography seeks to uncover the meanings of interactions and behaviours.
- Critical ethnographies investigate culture adopting a critical lens to identify internal and external power relationships that influence how the group behaves, with the aim to empower the cultural group by raising individuals' and the group's awareness.
- Understanding the world of cultures or cultural groups provides a rich tapestry for making sense of the knowledge that is integral to the culture of interests' collective identity.

- The centrality of the researcher as investigator, the cyclical nature of data generation and analysis and cultural immersion are fundamental characteristics that underpin ethnographic research.

- The collection of data for ethnographic studies aims to capture the social meanings and ordinary activities of members of the cultural group of interest (informants) in naturally occurring settings, or contexts (e.g. home, community, workplace, educational setting).

- Ethnographers traditionally generate data using a variety of techniques that include but are not limited to observation, interviews, focus groups, review of documentary evidence and keeping field notes.

- Ethnographic data are generally of: cultural behaviours (what members do); cultural artefacts (what members make and use); and cultural speech (what people say).

Critical review questions

1 Discuss the strengths and limitations of ethnographic research.

2 Discuss the ethical issues that ethnographers need to consider before entering the 'field'.

3 Identify and discuss the range of data generation methods that maybe adopted by ethnographers.

References

Allbutt, H. (2010). Ethnography and the ethics of undertaking research in different mental health settings. *Journal of Psychiatric and Mental Health Nursing*, 17, 210–215.

Allen, S., K. Francis et al. (2008). Examining the methods used for a critical ethnographic enquiry. *Contemporary Nurse* 29(2): 227–237.

Anderson, M.L. and H.F. Tayor (2009). *Sociology: The essentials*. Belmont, USA: Thomson Wadsworth.

Barton, D. (2008). Understanding practitioner ethnography. *Nurse Researcher* 15(2): 7–18.

Baumbusch, J.L. (2010). Conducting critical ethnography in long-term residential care: experiences of a novice researcher in the field. *Journal of Advanced Nursing* 67(1): 184–192.

Bland, M. (2006). Betwixt and between: a critical ethnography of comfort in New Zealand residential aged care. *Journal of Clinical Nursing* 16(937–944): 937.

Blogg, A. and C. Hyde (2008). The experience of spouses caring for a person on home haemodialysis: an ethnography. *Renal Society of Australasia Journal* 4(3): 75–80.

Burns, N. and S.K. Grove (2005). *The practice of nursing research: Appraisal, synthesis and generation of evidence*. St Louis, USA: Saunders Elsevier.

Carspecken, P. F. (1996). *Critical ethnography in educational research: A theoretical and practical guide*. New York and London, Routledge.

De Silva, B.S.S. (2008). An ethnography study of nurses cancer pain management in Sri Lanka. Nursing & Midwifery. Melbourne, Australian Catholic University. Master of Nursing.

Eberle, T.S. and C. Maeder (2011). Organizational ethnography. *Qualitative Research* D. Silverman. Los Angeles, Sage: 53–74.

Foley, D. and A. Valenzuela (2008). Critical ethnography: The politics of collaboration. *The Landscape Qualitative Research*. N.K. Denzin and Y.S. Lincoln. Los Angeles, Sage: 287–310.

Genzuk, M. (2003). A synthesis of ethnographic research. Retrieved 3 November 2012, from http://www-bcf.usc.edu/~genzuk/Ethnographic_Research.html.

Giampietro, G. (2011). Ethnography. *Qualitative Research*. D. Silverman. Padstow, UK, Sage: 15–34.

Hoare, K., S. Beutow et al. (2012). Using an emic and etic ethnographic technique in a grounded theory study of information use by practice nurses in New Zealand. *Journal of Nursing Research*: 1–12.

King, M., R. Hunt et al. (2007). The impact of a postgraduate diabetes course on the perceptions of Aboriginal health workers and supervisors in South Australia. *Contemporary Nurse* 25(1–2): 82–93.

Lambert, B., M. Glacken et al. (2011). Employing an ethnographic approach: key characteristics. *Nurse Researcher* 19(1): 17–24.

Leininger, M.M. (1985). *Qualitative research methods in nursing*. New York, Crune & Stratton

McMurray, A.J., R.W. Pace et al. (2004). *Research: a common sense approach*. Southbank, Victoria, Thomson.

Nagy, S., J. Mills et al. (2010). *Using research in healthcare practice*. Broadway, Wolters Kluwer, Lippincott, Williams & Wilkins.

National Health and Medical Research Council (2012). National approach to single ethical review. Retrieved 11 December 2012, from http://www.nhmrc.gov.au/health-ethics/national-approach-single-ethical-review.

Nawafleh, H., K. Francis et al. (2012). The impact of nursing leadership and management on the control of HIV/Aids: an ethnographic study. *Contemporary Nurse* 42(2): 247–257.

Nelson, L.D. (1998). Herbert Blumer's Symbolic Interactionism. Retrieved 12 November 2012, from http://www.colorado.edu/communication/meta-discourses/Papers/App_Papers/Nelson.htm.

Omohundra, J.T. (2008). *Thinking like an anthropologist: a practical guide to cultural Anthropology*. New York, McGraw Hill.

Pannowitz, H.K., N. Glass et al. (2009). Resisting gender-bias: insights from Western Australian middle-level women nurses. *Contemporary Nurse* 33(2): 103–119.

Polit, D.F., and C.T. Beck (2001). *Essentials of nursing research: methods, appraisal and utilization*. Philadelphia, Lippincott.

Roberts, T. (2009). Understanding ethnography. *British Journal of Midwifery* 17(5): 291–294.

Schneider, Z., D. Elliot et al. (2003). *Nursing research*. Sydney: Mosby.

Spradley, J.P. (1979). *The ethnographic interview*. New York: Rinehardt & Winston.

Strauss, A.L.S., J. Corbin et al. (1984). *Chronic illness and quality of life*. St Louis, C.V. Mosby.

Streubert, H.J. and D. Rinaldi Carpenter (2011). *Qualitative research in nursing, advancing the humanistic imperative*. Philadelphia, Wolters Kluwer, Lippincott, Williams & Wilkins.

Vandenberg, H. and W. Hall (2011). Critical ethnography: extending attention to bias and reinforcement of dominant power relations. *Nurse Researcher* 18(3): 25–30.

5

Phenomenology

Bev Taylor

In this chapter, we turn our attention to an early 20th-century philosophical tradition, which opened up for systematic and in-depth discussion, areas of inquiry relating to human consciousness and experience. The development of phenomenology as a methodology for research inquiry came about as a result of philosophical debates about the purposes and means for understanding phenomena, as potential answers to epistemological and ontological questions.

At the outset, I need to alert you to the possibility that you may begin to feel overwhelmed by the immensity and complexity of phenomenological thought, because it is the 'bread and butter' of philosophers, who are properly skilled in tackling epistemological and ontological puzzles. My first intention in this chapter, therefore, is to guide you through the essentials, so you can understand the fundamental ideas and make an informed choice about the type of phenomenology to suit your research project. Also, healthcare researchers have been criticized by contemporary philosophers for misapplying phenomenology. Therefore, my second intention in this chapter is to assist you in conceptualizing phenomenology sufficiently to ensure that your project is indeed phenomenological, not simply qualitative, and that its methods and processes reflect and apply as faithfully as possible, various selected phenomenological concepts.

As an introduction to phenomenology as a methodology, our initial focus in this chapter will be on definitions of phenomenology and some theoretical assumptions as proposed by its originators. Given that the field of phenomenology is vast and rich philosophically, we will then explore some common phenomenological concepts and methods. The chapter concludes with a discussion of some examples of phenomenological research in healthcare.

Defining phenomenology

Defining phenomenology can be a very simple or an extraordinarily complex task. At its simplest definitional level, phenomenology is the study of things (phenomena). Beyond that simple definition there are many ways of encapsulating phenomenology, depending on the type to which philosophers subscribe. However, the constant in definitions is located in the catch-cry of phenomenology from its Husserlian beginnings, to go: 'To the things!'

(*Zu den Sachen*). Given the common intention of phenomenologists, a definition of phenomenology is that is a philosophy which seeks to discover, explore and describe 'uncensored phenomena' (Spiegelberg, 1970, p. 21) of the things themselves, as they are immediately given.

Various definitions of phenomenology emerge, reflecting their types and the intention to 'go to the things themselves'. There are so many types of phenomenology that the historian Herbert Spiegelberg (1976) suggested that there is no school of phenomenology representing a rigid, uniform view, rather phenomenology is a movement. Spiegelberg (1970) provided a 'staggered approach' to finding common ground within the phenomenological movement, by compiling six types of phenomenology. He explained that the types of phenomenology are not mutually exclusive, rather they are unified in a common purpose of 'giving us a fuller and deeper grasp of the phenomena' (p. 19). Spiegelberg's types of phenomenology include descriptive phenomenology, essential (eidetic) phenomenology, phenomenology of appearances, constitutive phenomenology, reductive phenomenology and hermeneutic phenomenology.

Descriptive phenomenology is a direct description of phenomena aimed at maximum intuitive content. Essential (eidetic) phenomenology seeks to explain essences and their relationships. The phenomenology of appearances attends to the ways in which phenomena appear. Constitutive phenomenology studies the processes whereby phenomena become established in our consciousness. Reductive phenomenology relies on suspending belief in the reality or validity of phenomena. Hermeneutic phenomenology is a special kind of phenomenological interpretation used to reveal hidden meanings in phenomena. Each type of phenomenology is related in part to the others, through complex networks of philosophical debate. The binding concern that they share is the intention to explore phenomena directly, by going to them as immediately given, to explicate their 'truest' nature, or essence.

Other classifications of types of phenomenology have been suggested (e.g., van Manen, 2007). The lack of consensus about the specific types and the interrelatedness of the concepts, give researchers some inkling of the complexity and pitfalls they may face when trying to apply phenomenological philosophy as a research methodology to guide their phenomenological inquiry. When you add to this complexity the intricate philosophical adaptations and developments in phenomenology over the course of the last century, it is small wonder that researchers have been accused of misinterpreting and misapplying phenomenological concepts (e.g., Crotty, 1996). We turn next to an outline of the origins of phenomenology, and later on in the chapter we will examine some of the major criticisms of the application of phenomenological research in healthcare.

Origins of phenomenology

It is commonly agreed that phenomenology originated with Husserl's eidetic concepts. Thereafter, other 'primary' phenomenologists added their inputs. (I refer to 'primary' phenomenologists as the originators of phenomenology, such as Husserl, Heidegger, Gadamer and Ricouer.) Some of Husserl's, Heidegger's and Gadamer's key ideas are discussed in this section. For Ricoeur's main ideas, please refer to some of his foundational works (1976, 1981).

Husserl

Husserl (1970) criticized Descartes for introducing into philosophy the separation between thinking substance (*res cogitans*) and extended substance (*res extensa*), thereby promoting Cartesian dualism. Instead of using Cartesian doubt to explore human knowing and being, which he argued would ultimately deny the world itself, Husserl advocated a method of eidetic reduction. Husserl extended the investigation of experiencing past things known by sense perception, as suggested by Descartes and demanded by empirico-analytical analytic methods, to anything of which one was conscious. In this way, Husserl advocated a return to philosophical questions about human subjectivity and consciousness, which as unseen and immeasurable phenomena, were nevertheless still legitimate matters for philosophical exploration.

Husserl's commitment to the idea of transcendental phenomenology (Husserl, 1980) came from his search for a science of essences, an 'apodictic beginning point, for an indubitable epistemic foundation', which in itself discovers Being' (Stapleton, 1983, p. 4). In other words, Husserl sought to understand the home of knowing and being, from which all things sprang. Husserl used the word *transcendental* in the Kantian sense, to mean the necessary conditions for experience. In his view, the transcendental was neither subject nor object, rather it formed the conditions that make subjective and objective experience possible and knowable.

Husserl's phenomenological method required that one suspend one's unquestioning acceptance of the pre-philosophical or natural attitude, which is situated in a web of relationships to things and people in the natural world. This means he wanted philosophers to suspend what they already knew about anything when they were focusing phenomenologically on an area of interest. Instead, he advocated taking on the philosophical attitude, which demands to know the reasons why things are as they are. The transition from the pre-philosophical to the philosophical attitude was through a method of phenomenological reduction, which narrowed one's attention in such a way as to be able to discover rational principles underlying the phenomenon of concern. Therefore, in exploring consciousness and subjectivity, Husserl was advocating an objective phenomenological process.

This narrowing of focus was through phenomenological reduction, otherwise known as the phenomenological epoché. The narrowing of focus was achieved by suspending judgement by questioning and laying aside all previous presuppositions until further investigation was possible. Being a mathematician, Husserl gave the name 'bracketing' to this process of leaving something (in this case, ideas) to one side in parenthesis. Keen to make his meaning clear for this important step in gaining phenomenological understanding, Husserl used the words phenomenological reduction, epoché and bracketing simultaneously, as different metaphors explaining the same philosophical attitude for 'getting to the things themselves'.

Husserl claimed that after bracketing a residue remained, which was the ego itself. In order to escape the subject–object dualism of Cartesian thought, Husserl referred to this ego as 'transcendental consciousness', because it embraced both subjective and objective elements. He contended that ego could not be conceived apart from conscious life, thus consciousness was always intended towards ego. Therefore, phenomenological epoché was a means by which the natural world could be reduced to 'a transcendental consciousness or transcendental subjectivity', through which 'consciousness' was purified and only the phenomena remained, as essences, unburdened by preconceptions. Analysing the phenomena, in turn, revealed the basic structure of consciousness itself (Husserl, 1980).

Husserl argued that every experience could be transformed into its essence, or eidos. Eidetic intuition meant seeing into the essence of a thing. Stapleton (1983, p. 40) clarified that Husserl meant eidos or essence as

> a priori, but by this he did not mean that it was supplied solely by the mind prior to empirical experience, but rather that it is an ability to have an insight prior to empirical experience, which is then fulfilled or 'fleshed out' by experience. In short, the eidos is the 'essential possibility', without which experience would be impossible.

In response to his critics, who claimed that his theory of eidetic phenomenology was taking him away from the world of everyday experience, Husserl defended his concept of the lived world (*Lebenswelt*) (1960; 1964). Husserl insisted that *Lebenswelt* is the lived world, which is the context for all experience. This context, or 'horizon' included everything in which one experiences things, such as time, space, surrounding people and the world itself. He reiterated that one could not be separate from the world, but that it was always there as background for all human endeavours, regardless of whether they could be judged as real or illusory.

Martin Heidegger, one of Husserl's students, extended and adapted Husserl's phenomenology and various authors (Kockelmans, 1967; Spiegelberg, 1970, 1976; Stapleton, 1983; Sukale, 1976) have elaborated on their personal and philosophical differences. Sukale (1976, p. 101) concluded that the basic difference between Husserl and Heidegger

> boils down to their different interpretations of the concept of 'world'. It was as though there were two different levels; the level of the natural world and the level below the natural world from which all things sprang. Husserl was intent on reaching the world below, whilst Heidegger was concerned with Being-in-the-world, therefore, instead of trying to lay presuppositions to one side, Heidegger explored them as legitimate parts of Being.

Heidegger

Heidegger's main departures from Husserlian phenomenology were explicated in Heidegger's (1962) book *Being and Time,* which began with a question about Being. Heidegger's phenomenology (1962, p. 22) was essentially hermeneutical, because he established 'Being [as] the most universal concept' (p. 22). Heidegger (1962, p. 24) then argued that 'the question of Being must be *formulated.* If it is a fundamental question, or indeed *the* fundamental question, it must be made transparent and in an appropriate way.'

Heidegger sought to establish the basis of philosophy as a historical analysis of existence, raising questions about Being and hermeneutical enquiry. Thus, Heidegger (1962) saw the task of philosophers as ontologists, seeking to unravel 'the universal structures of Being as they manifested themselves in the phenomena' (p. 277). Herein lies a major departure from Husserl's work, because Heidegger 'overcame the obsession with epistemology that characterises much of nineteenth and twentieth century approaches' (Hekman, 1986, p. 112), to pursue understanding through ontological inquiry.

In using hermeneutical inquiry to pursue the question of Being, Heidegger effectively demonstrated the nature of *Dasein,* translated directly as there (*Da*) being (*Sein*). Dasein is the ontological nature of human entities, who have some awareness of how to ask questions about Being, in as much as their Being-in-the-world (there being, or being there) as humans gives them some clues to the existence and the essential nature of Being (with a capital B). When first introduced into the text, Heidegger (1962, p. 27) explained Dasein in this way:

> Thus to work out the question of Being adequately, we must make an entity – the enquirer – transparent in his [*sic*] own Being. The very asking of this question is an entity's mode of *Being*; and as such gets its essential character from what is enquired about – namely, Being. This entity which each of us is himself [*sic*] and which includes enquiring and the possibilities of its Being, we shall denote by the term '*Dasein.*'

Heidegger began his hermeneutical enquiry into Being by examining the formal structures of questioning itself, before considering the behaviours of the questioner. In this analysis, Heidegger shifted from the question to the essential act of questioning itself. In so doing, Heidegger uncovered certain a priori objective and subjective forms. Heidegger's final step was arguing that, in order to raise a question, the questioner must have some idea of what to ask. In this way, Heidegger created a hermeneutical circle that demonstrated the need of a knowing questioner.

Heidegger's ontological use of the hermeneutic circle transformed the scope, meaning and significance of it as described by Scheiermacher (1977) and Dilthey (1976), by moving hermeneutics away from its sole focus on the interpretation of texts, to the wider scope of interpreting human existence through the understanding of Being implicit in Dasein. In this way, Heidegger (1962) effectively extended the hermeneutic circle to the ontological expression of Dasein, so that a fundamental ontology could be developed by a hermeneutic interplay between entities (expressions of Being) and sense (concern about Being).

For Heidegger, the hermeneutic circle aided in the interpretation of 'Dasein' itself as a understanding, caring mode of Being. Dasein tied to the world the one who questioned, in a place from which no conscious separation was possible, given the nature of Being-in-the-world. For Husserl, the 'ultimate intentional connection between the act of knowing and the thing as known, abided in "pure consciousness" or in transcendence of the natural attitude', whereas, for Heidegger, it was in the whole of people's precognitive awareness, by virtue of their prior understanding of Being, by being immersed inextricably within it.

Schrag (in Kockelmans, 1967, pp. 283–284) summarized it thus:

> 'Dasein' … is a being who is intentionally related to his world in his [sic] pre-theoretical preoccupations and concerns. In all of man's [sic] practical and personal concerns a world is presupposed. To exist is to find oneself in a world to which one is related in one or several of the manifestations of care (*Sorge*) in one's construction and use of tools, in one's understanding and ordering of projects, or in one's encounter and dealings with other selves.

Heidegger conceptualized Dasein as the kind of Being that had *logos*, or the potential to make manifest phenomena as they were, not so much through reason or speech, but as the power it had within itself to gather and preserve the things that were manifest in its Being. For people living their day-to-day lives, this gathering happens already in a fundamental yet unobtrusive way in their everyday dealings. Hence, for Heidegger, Being was not gained through Husserl's method of eidetic reduction, it was already present in the concrete existence of things and people in the world, a concept Heidegger named Being-in-the-world.

Heidegger's ontological phenomenology was concerned with existence, specifically human existence, or Dasein, so in that sense it was existential. However, the point of departure with his approach as existential phenomenology as such, was in his emphasis on a hermeneutic, which analysed the historically-situated self as a Being-in-the-world, thus it became an existential-ontological hermeneutic. For Heidegger, people were always arriving out of their past, deciding on their present and anticipating their future, the ultimate reality of which is death, thus the seeds to understanding Being itself and its phenomena, were in the historicity and temporality of people's Being-in-the-world.

Gadamer

Gadamer's major work, *Truth and Method* (1975) addressed the task of hermeneutics to explore philosophically the conditions of all understanding.

Attempting to find out what the human sciences really were, that is, 'what kind of insight and what kind of truth' could be found in the human sciences (p. xi), he set up a conflict between truth and method. Gadamer sought to address the question: If human sciences went beyond method and still had truth, then was truth itself beyond the question of method?

By exploring basic humanistic concepts and by making an analysis of the experience of art, Gadamer sought to discover how understanding was possible. Gadamer (1975, p. xxii) decided that all understanding is hermeneutical, because hermeneutics is the 'basic being-in-motion of There-being, which constitutes its finiteness and historicity and, hence, includes the whole experience of the world'. For Gadamer, the study of hermeneutics was ontological, being ultimately connected to the study of language, wherein Being could be understood. He resolved that the nature of the human sciences was in appreciating that all understanding is linguistic and can be thus examined through language. Like Heidegger before him, Gadamer was convinced that understanding was not an epistemological problem, but that rather it was an ontological one. In avoiding Heidegger's tendency towards ontological absolutism, however, Gadamer discussed ontology in terms of the linguisticity of all understanding and historicity.

Gadamer adopted Heidegger's view of the hermeneutic circle, that it was necessary in the ontology of understanding as an 'interplay of the movement of tradition' and its consequences (Gadamer, 1975. p. 261). He determined that the tendency of the Enlightenment to attempt to eradicate prejudice was prejudicial in itself and that truth could be pursued by identifying the connections between truth and prejudice. He contended that it was the task of hermeneutics to make distinctions between true and false prejudices, by a process of effective historical consciousness. Gadamer suggested that effective historical consciousness was analogous to the I–Thou relationship (1975, p. 323), in which openness to the other and willingness to be modified, created a dialogical relationship.

Using the concept of horizon described by Husserl, as the 'range of vision that includes everything that can be seen from a particular vantage point', Gadamer (1975, p. 269) determined that a 'fusing of horizons' occurs 'in effective historical consciousness. One's own horizon is understood in order to understand another's and the conscious act of fusion of the two horizons is through an act of understanding, as the task of effective historical consciousness'.

Gadamer (1975, pp. 350–351) used conversation as an example of the fusion of horizons, by noting the merging of meaning that goes on in a conversation is an instance of the linguisticality of understanding, as the 'concretation of effective historical consciousness'. This means that we have flow and understanding in conversations, because we bring to them our readily available understanding of lived contexts and meanings we have built up over time. We understand each other and the messages we are communicating in conversations when meanings merge successfully. The correctness of our interpretations is decided by examining the degree of 'conformity to the horizon from which the interpretation is made and the prejudices that constitute the horizon' (Hekman, 1986, p. 115). Thus, for Gadamer and for Heidegger, understanding is ontological, having its basis in language, which is the 'House of Being'. In other words, ontology is the basis of epistemology, meaning knowledge and knowing arises from, and is inextricably linked to, being communicating, context-dependent humans.

Summary

As the first philosopher to expound on matters relating to phenomenological reduction, Husserl provided a basis on which other phenomenologists could build. Using some of Husserl's concepts of horizon and lived experience, Heidegger set up the pursuit of understanding as an ontological problem. Heidegger emphasized that being within the world of people and things is fundamental to epistemology. Gadamer continued Heidegger's ontological explorations by conceptualizing effective historical consciousness, gained through a fusion of horizons of the interpreter and the text. While these ideas as outlined in this section are just a drop in a vast ocean of phenomenology, I hope you can begin to see the origins and intentions of phenomenology, in expounding a philosophy about illuminating human consciousness and lived experiences.

Applying phenomenological concepts

Although philosophers have adapted various types of phenomenology, certain key concepts keep popping up in their discussions, as developed in the literature. In view of the potential for you to feel overwhelmed by the philosophy, I suggest that you consider an 'applied approach' to your phenomenological research. By this I mean that you explore various types of phenomenology and select some core concepts within that type, to inform your project. For example, in my PhD research, I was informed by Heideggerian phenomenology, so I applied the concepts of lived experience (Dilthey, 1985; Heidegger, 1962; Husserl, 1965, 1970, 1980; Gadamer, 1975); Dasein (Heidegger, 1962); Being-in-the-world (Dreyfus, 1991; Heidegger, 1962) and fusion of horizons (Gadamer, 1975) as a theoretical framework, to illuminate the phenomenon of ordinariness in nursing. In this section I introduce these enduring phenomenological concepts, as possibilities for your potential phenomenological project in healthcare.

Lived experience

Lived experience is awareness of life without thinking about it, a pre-reflexive consciousness of life (Dilthey, 1985), that when remembered, gathers interpretive significance. Gadamer (1975) claimed that the value of lived experience is in its potential to join together universal and personal aspects of people's worlds. Humans live and work together in their daily worlds and it

Food for thought

Try making sense of some basic phenomenological concepts, by using the phenomenological terms introduced within this chapter, to respond to the following questions:

- Who am I? (For example, you might respond: I am a Being-in-the-world, with lived experiences …)

- How do I know anything?

- What humans are my best source of research data?

You need to begin by reading the basic theoretical assumptions of phenomenology. This chapter is by way of *introduction only* to phenomenology. Although I have as proposed some ideas within this chapter, you will need to read many other sources to get a firmer grasp on phenomenological basics. I recommend you read a wide range of books (e.g., Lewis and Staehler, 2010; Moran and Mooney, 2002; Svenaeus, 2001) and also research articles purporting to use phenomenology (e.g., Afrell, Biguet and Rudebeck, 2007; Erichsen, Danielsson and Friedrichsen, 2010; Heravi-Karimooi, Anoosheh, Foroughan, Sheyki and Hajizadeh, 2010). You can also read published phenomenological methods and apply one of these to your project. Be particularly mindful of the types of phenomenology, to find one to suit your research inquiry. For example, some useful resources for methods are Giorgi, 2009; Moustakas, 1994, van Manen, 1990, 1997, 2007.

In summary, if phenomenological philosophy seems so complex and abstract to you that it is difficult to imagine how to undertake phenomenological research, one suggestion is to apply selected concepts to your project's aims and objectives. You need to begin by reading the basic theoretical assumptions of phenomenology, as proposed within this chapter, and in other sources you locate through database searches. When you locate a type of phenomenology that is suited to your project, select key concepts from that approach to inform your project's methods and processes. Alternatively, you can choose to read published phenomenological methods and apply one of these to your project.

is through this living that they amass and make sense of their experiences. In cognitively aware individuals, lived experiences last for a lifetime. We live our experiences within the total context of our lives, that is, within the time and space of our existence, from our birth until our death. Therefore, the concept of lived experience is integral to any phenomenon of human experience. In phenomenological research, we get to people's lived experiences through experiential accounts. Through sharing their accounts of lived experiences, people tell us about their amassed impressions of their living in their worlds, relevant to the phenomenon of research interest.

Dasein

Heidegger (1962) used the term Dasein (there being) to denote the exploration of an entity (phenomenon), as a means of finding Being (the essence of existence). Although phenomenology can search for Being in all phenomena, ontological searches in the human sciences use the human being as a linguistic entity, through whom to understand Being. For Heidegger, the Dasein of the questioning inquirer was the beginning point of discovery of Being within any aspect of inquiry. Dasein connects to the concept of lived experience, because the 'there-being' of people is always within the context of their life, so as ontological beings they hold the keys to unlock the doors to epistemological discoveries. Therefore, in phenomenological research the researcher explores Dasein (as a focused area of inquiry) with human participants, to access the nature of a phenomenon.

Being-in-the-world

As people living within the world (meaning any part of our personal world or the larger planet) we are fashioned and affected by it, so we cannot claim to ever be free of it, while we are breathing and consciously aware. Our Being-in-the-world connects all that we are and know, and to the explication of Being within us. As a historically-situated person, with your own life stories, you are a Being-in-the-world, connected to your past, deciding on your present and anticipating your future. As a Being-in-the-world, you are held in time (historicity) and space (temporality) until your ultimate death. However, your Being-in-the world gives you immediate access to your embodied knowing, thus your ontological (experiencing, being) self is at the same time your epistemological (inquiring, knowing) self. In phenomenological research, people as participants give us access to their Being-in-the-world of the phenomena of interest to us.

Fusion of horizons

Taking into account the effects of Being-in-the-world and the ways in which we understand ourselves and other people and things through our lived experiences and language, the Gadamerian concept of fusion of horizons allows us to integrate the meaning of our experiences. When inquirers immerse themselves in the analysis of texts (representations) of all kinds (written or verbal language, images, symbols and so on) and allow the horizon of the selected text(s) to fuse with the horizon of their own awareness, a 'fusion of horizons' (Gadamer, 1975) occurs. In phenomenological research, the concept of fusion of horizons is reflected in a project's methods and processes to collect, analyse and interpret information about lived experiences. The fusion of horizon occurs when interpretations merge into meaningful whole representations that give insights into the phenomenon of research interest.

Phenomenological methods

Phenomenological methods differ according to the theoretical assumptions on which they are based. For example, some authors advocate that there should be no structured steps in a method (Psathas 1973; Morris 1977; Schwartz and Jacobs, 1979). Others, such as Patton (1980), suggest that the inquiry must proceed as the experience unfolds, with the only methodological consideration being that inquirers use some form of bracketing to minimize presuppositions. Bracketing means acknowledging and setting aside what you already know about a research interest, so that you do not impose your prejudices on what emerges from the research methods and processes.

Spiegelberg (1976) suggests that researchers use a framework for exploring particular phenomena, such as intuiting, analysing and describing (Spiegelberg 1976). Some other frameworks include the Van Kaam method (1959), the Giorgi method (Giorgi et al. 1975) the Colaizzi method (1978) and a method of transformation of interpretations (Langveld 1978). These methods suggest various steps in guiding the researcher in a method to uncover the nature of a phenomenon of interest.

van Manen's method

Max van Manen (1990) is a contemporary phenomenologist, who developed a method that may be useful to you in understanding how to go about phenomenological research. van Manen's approach is sufficient methodologically to provide a robust theoretical framework for any postgraduate project, including a PhD. Essentially, van Manen takes an eclectic view of phenomenology, by applying various concepts, but his main emphasis is on lived experience. Not only is van Manen's view of phenomenology accessible as a straightforward and uncomplicated exposition of phenomenology, he also maintains a very useful website (Phenomenology Online) through which he generously shares his phenomenological resources.

van Manen's (1990) phenomenological method involves:

1 Turning to the nature of the lived experience

2 Investigating experience as we live it, rather than as we conceptualise it

3 Reflecting on the essential themes, which characterise the phenomenon

4 Describing the phenomenon through the art of writing and rewriting

5 Maintaining a strong and oriented relation to the phenomenon

6 Balancing the research context by considering the parts and the whole.

It may not be immediately apparent to you, just what to 'do', to follow van Manen's method. In effect, he leaves you to interpret the method yourself, so creativity is encouraged, as you seek the phenomenon. A very simple reading of this method, is:

1 Turning to the nature of the lived experience

Ask yourself: What experience do I want to research? Access the people who can tell you about it from their lived experience. Your lived experience may also be relevant to the research topic. Focus on the phenomenon and leave yourself open to what comes to you through discussions, reading, personal reflective moments, and so on.

2 Investigating experience as we live it, rather than as we conceptualize it

The emphasis here is on researching experiences as lived by participants and/or yourself, rather than treating the project as an objective theorizing activity. The experience is to be told, as it is lived, so it needs to come from a spontaneous source, as a free-flowing account, with little or no rehearsals or self-editing. In this step you gather spontaneous accounts of the phenomenon of interest, by the best methods you can use, such as conversations, interviews, reflective writing, and so on.

3 Reflecting on the essential themes, which characterize the phenomenon

This is where you start to make sense of the collected information (data, images, and so on). To maintain your focus, keep your aims and objectives in mind, as you ask yourself: What do these experiential accounts (images, and so on) tell me about the nature of the phenomenon I am exploring? Search the visual data sources such as transcripts, creative writing, photographs, and so on, for illumination on the essence of the directly expressed phenomenon (thing about which you want to know).

4 Describe the phenomenon through the art of writing and rewriting

This step allows you to provide deeper, richer insights into the phenomenon by writing and rewriting in any way you see as useful. It might mean working with participants' transcripts to create themes or exemplars, or you may introduce poems or synopses of reflective writing to make the phenomenon fuller and clearer.

5 Maintaining a strong and oriented relation to the phenomenon

The phenomenon can only be itself, so ensure you keep focused on the research inquiry, so it illuminates itself. Keep your thoughts and attention on the phenomenon for richer and deeper insights, so they come with eloquent clarity of simplicity and directness to illuminate the research interest.

6 Balancing the research context by considering the parts and the whole

All things (phenomena) exist in relationship with other phenomena, so keep this in mind when considering all of the features of the research, to which this phenomenon relates. Have you illuminated the phenomenon? Do the experiential accounts and so on reflect the nature of the phenomenon you set out to illuminate? Can you recognize the phenomenon from its various parts?

If you look closely at van Manen's steps, you will see that they are analogous to the steps in undertaking a qualitative research project of any kind. You may think of Step 1 as being equivalent to the early part of the project, where you focus in on the specific research interest, by clarifying the research background, aims, objectives, potential significance, and by reading literature and so on. Step 2 is the data collection phase of the research, in which you use congruent methods, such as observations, creative writing, art works and interviews, to expose fresh, immediate insights. Step 3 is tantamount to the analysis phase of a project, where you use analysis methods, such as thematic analysis, narrative analysis, and so on. In the totality of your project, Steps 4 and 5 could be aligned with the interpretation phase of the research. Step 6 can be considered as the discussion part of a thesis, in which you tie in all of the aspects of research, bringing in literature in relation to your project's findings and so on, to bring the research to a conclusion.

There are no absolutes when it comes to phenomenological methods, because the very nature of phenomenology makes it a nebulous task that defies sure and certain methods for grasping and representing the phenomena. For example, Heidegger (1962) focused on the meaning of Being (existence) and after the infinite regress of circularity in his ideas, he came to the conclusion that: 'It is itself!' So, if you are embarking on phenomenology, use the type of phenomenology you prefer, but be very careful about claiming you are a phenomenologist or that you have '*done* phenomenology'. Unless you are trained in philosophical traditions and can rightly claim the title of philosopher, you can only claim that your research has *been informed* by phenomenological thought.

Phenomenological research projects in the health sciences

Any research questions, which ask: 'What is the nature of ...?' and 'What is it like to experience ...?' can be considered to be research interests that may be illuminated by a phenomenological approach. As phenomena are the foreground and context of human life, this allows you plenty of scope for being informed by phenomenology in your healthcare research. For example, you may choose to raise questions about the nature and effects of your profession or of your work within your profession. For example, research questions may be posed broadly, such as: 'What is a caring practice?' or specifically, such as 'What is the caring practice of X?' You may ask: 'How do clients perceive caring intentions?' or 'How do clients perceive the caring intentions of X?'

You might also want to explore how certain people experience various phenomena, such as patients' experiences of particular illnesses, caring professionals' experiences of specific clinical practices, and/or relatives' perceptions of all phenomena with which they are concerned, in any healthcare setting. For example, questions may be asked like: 'What is the nature of waiting for a diagnosis?' or 'What is it like to experience chemotherapy?' There are so many opportunities for using phenomenological research in healthcare, so if your questions relate to the nature of experiential phenomena, they can be informed by a phenomenological approach.

Food for thought

Imagine you are interested in knowing more about the phenomenon of hope for survival from cancer. Write a title for the research, using a phenomenological approach. Write an aim, at least two objectives, and one phenomenological method for data collection and analysis. Identify three phenomenological concepts connected to the method you have selected.

It is advisable that you spend time reading as many projects as you can, which claim to be phenomenological. In view of the criticisms of phenomenological research (Crotty, 1996; Norlyk and Harder, 2010), you need to be able to recognize projects that might reasonably call themselves phenomenological and those that are simply qualitative in an interpretive, descriptive sense. For example, Healey-Ogden and Austin (2011, p. 85) undertook a hermeneutic phenomenological study of well-being, because they wanted to shed more light on its nature, given that 'words well-being, health, and wellness are commonly used in an interchangeable manner by healthcare professionals and the lay public'.

Healey-Ogden and Austin (2011) sought accounts from five Canadians, aged from 40 to 60, on the basis that they were exemplary of well-being. The participants 'told their stories in individual, conversational interviews' either face-to-face or by telephone. The researchers claimed they used hermeneutic phenomenology, informed by the work of Heidegger, Gadamer and van Manen, 'to understand everyday human experience that is hidden from view, yet shows itself within the tensions of life' (Healey-Ogden and Austin, 2011, p. 86). They selected as key concepts the lived experience, the hermeneutic circle and fusion of horizons to illuminate the phenomenon of well-being.

The data analysis used van Manen's (1997) six activities, with special attention to van Manen's (1997, p. 34) process of having an 'inventive thoughtful' attitude (p. 34), to move back and forth in reflecting, writing and rewriting. The researchers began with an etymological search of the definitions of the word well-being and continued with a thematic analysis of participants' accounts, to highlight their 'words, phrases, and full stories of their experiences of well-being' (Healey-Ogden and Austin, 2011, p. 87).

The emergent themes were seeing differently, letting go to experience well-being, dwelling spaces, the sustaining nature of rhythmic flow, balanced tension, rhythmic interchange in the space of difference, the fluctuating nature of well-being, quietude of voice and becoming oriented toward a new identity. Seeing differently refers to 'a shift in view from a self-focused perspective to looking beyond themselves' (Healey-Ogden and Austin, 2011, p. 88). Letting go to experience well-being related to being 'in the moment for well-being to exist' (Healey-Ogden and Austin, 2011, p. 88). Dwelling spaces 'opens people to well-being in four significant relational spaces: play space, creative space, nature's space, and spiritual space' (Healey-Ogden and Austin, 2011, p. 88). The sustaining nature of rhythmic flow relates to 'people moving toward well-being' (Healey-Ogden and Austin, 2011, p. 90). Balanced tension 'arises in the space of difference between dwelling spaces of well-being and living in the day-to-day world' (Healey-Ogden and Austin, 2011, p. 91). Rhythmic interchange in the space of difference 'occurs in a space of overlapping relationships, where differences exist between people' (Healey-Ogden and Austin, 2011, p. 91). The fluctuating nature of well-being describes how 'well-being does not achieve a steady state. It fluctuates over time' (Healey-Ogden and Austin, 2011, p. 92). Quietude of voice refers to how participants 'came to experience a newfound voice within their well-being experiences. Voice, here, is not meant as vocal tone, pitch, or volume. It is meant as a strength that allowed them to enter into and speak of their well-being' (Healey-Ogden and Austin, 2011, p. 92). Becoming oriented toward a new identity refers to how participants adjusted at deep personal levels to changing life roles.

The researchers (Healey-Ogden and Austin, 2011, p. 93) concluded

> We did not find well-being in the science of how the body functions or in medical approaches to illness and recovery. Instead, by exploring this experience and by engaging in writing a description of it, we found well-being to be inherent in life and therefore lived. We discovered that coming to experience well-being arose from being open to this phenomenon in a space where people embraced the wonder of the moment and of their connections with life in and around them. The lived experience of well-being was in their dwelling and moving forward on the journey toward and within this space. Regardless of the degree of emotional pain people endured, their journeys toward well-being led to the same place, toward this shared phenomenon. Through people's well-being journeys, they came home to themselves by losing themselves to a new way of dwelling and being.

It is difficult to gauge the extent to which Healey-Ogden and Austin's (2011) project is phenomenological. Given the word limit considerations in refereed journals, the article reads well enough, in relation to the methodology section. The authors identify a type of phenomenology and several key concepts. However, as readers, we are not party to the philosophizing that went on to focus the project's preliminary phases, nor are we witness to the writing and rewriting during the data analysis and interpretation. Like so many other projects, we only have before us in a refereed article, a synopsis at best of a much longer project. We have to take on face value, according to a set of agreed criteria that this project is not just an interpretive qualitative project, but that it speaks of well-being with phenomenological validity. Even if the project stands up to our methodological scrutiny, will it also be acceptable to a philosopher educated fully in the nuances of phenomenology?

What makes a study phenomenological?

As a PhD candidate, I was very concerned to answer the question: What makes a study phenomenological? Even before Crotty (1996) criticized nurse researchers for misinterpreting phenomenology, I could see my potential for huge blunders, and I was worried that my PhD would fall at its first hurdle – to be 'phenomenological'. I took my question to a philosopher, who had been employed by the Faculty of Nursing at Deakin University in Australia to teach philosophy to Registered Nurses bridging their hospital certificate to a Bachelor award. He was a tall, lanky man in his 30s, with a love of philosophy and a very accessible way of introducing to novices the puzzles of epistemology and ontology, such as the nature of 'truth', Cartesian dualism, and so on. His very simple, considered response to my earnest question was: 'A project is phenomenological if it attempts to explicate Being (with a capital B).' While I do not wish to present his answer as the only and ultimate response, it had the effect on me at that time of releasing me from my transient methodological paralysis.

I went back to my PhD project and looked again at the analysis and interpretation phase while keeping in mind the focusing question: 'Does this account attempt to explicate Being?' At that point in the analysis, I had brought forward themes, which I realized would have been just as easily extracted by a standard thematic analysis method under the umbrella of many other qualitative methodologies. I (Taylor, 1991) acknowledged that

> the nature of the phenomenon was still not explicated as the 'Beingness' of ordinariness in nursing. All phenomenological methods assert an intention to go 'to the thing itself', by seeking the nature of Being within the being (entity), so a further re-immersion in the text with the insights already gained, created a fusion of horizons, which emerged as '-ess' words, that portrayed the 'innerness' of each of the aspects, these being 'allowingness', 'straightforwardness', 'self-likeness', 'homeliness', 'favourableness', 'intuneness', 'lightheartedness' and 'connectedness'.

Quite frankly, I do not put forward to you as philosophically sound my interpretations of how I decided my project was phenomenological, even if the thesis examiners seemed to accept they were. However, I took some comfort in the fact that in trying to explicate Being, I arrived at much the same point as Heidegger did, in that I realized that the phenomenon 'is itself', and that I too was caught in the circularity of words and language as the only mode I had to express what the phenomenon of ordinariness might be.

Time has moved on and we are now in the era of evidence based practice, determined often by the findings of systematic reviews of research projects. Norlyk and Harder (2010) asked a similar question to me, but they sought to justify their answer with a systematic review of research. Aware that the 'critique of phenomenological nursing research was raised in 1996 and 1997', they analysed peer reviewed articles published 10 years later, reasoning that a decade would have been sufficient to see if the situation had been addressed. Norlyk and Harder (2010) reviewed published empirical studies 'from January, 2006, to June, 2007 ... with nurse researchers listed as first or corresponding author, and limited to publications in English'. A total of 88 articles met the inclusion criteria, representing 41 periodicals. All articles were included in the initial phase of the study, and 37 were chosen for further analysis.

To review the projects, Norlyk and Harder (2010, p. 423) constructed a comprehensive reading guide for the systematic review, including the authors' presentation of: the 'stated phenomenological approach (e.g., philosophical ground, methodological keywords)'; the 'design and the analysis (e.g., purpose/research question, investigated phenomenon, sampling procedure and data collection, analysis process, and researcher role)'; the 'findings (e.g., explication of the phenomenon)'; and the 'justification of the study (e.g., criteria addressed)'. The projects scored low on all criteria and Norlyk and Harder (2010, p. 420) concluded that the review revealed

> considerable variation, ranging from brief to detailed descriptions of the chosen phenomenological approach, and from inconsistencies to methodological clarity and rigor. The variations, apparent inconsistencies, and omissions make it unclear what makes a phenomenological study phenomenological.

Norlyk and Harder's (2010) analysis pointed to the need for understanding differences in phenomenological research approaches and distinguishing them more clearly. Norlyk and Harder (2010, p. 429) suggested that it

> is not enough to refer to phenomenology as a research approach. It is important to clarify how the principles of phenomenological philosophy are implemented in the particular study. Published empirical studies based on phenomenology should include a minimum of scientific criteria such as articulation of methodological keywords, articulation of the investigated phenomenon, and description of how an open attitude was adopted throughout the research process ... Nurse researchers are faced with the difficulties inherent in offering adequate philosophical and methodological explication and still keeping within the word limits of journals. But there is room for improvement, and we must continue to critically examine applications of stated phenomenological approaches.

I suspect that the problems besetting nurse researchers are no different to those that can be encountered in other healthcare professions, when it comes to ensuring methodological correctness and thoroughness. Without formal education in philosophy, researchers can easily fail to reach philosophical credibility in relation to phenomenological thought. However, we need to differentiate between researcher sloppiness in general (failure to articulate methodological keywords, the investigated phenomenon, and an open attitude) and major breaches of methodological concepts (methodological misconceptions, with subsequently flawed methods and processes).

When you go to the databases and search for phenomenological projects in your healthcare profession, there is a very good chance many will come up. Some examples of recent additions to phenomenological enquiry are Izumi (2010) and Steinvall, Johansson and Bertero (2011). I suggest you read as many phenomenological research examples as possible, to get a sense of the approaches and the extent to which they have been able to illuminate healthcare phenomena with methodological merit.

Chapter summary

In this chapter, we turned to phenomenology as a methodology for research inquiry for understanding phenomena, as potential answers to epistemological and ontological questions. I alerted you to the possibility that you may feel overwhelmed by the immensity and complexity of phenomenological thought, because it is in the realm of philosophers, properly skilled in tackling epistemological and ontological puzzles. The initial focus in this chapter was on definitions of phenomenology and some theoretical assumptions as proposed by its originators. A definition of phenomenology can be very simple, as in the study of things (phenomena), however, definitions vary according to the types of phenomenology. Even so, the common intention of phenomenologists is to go to the things themselves, to discover, explore and describe 'uncensored phenomena' (Spiegelberg, 1970, p. 21) of the things themselves, as they are immediately given.

We turned next to the origins of phenomenology, by exploring some of Husserl's eidetic concepts. Husserl advocated a method of eidetic reduction to return to philosophical questions about human subjectivity and consciousness. Husserl sought to understand the home of knowing and being, from which all things sprang as the necessary conditions for experience. Husserl's bracketing required philosophers to suspend what they already knew about anything, to narrow their attention to discover rational principles underlying the phenomenon of concern. Husserl also introduced the concept of the lived world (*Lebenswelt*) (1960; 1964) as the context, or 'horizon' in which one experiences things, such as time, space, surrounding people and the world itself.

After Husserl, Heidegger (1962) saw the task of philosophers as ontologists. In using hermeneutical inquiry to pursue the question of Being, Heidegger effectively demonstrated the nature of Dasein as the ontological nature of human entities. Heidegger examined the formal structures of questioning itself, before considering the behaviours of the questioner, thereby shifting from the question to the essential act of questioning itself. Heidegger (1962) extended the hermeneutic circle to the ontological expression of Dasein, as a hermeneutic interplay between entities (expressions of Being) and sense (concern about Being). Heidegger's emphasis on a hermeneutic, which analysed the historically-situated self as a Being-in-the-world, thus it became an existential-ontological hermeneutic.

Gadamer addressed the task of hermeneutics by exploring basic humanistic concepts by making an analysis of the experience of art. Gadamer decided that all understanding is hermeneutical, being ultimately connected to the study of language. Gadamer extended the concept of horizon described by Husserl, to a 'fusing of horizons' in effective historical consciousness.

In view of the potential to feel overwhelmed by these philosophical ideas, I suggested that you consider an 'applied approach' to your phenomenological research. By exploring various types of phenomenology you can select some core concepts within that type, to inform your project. I then provided simplified explanations of key concepts, such as lived experience, Dasein (there being), Being-in-the-world and fusion of horizons.

We then turned to various phenomenological methods, noting that there are as many as there are types of phenomenology. As a useful contemporary method, I recommended to you the work of Max van Manen, to provide a robust theoretical framework for any postgraduate project. Many healthcare projects have claimed to be phenomenological, but you need to be able to recognize projects that might reasonably call themselves phenomenological and those that are simply qualitative in an interpretive, descriptive sense. I used Healey-Ogden and Austin's (2011) hermeneutic phenomenological study of well-being, to raise questions about the methodological credibility of projects. As Norlyk and Harder (2010) found in their systematic review of published empirical studies in nursing, there are many deficiencies in research projects purporting to be phenomenological. The problems besetting nurse researchers are no different to other healthcare professionals and researchers who can easily fail to reach philosophical credibility. Therefore, I suggested you read as many phenomenological research examples as possible, to use phenomenology well in your healthcare research.

Key points

- At it is simplest definitional level, phenomenology is the study of things (phenomena).

- Phenomenology is a philosophy which seeks to discover, explore and describe 'uncensored phenomena' of the things themselves, as they are immediately given.

- Spiegelberg's types of phenomenology include descriptive pheno-menology, essential (eidetic) phenomenology, phenomenology of appearances, constitutive phenomenology, reductive phenomenology and hermeneutic phenomenology.

- As the first philosopher to expound on matters relating to pheno-menological reduction, Husserl provided a basis on which other phenomenologists could build.

- Using some of Husserl's concepts of horizon and lived experience, Heidegger set up the pursuit of understanding as an ontological problem.

- Gadamer continued Heidegger's ontological explorations by conceptualizing effective historical consciousness, gained through a fusion of horizons of the interpreter and the text.

- In view of the potential to feel overwhelmed by the philosophy, consider an 'applied approach' to your phenomenological research, by exploring various types of phenomenology and selecting some core concepts to inform your project.

- Lived experience is awareness of life without thinking about it, a pre-reflexive consciousness of life, that when remembered, gathers interpretive significance.

- Heidegger used the term Dasein (there being) to denote the exploration of an entity (phenomenon), as a means of finding Being (the essence of existence).

- As historically-situated people living within the world, our Being-in-the-world connects all that we are and know, and to the explication of Being within us.

- The Gadamerian concept of fusion of horizons integrates the meaning of our experiences, when inquirers immerse themselves in the analysis of texts (representations) of all kinds (written or verbal language, images, symbols and so on) and allow the horizon of the selected text(s) to fuse with the horizon of their own awareness.

- Read many sources to get a firmer grasp on phenomenological basics.

- Phenomenological methods differ according to the theoretical assumptions on which they are based.

- Any research questions, which ask: 'What is the nature of …?' and 'What is it like to experience …?' can be considered to be research interests that may be illuminated by a phenomenological approach.

- As phenomena are the foreground and context of human life, there is plenty of scope for being informed by phenomenology in healthcare research.

Critical review questions

1 In what ways is it possible for phenomenological research to inform healthcare practice?

2 To what extent can phenomenological research offer insights into your clients' experiences of health and illness?

References

Afrell, M., Biguet, G., & Rudebeck, C.E. (2007). Living with a body in pain – between acceptance and denial. *Scandinavian Journal of Caring Science*, 21(3), 291–296.

Colaizzi, P. (1978). Psychological research as the phenomenologist views it. In R.S. Valle & M. King (Eds.) *Existential phenomenological alternatives for psychology*. New York: Oxford University Press.

Crotty, M. (1996). *Phenomenology and nursing research*. Melbourne: Churchill Livingstone.

Dilthey, W. (1976). In H.P. Rickman (Ed.) *Dilthey: Selected writings*. Cambridge: Cambridge University Press.

Dilthey, W. (1985). *Poetry and experience. Selected works. Vol V*. New Jersey: Princeton University Press.

Dreyfus, H. (1991). *Being-in-the-world: A commentary on Heidegger's being and time*. Cambridge, MA: MIT Press.

Erichsen, E., Danielsson, E.H., & Friedrichsen, M. (2010). A phenomenological study of nurses' understanding of honesty in palliative care. *Nursing Ethics*, 17(1) 39–50.

Gadamer, H.-G. (1975). *Truth and method*. G. Barden & J. Cumming (ed. and trans.). Seabury: New York.

Giorgi, A. (2009). *The descriptive phenomenological method in psychology: A modified Husserlian approach*. Pittsburgh, PA: Duquesne University Press.

Giorgi, A., Fischer, C.L., & Murray, E.L. (1975). *Duquesne studies in phenomenological psychology*. Pittsburgh, PA: Duquesne University Press.

Healey-Ogden, M.J., & Austin, W.J. (2011). Uncovering the lived experience of well-being. *Qualitative Health Research*, 21(1) 85–96.

Heidegger, M. (1962). *Being and time*. J. Macquarrie & E. Robinson (trans.). New York: Harper and Row.

Hekman, S.J. (1986). *Hermeneutics and the sociology of knowledge*. Cambridge: Polity Press.

Heravi-Karimooi, M., Anoosheh, M., Foroughan, M., Sheykhi, M.T., & Hajizadeh, E. (2010). Understanding loneliness in the lived experiences of Iranian elders. *Scandinavian Journal of Caring Science*; 24(2), 274–280.

Husserl, E. (1960). *Cartesian meditations: An introduction to phenomenology*. D. Cairns (trans.) The Hague: Matinus Nijhoff.

Husserl, E. (1964). *The idea of phenomenology*. W.P. Alston & G. Nakhnikian (trans.) The Hague: Martinus Nijhoff.

Husserl, E. (1965). *Phenomenology and the crisis of philosophy*. Q. Lauer (trans.) New York: Harper and Row.

Husserl, E. (1970). *The crisis of the European sciences and transcendental phenomenology*. Evanston: Northwestern University Press.

Husserl, E. (1980). *Phenomenonology and the foundations of the sciences*. T.E. Klein & W.E. Pohl (trans.) The Hague: Martinus Nijhoff.

Hyang, J. (2011). Alternative view of health behavior: The experience of older Korean women. *Qualitative Health Research*, 21(3), 324–332.

Izumi, S. (2010). Ethical practice in end-of-life care in Japan. *Nursing Ethics*, 17(4), 457–468.

Kockelmans, J.J. (1967). (Ed.) *Phenomenology: The philosophy of Edmund Husserl and its interpretation*. New York: Anchor Books, Doubleday and Company.

Langveld, M.J. (1978). The stillness of the secret place. *Phenomenology and Pedagogy*, 1(1), 181–189.

Lewis, M., & Staehler, T. (2010). *Phenomenology: An introduction*. New York: Continuum International Publishing Group.

Moran, D., & Mooney, T. (Eds) (2002). *The phenomenology reader*. New York: Routledge.

Morris, M. (1977). *An excursion into creative sociology*. New York: Columbia University Press.

Moustakas, C. (1994). *Phenomenology research methods*. Thousand Oaks: Sage.

Norlyk, A., & Harder, I. (2010). What makes a phenomenological study phenomenological? An analysis of peer-reviewed empirical nursing studies. *Qualitative Health Research*, 20(3) 420–431.

Patton, M.G. (1980). *Qualitative evaluation methods.* Thousand Oaks: Sage.

Psathas, G. (1973). *Phenomenological sociology: Issues and applications.* New York: John Wiley.

Ricoeur, P. (1976). *Interpretation theory: Discourse and the surplus of meaning.* Fort Worth: Texas Christian University Press.

Ricoeur, P. (1981). *Hermeneutics and the human sciences.* Cambridge: Cambridge University Press.

Scheiermacher, F. (1977). *Hermeneutics: The handwritten manuscripts.* H. Kimmerle (ed.) and J. Duke & J. Fortsman (trans.) Atlanta: Scholars Press.

Schwartz, H., & Jacobs, J. (1979). *Qualitative sociology: A method to the madness.* New York: Free Press.

Spiegelberg, H. (1970). On some human uses of phenomenology. In F.J. Smith (Ed.) *Phenomenology in perspective.* The Hague: Martinus Nijhoff.

Spiegelberg, H. (1976). *The phenomenological movement (Vols 1 and 11).* The Hague: Martinus Nijhoff.

Stapleton, T.J. (1983). *Husserl and Heidegger: The question of a phenomenological beginning.* Albany: State University of New York Press.

Steinvall, K., Johansson, H., & Bertero, C. (2011). Balancing a changed life situation: The lived experience from next of kin to persons with inoperable lung cancer. *American Journal of Hospice & Palliative Medicine, 28*(2) 82–89.

Sukale, M. (1976). *Comparative studies in phenomenology.* The Hague: Martinus Nijhoff.

Svenaeus, F. (2001). *The hermeneutics of medicine and the phenomenology of health: Steps towards a philosophy of medical practice.* Denmark: Kluwer Academic.

Taylor, B.J. (1991). *The phenomenon of ordinariness in nursing.* Unpublished PhD (Nursing) thesis, Deakin University, Geelong.

Van Kaam, A.L. (1959). The nurse in the patient's world. *American Journal of Nursing, 59*(12), 1708–1710.

van Manen, M. (1990). *Researching lived experience: Human science for an action sensitive pedagogy.* New York: State University of New York.

van Manen, M. (1997). From meaning to method. *Qualitative Health Research, 7*(3), 345–369.

van Manen, M. (2007). Phenomenology of practice. *Phenomenology & Practice, 1*(1), 11–30.

6

Narrative inquiry

Bev Taylor

Narrative inquiry as a research methodology is as broad and wide as the human imagination and our ability to tell stories about our lives. Humans narrate their lives by recounting their experiences and they make sense of their existence through reflecting on their life narratives. Being able to tell stories makes our lives interpersonal and meaningful, as we cooperate linguistically in finding our places and purposes as human beings. Qualitative researchers use words and language as data from which to create meaning about human experiences. Given that there are potentially no bounds to the human imagination and our natural propensity for telling stories, narrative inquiry as a research methodology keeps on evolving and expanding outwards in every direction, like the Universe after the Big Bang.

In this chapter, I present various definitions of narrative inquiry and opinions as to its genesis. I then describe some of the main theoretical assumptions underlying narrative inquiry and some common narrative inquiry concepts. Narratives are gathered by researchers by capturing participants' accounts of their experiences. There are many narrative inquiry methods for data collection and analysis, so I introduce some questions related to them here, and these questions and more will be taken up in Chapter 14 of this book. In the final part of the chapter, we look at two narrative inquiry research projects that have been undertaken in the health sciences. By reading through to the end of this chapter and 'chewing over' the food for thought prompts, you should have a good understanding of the potential of narrative inquiry for providing insights into some of your qualitative research interests.

Defining narrative inquiry

The definitions of narrative analysis and inquiry have changed over time. Originally, as a serious academic pursuit, narrative analysis of stories in books and articles began in the social sciences, as a systematic means of literary critique. Literary works do not necessarily need to be truthful, nor did they deign to be, because their appeal and insights come through the imagery of metaphor and the flow and impact of the story. Literary criticism did not stray into the arena of objective (scientific) human research, because the positivist paradigm establishing itself at the end of the 19th century did not allow for subjectivity and the relativity of truth claims, or value knowledge bound to the context of people's times, places and situations. Only since the emergence of qualitative research approaches, as valid epistemological choices for researching human experiences, has narrative inquiry been considered as appropriate for researching the human condition.

Interestingly, definitions for narrative inquiry are fairly similar, even though the attempts to categorize narrative inquiry are many and varied. While definitions are similar, a fair amount of confusion has been generated by researchers tending to use the words 'story' and 'narrative' interchangeably. For example, in healthcare research, the terms 'story', 'narrative' and 'voice' have been used synonymously in relation to telling stories with therapeutic dimensions (Wiltshire, 1995, p. 75). Polkinghorne (1988) attempted to create some definitional clarity, by differentiating a story as a single account reviewing life events in a true or imagined form, and a narrative as a series of multiple stories 'that organises events and human actions into a whole' (p. 18). I agree with Polkinghorne's differentiation, so when I refer to narrative in this chapter in relation to research, I mean a series of stories.

On the face of it, narrative inquiry suggests a systematic exploration of a series of stories with a specific focus or set of foci. Definitions of narrative inquiry spin around the central, three-pronged axis of the importance of the story, the storyteller and the listener. Firstly, narratives are a series of stories depicting people's lived experiences (Bell, 2009; Riessman, 2008). Secondly, researchers are interested in how storytellers narrate their experiences, thereby constructing meaning for themselves and their audiences (Chase, 2010; Hole, 2007). Thirdly, in narrative inquiry, the researchers become the listeners, focusing on the reflexive interplay between the narrative practices and environments (Gubrium and Holstein, 2009), and sometimes finding deeper meaning by aligning themselves experientially within participants' stories (Myerhoff, 1979; Behar, 2007).

The three-pronged axis of narrative inquiry creates the potential for various definitions of narrative inquiry, essentially saying similar things, but from different views of the same entity. Chase's (2011) definition of narrative inquiry is helpful in pulling together many disparate views of narrative and how they serve as data sources in human research. She suggests that

> Narrative inquiry revolves around an interest in life experiences as narrated by those who live them. Narrative theorists define narrative as a distinct form of discourse: as meaning making through shaping or ordering of experience, a way of understanding one's own and other's actions, of organizing events and objects into a meaningful whole, of connecting and seeing the consequences of actions and events over time. Narrative researchers highlight what we can learn about anything – history and society as well as lived experience – by maintaining a focus on narrated lives.
>
> (Chase, 2011, p. 421)

> **Food for thought**
> If we accept the idea that a narrative is a series of stories and that storytellers shape their stories for listeners, how can we make the shift from stories as fiction to stories as research data?

Another important point to remember, as you search for a unifying definition of narrative inquiry, is that some researchers think of narrative inquiry as a methodology, with a matching set of congruent methods and processes, while others see stories as data sources only. For example, researchers may be using a phenomenological approach as a methodology and choose as a method for sourcing data, people's stories of their lived experiences. Similarly, if you think across the whole range of interpretive qualitative, critical qualitative and postmodernist research approaches, when researchers need full-bodied accounts of people's lived experiences, they may quite reasonably use stories gathered from in-depth interviews as data sources. This does not necessarily mean that they would label their project as narrative inquiry overall, but they have nevertheless used the power of storied accounts as the main source of information in exploring their research interests. So, read research articles or reports carefully, to see if the researchers are claiming they are using narrative inquiry as a methodology (with congruent methods), or if they are using stories and narratives as data collection methods only.

In summary, the definitions of narrative analysis and inquiry have changed over time from their sole focus on literary critique, to the emergence of qualitative research approaches for researching human experiences. Definitions for narrative inquiry are fairly similar, even though a fair amount of confusion has been generated by researchers using the words 'story' and 'narrative' interchangeably. Narrative inquiry is a systematic exploration of a series of stories with a specific focus or set of foci. The story, the storyteller and the listener are important in narrative inquiry, because they encompass narrated life experiences as forms of discourse, from which we can learn about human knowledge and existence.

Origins of narrative inquiry

Accounts vary as to the origins of narrative inquiry. While all agree that the oral tradition of telling stories had its genesis in language-based humanity, there is less consensus on the actual starting point of narrative inquiry as human science research. Elliott (2005) suggests that narrative analysis began in the 1920s in social science research, as a systematic means of analysing literature. The French literary critic Barthes (1977), a strong advocate of narratives, promoted their ability to cross human differences in ages, places, societies, and classes, to become valid international, transhistorical and transcultural accounts of experience. As a literary critic, Martin (1986) suggested that Barthes and other literary analysts provided social science strategies for others to use and adopt as narrative inquiry evolved into a means of researching accounts of lived human experiences.

The history is unclear of the move from narrative analysis as literary critique to narrative inquiry into human experiences for research purposes. Clandinin and Rosiek (2007) suggest that the history of narrative inquiry as a research methodology varies according to the disciplinary group giving the account. For example, one view is that narrative inquiry emerged as a result of the decline of the dominant positivist paradigm in social science research (Leiblich, Tuval-Mashiach, and Zilber, 1998), with its intellectual roots anchored in the humanities in the form of narratology (Connelly and Clandinin, 1990). The discipline of medicine traces the emergence of narrative inquiry to the ethical scandals of the 20th century, when medicine lost some of its invincibility with patients and the general public (Hurwitz, Greenhalgh, and Skultans, 2004). In contrast to medicine, oral narrative research in women's studies traces its historical roots to the oppression of Africana women struggling against patriarchy and colonialism (Vaz, 1997).

Other attempts to trace the history of narrative inquiry have focused on the history of ideas as the philosophical influences on research methodologies, methods and processes. The history of ideas is a wide open field of inquiry, built up in various traditions of philosophy. Clandinin and Rosiek (2007) acknowledge the vastness of philosophical inquiry and use three paradigms to provide an impressive map of the landscape of narrative inquiry, by exploring the key markers of borderland spaces and tensions between post-positivism, Marxism, and post-structuralism. Given that narratives are essentially about recounting human experiences, they use as a starting point Dewey's (1938) pragmatic philosophy, which is transactional, as 'a changing stream that is characterized by continuous interaction of human thought with our personal, social, and material environment' (Clandinin and Rosiek, 2007, p. 39). The authors assert that Dewey's conceptualization of experience is a good starting point to map the landscape of narrative inquiry, because:

> In this pragmatic view of knowledge, our representations arise from experience and must return to that experience for their validation … There are several features of this ontology of experience that make it particularly well suited for framing narrative inquiry … First, the temporality of knowledge generation is emphasized. Experience, for the pragmatist, is always more than we can know and represent in a single statement, paragraph, or book. Every representation, therefore, no matter how faithful to that which it tries to depict, involves selective emphasis of our experience.
>
> (Clandinin and Rosiek, 2007, p. 39)

Clandinin and Rosiek (2007, p. 58) use the metaphor of borders, pointing out that they are abstractions, which 'exist as clear demarcations of territory only on maps, but do not show up so clearly in the real world'. Similarly, they make the point that trying to trace the history of narrative inquiry through an overview of major traditions is akin to travelling in philosophical territory with no clear-cut borders. They make the observation that in

> the practice of research, however, such philosophical exactness is often a luxury. The actual business of interpreting human experience is messier. As researchers we find ourselves drifting, often profitably, from one paradigm of inquiry into another. We do not cross borders as much as we traverse borderlands.
>
> (Clandinin and Rosiek, 2007, p. 58)

This degree of paradigmatic honesty gets to the heart of the philosophical dilemma of trying to record a concise history of narrative inquiry. The history of narrative inquiry changes according to the storyteller and to the emphasis he or she places on chronological events within their own disciplinary context and paradigmatic position. For example, the 'post-positivists seek a description of a reality that stands outside human experience, (whereas) the narrative inquirer seeks a knowledge of human experience that remains within the stream of human lives' (Clandinin and Rosiek, 2007, p. 44). Marxist, critical ideologies analyse the 'large-scale social arrangements [that] conspire not only to physically disempower individuals and groups, but also to epistemically disempower people' (Clandinin and Rosiek, 2007, p. 47). In contrast, narrative inquiry values lived experiences as sources of human inquiry and humanism as a mode of being, which critical ideologies reject as false consciousness for failing to deal with the oppressive, macrosocial conditions of life.

Post-structuralism and postmodernism extend beyond critical theories of knowledge generation and validation and critiques of large, disempowering forces, to focus on the linguistic and narrative structure of knowledge. They place epistemological value on ultra relativity, subjectivity, the partiality of truth, difference and context, and raise 'fundamental and highly technical questions about the ways we represent the world and makes compelling arguments for encouraging epistemic and methodological diversity in the social sciences' (Clandinin and Rosiek, 2007, p. 52). In Clandinin and Rosiek's (2007, p. 55) opinion, poststructuralism and postmodernism are at odds with narrative inquiry, because:

> For the post-structuralist ... signs can only rely on other signs for their meaning, and thus inquiry does not deal with lived experience itself. Such experience may exist. But as soon as we speak or write about it, we have moved into the process of re-presentation. Representations depend on other representations and discursive systems for their meaning. Consequently, the post-structuralist researcher may listen to stories that individual persons tell her or him. But in so doing she or he will not be interpreting those experiences as immediate sources of knowledge and insight; instead, she or he will be listening through the person's story to hear the operation of broader social discourses shaping that person's story of their experience. Narrative inquiry, by way of contrast,

begins with a pragmatic ontology that treats lived experience as both the beginning and ending points of inquiry

In summary, while it would be ground-breaking to provide you with a concise history of narrative inquiry as research into human experience, it is not possible. To untangle the history of narrative as a series of topical stories we tell one another, from the formalized system of literary critique, and from the exact moment narrative inquiry came into being as a research methodology for exploring human experience, would be tantamount to extracting the milk from a cafe latte. We start to sip the history of narrative inquiry at the point at which it feels right for us. We may see it as originating in caves around camp fires, or in the 1920s with social science and literary critique, or we may rely on *her* or *histories* from our own disciplinary roots – it does not really matter. What matters is that we acknowledge the importance of human experience, the storied accounts of which help us to understand our human existence and knowledge. Through the application of narrative inquiry we gain access to ontological and epistemological insights that may not otherwise have been possible.

Theoretical assumptions of narrative inquiry

Narratives are commonplace in human communication, because we share our ontological experiences through contextualizing our life events. Our existence matters enough to us to tell someone else about it. Telling stories to one another is a social medium through which we exchange our life experiences and make sense of our own existence, but is it actually a way of generating new knowledge through research?

Opinions vary as to the epistemological worth of telling and making sense of a series of stories. There has been a proliferation of books about narrative inquiry (Bamberg, 2007; Clandinin, 2007; Denzin and Lincoln, 2011; Gubrium and Holstein, 2009; Knowles and Cole, 2008; Riessman, 2008), and the journal *Narrative Inquiry* continues to be popular, but critiques of narrative inquiry are emerging about its widespread, uncritical and non-systematic use as qualitative research (Atkinson and Delamont, 2006); the limits of its research potential given that it is based on flawed epistemological assumptions (Hammersley, 2008) and the potential for validity issues when stories are treated as truth, not representations (Polkinghorne, 2007). Another area of critique is that of the ethical risks–benefits ratio for participants, especially if they are asked to recount stories of trauma and social suffering (De Haene, Grietens and Verschueren, 2010). Even with its limitations and possible misapplications, narrative inquiry is flourishing as a form of research with the potential to provide insights into people's lived experiences.

The potential value of lived experiences as sources of ontological and epistemological insights positions narrative inquiry paradigmatically as an interpretive qualitative methodology (e.g., Lindsay, 2011). However, when stories as interview data are gained through other lenses and for other purposes, such as for critiquing the status quo and providing political analyses of dominant social forces, narrative inquiry shifts paradigmatically to critical qualitative end of the absolute–relative philosophical continuum (e.g., Hall, 2011). In its most relativistic form, where it is valued for the subjective worth of highly contextualized individual, personal life stories, narrative inquiry positions itself beyond critical qualitative methodologies, shifting towards poststructuralist/postmodernist perspectives (e.g., McAllister, 2001). Consequently, the theoretical assumptions of narrative inquiry are grounded in the value of telling a series of life stories to capture lived experiences and their insights into human knowledge and existence, but the theoretical emphasis varies according to the influences of key assumptions characteristic of its particular paradigmatic positioning.

Key concepts relating to narrative inquiry vary according to their type. Deciding on the types of narrative inquiry is a difficult task, because of its ever increasing popularity. Even though prominent writers in the field (Bamberg, 2007; Mishler, 1995; Polkinghorne, 1995; Riessman, 2008) have offered typologies, I use Chase's (2011) approaches to contemporary narrative inquiry in this chapter. Chase (2011) suggests four main approaches to narrative inquiry: the story and the life; storytelling as lived experience; narrative practices and narrative environments; and the researcher and the story. For each of these types, key writers offer their key concepts of narrative inquiry.

The story and the life approach to narrative inquiry focuses on 'the relationship between people's life stories and the quality of their life experiences', so researchers emphasize '*what* people's stories are about – their plots, characters, and sometimes the structure or sequencing of their content' (Chase, 2011, p. 421). This type of narrative inquiry explores the potential of stories to enlighten people and improve their experience. Chase (2011) puts into this type, pragmatic and applied approaches (e.g., Clandinin and Rosiek, 2007); and personal growth of 'narrative identity' through psychologists' use of narrative therapy (e.g., White and Epston, 1990).

Researchers using the storytelling as lived experience approach to narrative inquiry are 'interested in *how* people narrate their experiences' to use narration as 'the practice of constructing meaningful selves, identities and realities' (Chase, 2011, p. 422). This type of narrative inquiry is interested in the cultural discourses narrators use to make sense of their experiences. The stories of lived experience can also be liberatory, by helping to locate and transform 'oppressive discourses' (p. 422). Chase (2011) includes in this type, research by Bell (2009) and Hole (2007).

Narrative practices and narrative environments is a type of narrative inquiry interested in the 'reflexive interplay' of how 'people's narrative practices are shaped by and shape their narrative environments' (Chase, 2011, p. 422). Researchers within this type are interested in 'narrative reality' of contexts, as shared in in-depth interviews, backed up by 'ethnographic understanding of local contexts and interactional circumstances' (Chase, 2011, p. 422). Writers and researchers in this type of narrative inquiry are Gubrium and Holstein (2009) and Weinberg (2005).

The last type of narrative inquiry described by Chase (2011) is the researcher and the story. In this type, the researcher becomes part of the research, by treating '*their* stories about life experience (including research itself as a life experience) as a significant and necessary focus of narrative inquiry' (p. 423). Also, narrative inquiry researchers in this type may seek an equitable researcher–researched relationship by being subjected to the research analysis along with the participants, and by sometimes including their own storied experiences in the research. Researchers using this type of narrative inquiry include Myerhoff (1979) and Behar (2007).

> **Food for thought**
> In this chapter, there is a brief overview of the four main approaches to narrative inquiry: the story and the life; storytelling as lived experience; narrative practices and narrative environments; and the researcher and the story (Chase, 2011). For each of these types, locate a least one example of a narrative research article and explore the author(s)' key narrative inquiry concepts. When you compare Chase's (2011) typologies of narrative inquiry with other authors (Bamberg, 2007; Mishler, 1995; Polkinghorne, 1995; Riessman, 2008), do you think Chase's four types are comprehensive enough to take in all the various approaches to narrative inquiry? Which typology do you prefer? Why?

Narrative inquiry methods

Narrative inquiry methods encompass how data are gathered and analysed and how the overall research is judged to be rigorous/trustworthy/good quality. The data collection and analysis methods chosen for any type of narrative inquiry project are subsumed within various approaches to inquiring into people's narratives, and they are chosen to suit the particular emphases on the central, three-pronged axis of the story, the storyteller and the listener. The layering of data collection and analysis methods into the selected concepts relating to the value of people's lived experiences, the ways storytellers narrate their experiences, the construction of meaning, the reflexive interplay between the narrative practices and environments, and the ways researchers find deeper meaning in participants' stories, all combine to create a wide variety of choices researchers can make when they are contemplating using narrative inquiry approaches.

Beginning with the story, or series of stories, choices need to be made about: what stories will be collected, with what focus, for what purposes, by what means? Will the storyteller be providing an unsolicited autobiographical experiential account, or will the storyteller be recruited for research purposes, by a researcher? Who will listen, with what focus, for what purposes, by what means? What is the role of the researcher as listener? To what extent will the listener contribute to the stories? Will the listener add in their own storied experience to the research? Once collected, how will the stories be analysed?

Once analysed, how will the overall quality of the project be ascertained? These questions and more will be addressed in Chapter 14 of this book.

Narrative inquiry research projects in the health sciences

Narrative inquiry has a broad appeal to a wide range of human health science practitioners, such as health economists (Smith, Mitton and Peacock, 2009), medical practitioners (Bradley, 2006; Sappol, 2009; Solomon, 2008; Thomas, 2006), midwives (McCourt, 2010; Pairman, Tracy, Thorogood and Pincombe, 2010), nurses (Hall and Powell, 2011; Holloway and Freshwater, 2007), health promotion practitioners (Larkey and Hecht, 2010; Riley and Hawe, 2005), risk communication researchers (McComas, 2006), psychologists (Berkley-Patton, Goggin, Liston, Bradley-Ewing and Neville, 2009) and social workers (Larsson and Sjöblom 2010). A search of key health science databases using keywords 'narrative research/inquiry' and any health discipline will bring up multiple listings for articles and books relating to this type of research. I suspect that the broad appeal of narrative inquiry to so many health science disciplines lies in our shared imperatives to understand and provide caring services for humans encountering health-related experiences.

There are many examples of health research using narrative inquiry, for the purposes of understanding human experiences, in order to care for people more effectively. For instance, nurse researchers in Hong Kong (Chan, Cheung, Mok, Cheung and Tong, 2006, p. 301) undertook a narrative inquiry into the Hong Kong Chinese adults' concepts of health through their cultural stories, in order to understand how participants perceived the meaning of health so that the insights would 'help health-care professionals to revisit the meaning of health promotion within the context of an individual's life situation'.

Data were collected through a series of audio-taped unstructured interviews and conversations from five participants, who were recruited by convenience sampling. The guiding questions for the interviews were: 'Describe what it is like to be healthy.'; 'In your view, have there been any changes to your health?'; and 'How do you know you are healthy?' The researchers listened attentively during participants' responses, allowing informal conversations in between the focusing research questions. Several interviews with each participant ensured that the researchers were clear about participants' responses and that the participants validated their own accounts.

The description of the analysis and interpretation of the participants' stories showed the researchers' creativity and their best intentions to be guided by narrative inquiry concepts and rigorous means of previous narrative researchers. Chan, Cheung, Mok, Cheung and Tong (2006, p. 303) reported that the

> research team met regularly to share their initial analysis, which dealt with matters such as character, scene, tension, and context. Prior to the meetings, each of the five research team members read and reread their

transcriptions and field notes. Through relentless rereading, narrative codings were used to identify possible plotlines, how they interconnected, the tensions that emerged, the settings of the events and the contexts (Tappan and Brown, 1989). Diverse events were also examined along a temporal dimension and the effects of one event on another were identified (Polkinghorn [sic], 1988). The team shared relevant literature to support, extend, or clarify the identified narrative themes at the researchers' meetings. Each researcher later prepared a written summary of the texts including identified common meanings, excerpts from the text to support the themes, and the reader's interpretation of the themes. The corresponding author of this paper read the summaries to discern patterns and meanings within and across the texts. A chronicled account was summarized from the different sets of field texts. Different texts were also compared and contrasted in relation to other field texts. After the analyses, feedback from the research team was solicited and incorporated into the final manuscript.

Data analysis of the participants' stories revealed the influences on their thinking of Confucian teachings, an Eastern view of self, the effects of Western biomedical, and Hong Kong's unique work culture. The researchers noted that responses showed participants' 'constructed identities' expressed through their attitudes and behaviours. From the participants' accounts, the researchers were able to conclude that, for these people:

> concepts of health evolved over time according to the personal meanings attached to them at various life stages. While participants recognized the interconnectedness of the mind and body, the physical foci of traditional Western medicine remained salient in their health stories. Furthermore, there is a clear delineation of personal management of the psychological health and professional management of physical health.
> (Chan, Cheung, Mok, Cheung and Tong, 2006, p. 301)

The researchers went to great lengths to describe their narrative inquiry methodology and matching method and process, but it left me wondering whether their research would be judged by some readers as 'true' narrative inquiry, or simply as a qualitative project using stories as data. To make a reasoned decision on the methodological worth of the project, I re-read the section pertaining to methodology, noting that the underlying assumptions were based on Mishler's (1995) idea that 'telling stories is a primary way of making sense of an experience', plus Clandinin and Connelly's (2000) contention that 'stories of experience can be understood through the three dimensions of time, personal–social interactions, and place' (Chan, Cheung, Mok, Cheung and Tong, 2006, p. 302).

The judgement as to the worth of this project as narrative inquiry would draw different opinions from various readers. For example, Atkinson and Delamont (2006) have been vocal about their concern that narrative inquiry has become so fashionable that it has been misapplied and treated carelessly. While they 'acknowledge the significance of narratives in many aspects of social life', they 'sound a note of caution concerning the popularity of "narratives", and "testimony", not least among "qualitative" researchers'. Their main complaint is that 'too many authors are complicit in the general culture of "the interview society", and are too ready to celebrate narratives and biographical accounts, rather than subjecting them to systematic analysis' (Atkinson and Delamont, 2006, p. 164). Would Chan, Cheung, Mok, Cheung and Tong's project (2006) be disciplined and systematic enough to fulfil Atkinson and Delamont's (2006) criteria for what constitutes good quality narrative inquiry? It is doubtful that Hammersley (2008) would be impressed, as he would disagree with narrative inquiry as legitimate human research, because he rejects the basic epistemological assumptions of qualitative research in general. Based on their selected narrative assumptions and their attention to other qualitative research principles, such as congruency between the methodological concepts and the methods chosen to gather and analyse the data, I consider Chan, Cheung, Mok, Cheung and Tong's (2006) project to be a sound example of narrative inquiry.

The second example is an interesting project relating to *Interdisciplinary Geriatric and Palliative Care Team Narratives: Collaboration Practices and Barriers* (Goldsmith, Wittenberg-Lyles, Rodriguez and Sanchez-Reilly, 2010). The researchers based their project on their observation that 'despite the development and implementation of team training models in geriatrics and palliative care, little attention has been paid to the nature and process of teamwork' (Goldsmith, Wittenberg-Lyles, Rodriguez and Sanchez-Reilly, 2010, p. 93). Even though literature extols the benefits of teamwork, power difficulties have been noted (Martin, O'Brien, Heyworth, and Meyer, 2008; Opie, 1998). Therefore, the aims of the research were to investigate 'interdisciplinary geriatric and palliative care team member narratives about dying patients, their families, and team process; and (employ) a functional narrative analysis to identify and interpret themes of content and group ordering to reflect on interdisciplinary collaboration practices and barriers' (p. 94).

The researchers used as their methodological rationale, the narrative paradigm concepts of the power of stories to shape and reshape interpretations, as espoused by Fisher (1987). The researchers justified their use of the narrative paradigm as the methodology of choice for their project, thus:

> Personal narratives serve as building blocks for public knowledge about public performance. The stories of individuals cannot be built and understood separately from public narrative. Critical care issues present a desire and necessity to make sense of health events. Narration is a way to organize, understand, make meaning, and reduce uncertainty; it is a communicative vehicle to perform these tasks. Narration provides those caring for individuals with serious illness a way to interpret, change, understand, manage, and respond to care.
>
> (Goldsmith, Wittenberg-Lyles, Rodriguez and Sanchez-Reilly, 2010, p. 95)

Participants were interdisciplinary members 'in 1-year fellowship placements, working in a combined consultation service in geriatrics and palliative care at a Veterans Affairs (VA) hospital in the southern United States' (p. 95). They included a psychologist, a social worker, a chaplain, a nurse, and two medical fellows. Two more medical fellows declined the invitation to participate, citing heavy workloads and time commitments.

Face-to-face, semi-structured interviews were conducted to gather accounts within two months of completing the one-year fellowship. The researchers had as prompts, eleven interview questions to assist participants in their reflection, including:

1 How did you get involved in the palliative care fellowship?

2 What previous experience did you have working in hospice and palliative care?

3 Describe your most memorable patient during your fellowship.

4 Describe one of your most challenging experiences from this year.

5 Who has taught you the most this year?

6 Who do you turn to when you have a problem?

7 Describe a bad experience as a fellow.

8 Did you enjoy working with medical students as part of their coursework?

9 What advice will you give the next fellow?

10 What do you still feel insecure about in this setting?

11 What are your thoughts on your own death?

The narrative analysis method was informed by Mishler's (1995) narrative functional analysis, to focus on 'what stories did, the setting in which they were told, and the effects they had' (Goldsmith, Wittenberg-Lyles, Rodriguez and Sanchez-Reilly, 2010, p. 96) and the narrative performance theory concepts of content ordering and group ordering (Langellier and Peterson, 2006).

The emergent themes were voice of the lifeworld, caregiver teamwork, alone on a team, and storying disciplinary communication. I will not go into a description of each theme here, suffice to say that the narratives revealed 'a divergence in team members' conceptualization of teamwork and team effectiveness', and participants did not 'easily recognize their role in achieving or producing successful teamwork' (p. 102). Even so, participants demonstrated their abilities 'to engage in the reflective process of teamwork' and they 'expressed strong ownership of team identity by group ordering work with caregivers' (p. 102). The benefits for these participants and for readers with whom these findings resonate, were in 'hearing each other's stories', so that 'team members can identify and evaluate team processes' (p. 103), leading to improvements in future teamwork efforts.

This project fits within an interpretive framing of narrative inquiry, because it sought to describe the concept of teamwork, as espoused and practised by various multidisciplinary health team members. I was interested in the number and range of prompt questions the researchers designed, to help the flow of the stories, if needed. Firstly, the number of questions presupposes the need for researchers to act as prompters of practice stories. While some people may be hesitant, or lack flow in recounting stories, I have found them for the most part to be 'natural' storytellers. If I listened closely and quietly with little or no interruptions, they invariably covered the terrain of my research objectives with very little prompting. Given they had the Explanatory Guide and Consent Form for the research, they already knew the questions they would be asked. Anticipating well-rounded narratives by a non-interrupting style has been described by Matthews and Ross (2010), who warn that too many questions and interruptions may result in the researcher restructuring the story.

The second aspect I noticed in the eleven prompts relates to their range of interest. The research aims focused on 'interdisciplinary geriatric and palliative care team member narratives about dying patients, their families, and team process' and 'interdisciplinary collaboration practices and barriers' (p. 94). While questions 1 and 2 were necessary to gather contextual information, and questions 3 to 10 deepened insights into teamwork, the last question, although important, does not appear to link in directly with the research aims. Thoughts on one's own death may be important for empathic and compassionate caring of the dying, but how do they relate to teamwork? Here again, the range of questions seems to suggest researcher anxiety, that participants may not be able to give full storied accounts, just by being given a simple invitation, such as: 'Tell me about your experiences of being part of a multidisciplinary health team. What was good? What was not so good?'

Conclusion

In this chapter, I presented various definitions of narrative inquiry and opinions as to its genesis. The definitions are connected to the origins and types of narrative inquiry. Essentially, narrative inquiry is a systematic exploration of a series of stories to highlight narrated life experiences as forms of discourse, from which we can learn about human knowledge and existence.

I then described some of the main theoretical assumptions underlying narrative inquiry and some common narrative inquiry concepts. While there is a general view that narrative inquiry is informative about human experiences, the theoretical assumptions and concepts differ according to the particular paradigmatic lens through which it is viewed and the particular focus on the story, the storyteller or the listener. In this chapter I raised some fundamental questions about narrative inquiry methods for data collection and analysis, leaving these questions and more to be addressed in Chapter 14 of this book. In the final part of the chapter, we looked at two narrative inquiry research projects that have been undertaken in the health sciences. These examples were just two of many other projects health science researchers are undertaking to explore the human experience of health and illness. By now, you should have a good understanding of the potential of narrative inquiry for providing insights into some of your qualitative research interests. Reading Chapter 14 will progress your insights into narrative analysis methods.

Key points

- Narrative inquiry is a systematic exploration of a series of stories to highlight narrated life experiences as forms of discourse, from which we can learn about human knowledge and existence.

- Given that there are potentially no bounds to the human imagination and our natural propensity for telling stories, narrative inquiry as a research methodology keeps on evolving and expanding outwards in every direction.

- Only since the emergence of qualitative research approaches, as valid epistemological choices for researching human experiences, has narrative inquiry been considered as appropriate for researching the human condition.

- Definitions of narrative inquiry spin around the central, three-pronged axis of the importance of the story, the storyteller and the listener.

- Narratives are commonplace in human communication, because we share our ontological experiences through contextualizing our life events, but opinions vary as to the epistemological worth of telling and making sense of a series of stories.

- The layering of data collection and analysis methods into the selected concepts relating to the value of people's lived experiences, the ways storytellers narrate their experiences, the construction of meaning, the reflexive interplay between the narrative practices and environments, and the ways researchers find deeper meaning in participants' stories, all combine to create a wide variety of choices researchers can make when they are contemplating using narrative inquiry approaches.

Critical review questions

1 In what ways is it possible for narrative research to inform healthcare practice?

2 To what extent can narrative research offer insights into your clients' experiences of health and illness?

References

Atkinson, P., & Delamont, S. (2006). Rescuing narrative from qualitative research. *Narrative Inquiry, 16* (1), 164–172(9).

Bamberg, M. (Ed.) (2007). *Narrative–state of the art*. Philadelphia: John Benjamins.

Barthes, R. (1977). *Introduction to the structural analysis of narratives*. Glasgow: Collins.

Behar, R. (2007). *An island called home: Returning to Jewish Cuba*. New Brunswick, NJ: Rutgers University Press.

Bell, S.E. (2009). *DES daughters: Embodied knowledge and the transformation of women's health politics*. Philadelphia, Temple University Press.

Berkley-Patton, J., Goggin, K., Liston, R., Bradley-Ewing, A., & Neville, S. (2009). Adapting effective narrative-based HIV-prevention interventions to increase minorities' engagement in HIV/AIDS services. *Health Communication*, 24, 199–209.

Bradley, L. (2006). Listening to Chekhov: Narrative approaches to depression. *Literature and Medicine*, 25(1), 46–71.

Chan, E.A., Cheung, K., Mok, E., Cheung, S., & Tong, E. (2006). A narrative inquiry into the Hong Kong Chinese adults' concepts of health through their cultural stories. *International Journal of Nursing Studies*, 43, 301–309.

Chase, S.E. (2010). *Learning to speak, learning to listen: How diversity works on campus*. Ithaca, NY: Cornell University Press.

Chase, S.E. (2011). Narrative inquiry: Still a field in the making. In N.K. Denzin and Y.S. Lincoln (Eds.) *The SAGE Handbook of Qualitative Research*, 4th edn. Thousand Oaks: Sage, 421–434.

Clandinin, D.J. (2007). *Handbook of narrative inquiry: Mapping a methodology*. Thousand Oaks: Sage.

Clandinin, D. J., & Connelly, F. M. (2000). *Narrative inquiry: Experience and story in qualitative research*. San Francisco: Jossey-Bass.

Clandinin, D.J., & Rosiek, J. (2007). Mapping a landscape of narrative inquiry: Borderland spaces and tensions. In Clandinin, D.J. (2007). *Handbook of narrative inquiry: Mapping a methodology*. Thousand Oaks: Sage, 35–75.

Connelly, F.M., & Clandinin, D.J. (1990). Stories of experience and narrative inquiry. *Educational Researcher*, 19(5), 2–14.

De Haene L., Grietens, H., & Verschueren, K. (2010). Holding harm: Narrative methods in mental health research on refugee trauma. *Qualitative Health Research*, 20(12) 1664–1676.

Denzin, N.K., & Lincoln, Y.S. (2011). *The SAGE handbook of qualitative research*, 4th edn. Thousand Oaks: Sage.

Dewey, J. (1938). *Experience and education*. New York: Collier Books.

Elliott, J. (2005). *Using narrative in social research: Qualitative and quantitative approaches*. London: Sage.

Fisher, W. (1987). *Human communication as narration: Toward a philosophy of reason, value, and action*. Columbia, CA: University of South Carolina Press.

Goldsmith, J., Wittenberg-Lyles, E., Rodriguez, D., & Sanchez-Reilly, S. (2010). Interdisciplinary geriatric and palliative care team narratives: Collaboration practices and barriers. *Qualitative Health Research*, 20(1): 93–104.

Gubrium, J.F. & Holstein, J.A. (2009). *Analyzing narrative reality*. Thousand Oaks: Sage.

Hall, J.M. (2011). Narrative methods in a study of trauma recovery. *Qualitative Health Research*, 21(1): 3–13.

Hall, J.M., & Powell, J. (2011). Understanding the person through narrative. *Nursing Research and Practice*, 2011, 1–10.

Hammersley, M. (2008). *Questioning qualitative inquiry: Critical essays*. Thousand Oaks: Sage.

Hole, R. (2007). Narratives of identity: A poststructural analysis of three deaf women's stories. *Narrative Inquiry*, 17, 259–278.

Holloway, I., & Freshwater, D. (2007). *Narrative research in nursing*. UK: Blackwell.

Hurwitz, B., Greenhalgh, T., & Skultans, V. (2004). *Narrative research in health and illness*. Oxford: Blackwell.

Knowles, J.G., & Cole, A.L. (Eds.) (2008). *Handbook of the arts in qualitative research: Perspectives, methodologies, examples, and issues*. Thousand Oaks: Sage.

Langellier, K., & Peterson, E. (2006). Narrative performance theory: Telling stories, doing family. In D. Braithwaite & L. Baxter (Eds.), *Engaging theories in family communication: Multiple perspectives*. Thousand Oaks: Sage, 99–114.

Larkey, L.K., & Hecht, M. (2010). A model of effects of narrative as culture-centric health promotion. *Journal of Health Communication, 15*, 114–135.

Larsson. S., & Sjöblom, Y. (2010). Perspectives on narrative methods in social work research. *International Journal of Social Welfare, 19*, 272–280.

Lieblich, A., Tuval-Mashiach, R., & Zilber, T. (1998). *Narrative research: Reading, analysis and interpretation*. Thousand Oaks: Sage.

Lindsay G.M. (2011). Patterns of inquiry: curriculum as life experience. *Nursing Science Quarterly 24*(3), 237–244.

Martin. W. (1986). *Recent theories of narrative*. Ithaca, NY: Cornell University Press.

Martin, D., O'Brien, J., Heyworth, J., & Meyer, N. (2008). Point counterpoint: The function of contradictions on an interdisciplinary healthcare team. *Qualitative Health Research, 18*, 369–379.

Matthews, B., & Ross, L. (2010) *Research methods: A Practical Guide for the Social Sciences*. Harlow: Pearson Publishers

McAllister, M.M. (2001). In harm's way: a postmodern narrative inquiry. *Journal of Psychiatric and Mental Health Nursing, 8*, 391–397.

McComas, K.A. (2006). Defining moments in risk communication research: 1996–2005. *Journal of Health Communication, 11*, 75–91.

McCourt, S. (Ed.) (2010). *Childbirth, midwifery and concepts of time*. Oxford: Berghahn Books.

Mishler, E. (1995). Models of narrative analysis: A typology. *Journal of Narrative and Life History, 5*(2), 87–123.

Myerhoff, B. (1979). *Number our days: Culture and community among elderly Jews in an American ghetto*. New York: Meridian.

Opie, A. (1998). 'Nobody's asked me for my view': Users' empowerment by multidisciplinary health teams. *Qualitative Health Research, 8*, 188–206.

Pairman, S., Tracy, S., Thorogood, C., & Pincombe, J. (2010). *Midwifery: Preparation for Practice* 2nd edn. Chatswood Australia: Elsevier.

Polkinghorne, D.E. (1988). Narrative Knowing and the Human Sciences, State University of New York, Albany.

Polkinghorne, D.E. (1995). Narrative configuration in qualitative analysis. In J.A. Hatch and Wisniewski (Eds) *Life history and narrative*. London: Falmer, 5–23.

Polkinghorne, D.E. (2007). Validity issues in narrative research. *Qualitative Inquiry, 13*, 471–486.

Riessman, C.K. (2008). *Narrative methods for the human sciences*. Thousand Oaks: Sage.

Riley, T., & Hawe, P. (2005). Researching practice: The methodological case for narrative inquiry. *Health Education Research, 20*(2), 226–236.

Sappol, M. (2009). The odd case of Charles Knowlton: Anatomical performance, medical narrative, and identity in antebellum America. *Bulletin of the History of Medicine, 83*(3), 460–498.

Smith, N., Mitton, C., & Peacock, S. (2009). Qualitative methodologies in health-care priority setting research. *Health Economics, 18*, 1163–1175.

Solomon, M. (2008). Epistemological reflections on the art of medicine and narrative medicine. *Perspectives in Biology and Medicine, 51*(3), 406–417.

Tappan, M., & Brown, L.M. (1989) Stories told and lessons learned: toward a narrative approach to moral development and moral education. *Harvard Educational Review* 59(2), 182–205.

Thomas, P. (2006). General medical practitioners need to be aware of the theories on which our work depends. *Annals of Family Medicine* 4(5), 450–454.

Vaz, K. (Ed.). (1997). *Oral narrative research with black women*. Thousand Oaks: Sage.

Weinberg, D. (2005). *Of others inside: Insanity, addiction and belonging in America*. Philadelphia: Temple University Press.

White, M., & Epston, D. (1990). *Narrative means to therapeutic ends*. New York: W.W. Norton.

Wiltshire, J. (1995). Telling a story, writing a narrative: Terminology in healthcare. *Nursing Inquiry*, 2(2), 75–82.

7

Case study research

Bev Taylor

The methodological versatility of case study research is so established that it spreads broadly and deeply across many human sciences and healthcare disciplines. The popularity of case study research relates to its accessibility as an easy-to-apply approach to investigate human interests. Over time, the proliferation of projects has led to considerable confusion in the demarcation of principles between disciplines and to the ways in which various authors apply case study methods. Therefore, in this chapter my brief is to ameliorate some of the methodological confusion, by providing some guidance in defining case study as research. The origins of case study research give rise to some common assumptions and key concepts, so I will trace these ideas. In the final sections of this chapter, I describe some case study research methods and exemplify them in projects that have been undertaken in the health sciences.

Defining case study research

Case study definitions vary. A case study can be considered as a methodology, design or method, according to the research perspectives of researchers and the disciplines they represent. Also 'muddying the methodological waters' potentially, is the common use of the term case study as an educational strategy to enhance teaching and learning (e.g., Salam, 2009; UNESCO, 2011), and as popular media and press references to specific topics of interest to listeners, readers and viewers. So, before you assume you are hearing, reading or seeing case studies as research approaches, check the context in which the words are used and for what purposes.

As a methodology – defined in this book as the theoretical assumptions underlying choices in research methods and processes – most definitions point to the value of the qualitative research paradigm either as a stand-alone set of epistemological approaches for generating and validating knowledge (Flyvbjerg, 2011), or integrated as mixed methods (Woodside, 2010). The methodological differences applied to the 'quant–qual divide' generally and to case study specifically, have lessened somewhat, now that we are witnessing the after-effects of the rise of EBP, in a conciliatory epistemological era characterized by some post-positivistic adjustments to extreme absolutist views, and increased acceptance of balanced paradigmatic arguments for mixed methods research (Creswell, 2011; Teddlie and Tashakkori, 2011). However, for researchers still leaning overtly towards the superiority of quantitative research assumptions, case study simply does not qualify as a methodology, because it does not adhere to the epistemological tenets of *the* scientific research method.

Even when case study is accepted as a valid qualitative approach, there may be still some reservation as to whether it constitutes a methodology. For example, Stake (2000, p. 435) tends to see case study as a method within a design, when he claims that

> Case studies have become one of the most common ways to do qualitative inquiry, but they are neither new nor essentially qualitative. Case study is not a methodological choice but a choice of what is to be studied. By whatever methods, we choose to study the case. We could study it analytically or holistically, entirely by repeated measures or hermeneutically, organically or culturally, and by mixed methods – but we concentrate, at least for the time being, on the case.

Stake (2008, p. 119) retained his view, that choices are made in a case study to identify and explore a specific case as a 'functioning specific' or a 'bounded system'. The emphasis here is not on the theoretical assumptions underlying the case study methods and processes, but rather on case study as the appropriate methods and processes choices to create a research design to explore a specific case or set of cases (system).

Yin (2003) agreed with Stake (2000), that case study is an all-encompassing research strategy, but Yin noted that definitional consensus has been difficult due to the scope and technical characteristics of case study. Yin (2003, pp. 13–14) (original emphasis) offered a 'technical definition', beginning with the scope of a case study:

1 *A case study is an empirical inquiry that*
- investigates a contemporary phenomenon within its real-life context, especially when
- the boundaries between phenomenon and context are not clearly evident.

2 *The case study inquiry*
- copes with the technically distinctive situation in which there will be many more variables of interest than data points, and as one result
- relies on multiple sources of evidence, with data needing to converge in a triangulating fashion, and as another result
- benefits from the prior development of theoretical propositions to guide data collection and analysis.

This technical definition attempts to grasp a wider view of case study, while being careful to differentiate it as a research method, not as an education strategy. The definition also shows Yin's view is that the case is studied by whatever means is necessary to gain the best information, thus he is open to mixed methods case study approaches. From my reading of Stake (2000, 2008) and Yin (2003), they both stop short of defining case study as a methodology.

For a case study to be a methodology it needs to have theoretical positions on epistemological questions. In other words, as a methodology, readers need to be able to discern theoretical assumptions about the nature and validity of knowledge claims of case study. Unsurprisingly, the failure of case study to be seen as anything more than a method or design springs often from those sources, who value the verification of knowledge by detailed, complex measures of reliability and validity, so variables can be controlled, in order for results to have predictive and generalizable potential (Woodside, 2010). For example, speaking from a marketing background, Woodside (2010, p. 1) defines case study as 'an inquiry that focuses on describing, understanding, predicting, and/or controlling the individual (i.e., process, animal, person, households, organization, group, industry, culture of nationality)'.

While totalizing definitions are difficult to articulate and possibly dangerous to decree, readers do tend to want to rest on a definition, especially in unfamiliar theoretical terrains, to give them some sense of conceptual safety. Unfortunately, readers' conceptual safety may not always be possible, and the quick answer to: 'What is case study?' may be flawed by a writer's unidentified assumptions and orientations. Writers offering definitions do not necessarily identify their paradigmatic origins and preferences, so it is up to readers to 'read between the lines' to recognize potential difficulties. Also, some definitions of case study have perpetuated an uncorrected, single view for decades. For example, Flyvbjerg (2011, p. 301) points out that the Penguin *Dictionary of Sociology* published an oversimplified definition of case study in the 1994 and 2006 editions, which 'promotes the mistaken view that the case study is hardly a methodology in its own right, but is best seen as subordinate to investigations of larger samples'.

> **Food for thought**
> Given that definitions of case study vary and may be outdated and problematic, what do you suggest is the way out of this definitional morass?

In summary, definitions of case study vary, because the approach can be considered as a methodology, design or method, according to the research perspectives of researchers and the disciplines they represent, and because case study is a term in common usage as an educational strategy and in the popular media and press. Stake's (2008, p. 119) view is that choices are made in a case study to identify and explore a specific case as a 'functioning specific' or a 'bounded system'. Yin (2003) agrees with Stake (2000, 2008), that case study is an all-encompassing research strategy, and that definitional consensus has been difficult due to the scope and technical characteristics of case study. While comprehensive definitions of case study are difficult to articulate, it is important not to oversimplify the approach, or to fail to update definitions in line with contemporary qualitative epistemological assumptions.

Origins of case study research

It is difficult to say with any degree of certainty, but it seems to me that case study as research arose in educational research and evaluation and its proliferation at that time and since has been propelled by the wave of qualitative research as a valid paradigm for exploring human interests. Unlike other methodologies in this book, such as grounded theory, phenomenology and narrative inquiry, I have not been able to locate a concise interpretation of the history of case study, rather I am relying on piecing together accounts from educational philosophy and the social sciences.

Simons (2009) links the evolution of case study research with the move to qualitative research. Her view of events originates in the late 1960s in the UK and the USA, when case study developed as a research approach for evaluating the experience of curriculum innovation. Qualitative research was also gaining ascendancy at that time, so it is the typical 'chicken and egg' conundrum as to which came first – the case study, which became evaluative research, or qualitative research approaches, which fitted well with case study. Simons (2009) suggested that the specific, innovative curricula programmes of the 1960s and 1970s needed broadened evaluative strategies from multiple perspectives and that Stake (1967a) in the USA was the first person to step into the breach and advocate rethinking evaluation by telling 'the programme story' (Stake, 1967b). Following on from Stake, many other authors have contributed to the discourse on case study as it applies to educational research (e.g., MacDonald and Walker, 1975; Simons, 1987).

In our broader disciplinary focus, the health sciences took up case study in various professions, at different times, for different purposes. For example, Anthony and Jack (2009) suggest that nursing took up case study research from its roots in the social sciences. They also note that the history of case study within the social sciences and nursing also reflects the dominance of quantitative criticisms of validity issues in qualitative research generally and case study research specifically.

Similarly, Greenwood and Lowenthal (2005, p. 181) connected case study to validity criticisms, when they traced the roots of social work's use of case study. Their article focused on 'exploring the differences between a case study approach that is influenced by a more scientific orientation to research compared with a method that places more emphasis on the description of the case and is less preoccupied with the need to provide proof in terms of empirical or statistical validation'. Proponents of case study and qualitative research have worked 'hand in hand' to answer the initial criticisms of so-called *scientific* research, to validate case study as a health science research methodology (Flyvbjerg, 2011). In the era of mixed methods, the integration of data findings as words and numbers in case studies has also answered some of these criticisms (Creswell, 2011; Teddlie and Tashakkori, 2011).

> **Food for thought**
> Go to your health science discipline's favoured databases and type in some keywords, including your profession's name, case study research, and history/origins. What comes up? Does your profession's acceptance/ rejection of case study parallel its acceptance/rejection of qualitative research? When? Who were the key writers at that time?

If you choose to undertake case study in your postgraduate research studies, you will need to explore your discipline's approaches to case study, in terms of their origins and adaptations over time. In this section, I described some possibilities for how and when case study originated and I highlighted the parallels between the emergence of case study and qualitative research. To continue this train of thought, we turn now to theoretical assumptions and key concepts in case study research.

Theoretical assumptions and key concepts in case study research

Given its origins and its alignment to qualitative research, writers have developed the theoretical assumptions of case study as a methodology, mainly through highlighting the characteristics it shares with qualitative theoretical assumptions. Having to justify case study as a valid form of qualitative research has helped to form case study into a methodology, not just a research method or design. Flyvbjerg's (2011) writing is an excellent example of countering the critiques of case study, based on its alignment with qualitative epistemological assumptions. To see the detail of the arguments he uses, please refer to (Flyvbjerg, 2011). You will see that he uses the theoretical assumptions of phenomenology, ethnography and the qualitative paradigm in general, to point out that perspectives other than empirico-analytical research methods exist and have methodological worth. To summarize Flyvbjerg's (2011, pp. 302–313) arguments, Table 7.1 provides a synopsis of five misunderstandings about case study and his responses to them.

Flyvbjerg's (2011) responses to the misunderstandings about case study rely not only on justifying long-held qualitative research assumptions about knowledge generation and validation, they also rest on his reading of current trends in case study research. He acknowledges that the paradigmatic wars between 'quant and qual' research are all but over, as a new generation of scholars is emerging 'trained in both quantitative and qualitative methods … (and) research is problem-driven and not methodology-driven, meaning that those methods are employed that for a given problematic best help answer the research questions at hand' (p. 313).

Case study embraces many methods for data collection and analysis, so it sits well as mixed methods research, but for those case studies seeking deep accounts of human experiences over time, case study can sit equally well as a 'stand alone' qualitative research methodology. Case study varies according

Table 7.1 A summary of Flyvbjerg's (2011, pp. 302–313) responses to methodological misunderstandings about case study

Misunder-standing	The methodological critique of case study reflected in the misunderstanding	Flyvbjerg's (2011) response to the misunderstanding
No. 1	General, theoretical knowledge is more valuable than concrete case knowledge.	Predictive theories and universals cannot be found in the study of human affairs. Concrete case knowledge is therefore more valuable than the vain search for predictive theories and universals (p. 304).
No. 2	One cannot generalize on the basis of an individual case; therefore, the case study cannot contribute to scientific knowledge.	One can often generalize on the basis of a single case, and the case study may be central to scientific development as supplement or alternative to other methods. But formal generalization is overvalued as a source of scientific development, whereas 'the force of example' and transferability are underestimated (p. 305).
No. 3	The case study is most useful for generating hypotheses; that is, in the first stage of the total research process, while other methods are more suitable for hypothesis testing and theory building.	The case study is useful for both generating and testing hypotheses but is not limited to these research activities alone (p. 306).
No. 4	The case study contains a bias towards verification, that is, a tendency to confirm the researcher's preconceived notions.	The case study contains no greater bias toward verification of the researcher's preconceived notions than other methods of inquiry. On the contrary, experience indicates that the case study contains a greater bias toward falsification of preconceived notions than toward verification (p. 311).
No. 5	It is often difficult to summarize and develop general propositions and theories on the basis of specific case studies.	It is correct that summarizing case studies is often difficult, especially as concerns case process. It is less correct as regards case outcomes. The problems in summarizing case studies, however, are due more often to the properties of the reality studied than to the case study as a research method. Often it is not desirable to summarize and generalize case studies. Good studies should be read as narratives in their entirety (p. 313).

to the foci chosen and research questions asked. The methodology can range from investigating a single person or phenomenon over time to investigating organizations and cultures. When research foci and questions are about how humans make sense of their lived phenomena and bring about change collaboratively in their cultural systems, case study can be wholly qualitative. Case study does not necessarily have to have quantitative components to make its knowledge claims legitimate. I watch with interest as one by one, the qualitative methodologies scramble to get into the mixed methods life-boats – my view is the ship is not sinking – qualitative methodologies are afloat and as resilient as ever, as relativistic, context-dependent approaches for exploring human interests.

Case study research methods

In this section, we look at the versatility of case study to embrace a wide range of data collection and analysis methods. If you realize at the outset that you have many choices when undertaking case study, you will see that you are facing a smorgasbord of possibilities, not selecting from a limited a la carte menu. If you are looking for prescriptive ways of undertaking case study research, you are apt to be disappointed. As there are no clear-cut ways of doing case study research, it is up to you as the researcher to set up a practical and systematic approach for gathering, recording, analysing and presenting information.

Let us agree that a general starting point is that case study methods gather data to describe as fully as possible, selected research interests, such as individuals, in groups, institutions, organizations and cultures. The researcher uses a case study approach to try to understand over time as much as possible about the area in focus, so the data collection methods gather data from which an intensive analysis of all the determinants involved will give rise to deeply considered answers to research questions. The first task then, is to decide on the research aims and objectives, and the next task is to identify the research questions, from which the data collection methods become apparent. These decisions are a logical consequence of needing a good research plan (research design).

Yin (2009, p. 27) puts it plainly when he contends that 'the main purpose of the design is to help to avoid the situation in which the evidence does not address the initial research questions'. To ensure congruence between the research questions, design and data, Yin (2009, p. 27) suggests that the five components of a case study research design are

1 a study's questions;

2 its propositions, if any;

3 its unit(s) of analysis;

4 the logic linking the data to the propositions; and

5 the criteria for interpreting the findings.

Even though it is up to you as the researcher to compile your own case study methods according to the specific research focus, aims, objectives and questions, there is help available to assist you in making well-reasoned choices. For example, locate Yin's (2009, 2012) books and read his comprehensive approach to designing case studies. They are useful books, because he helps you to see the broad overview of possibilities in designing a case study, including questions to ask yourself when choosing the methods best suited to your project's needs. Stake's (2006) book is excellent for multiple case study analysis. Also, for a comprehensive overview of case study designs and methods for the health sciences, refer to Crowe, Cresswell, Robertson, Huby, Avery and Sheikh (2011). In Crowe et al.'s (2011) article, the authors provide four examples of different case studies, tabled according to their research context, objectives, study design, cases, data collection and analysis methods, plus key findings and main limitations.

Rather than describe in full Yin's (2009), Stake's (2006) or Crowe et al.'s (2011) writing, to which you can refer as supplementary material, my approach in this chapter will be to raise key questions in every step of a case study project and direct you towards sources for deeper reading. My assumptions in taking this approach are that you are already conversant with foundational research concepts, you have some experience in undertaking your own projects, and that you are now at a postgraduate level in your professional studies and research. This is not to say that your research knowledge and skills are optimal, rather that you are building on what you already know to reach higher levels of understanding and application of research methods, in particular, case study. Table 7.2 should also be useful.

Like any research project, a case study approach is only as good as the methods it uses to gather and analyse data in relation to a project's aims, objectives and research questions. The success of case study research has caused such a proliferation of projects with so many different methods, that it may be difficult to collate them all into meaningful information for your health profession. Fortunately, the era of evidence based practice (EBP) in the health sciences (see Chapter 1) has ushered in systematic and integrative review processes for judging the overall worth of research projects. These comprehensive means for critiquing research projects provide careful and detailed overview strategies for amassing, analysing, and meta-synthesizing the findings of prolific research methodologies, such as case study approaches. Careful reading of systematic and integrative reviews of case studies in the health sciences will help you judge the scope and usefulness of methods used in case studies, to inform your particular healthcare discipline and practice.

For example, Anthony and Jack (2009) undertook an integrative review of the use of qualitative case study methodology in nursing research. The rationale for undertaking the project related to the growing use of case study in nursing research and increasing complexities in healthcare delivery. The authors searched data sources for case study research, published between 2005 and 2007, indexed in the CINAHL, MEDLINE, EMBASE, PsychINFO, Sociological Abstracts and SCOPUS databases. Forty-two case study research

Table 7.2 Case study research components, key questions and reading sources

Case study research component	Key questions	Reading sources in this book	Other useful reading sources
Preparatory work	Who/what is involved? the person, people, culture, organization, phenomenon, geographical location? Why? Are they relevant to your focus?	Chapter 11	Gerring (2007) Stake (2006) Yin (2009)
	What is the type of case? e.g. intrinsic, instrumental, collective?		Stake (1995)
	descriptive, interpretative, evaluative?		Merriam (1988)
	explanatory, descriptive, illustrative, exploratory, 'meta-evaluation'?		Yin (1994)
	theory-led, theory generated?	Chapter 2	Glaser and Strauss (1967) Charmaz (2006)
	other (within any interpretive or critical qualitative approach)?	Chapters 2–9	See reference list at end of each chapter
Working title of the research	What is the working title, including the: focus of the project? type of case study?		
Background	What is: your interest in the project? the literature informing you about the research to date?	Chapter 11	Booth, Papanioannou and Sutton (2012)
Aims, objectives, potential significance	What are the case study's: overall research intentions (aims)? subset of intentions (objectives)? likely important outcomes?	Chapter 11	
Methods and processes			
Ethical considerations	What are the: risks and benefits to participants? ethical safeguards? consent procedures? plans for data storage?	Chapter 11	
Participant recruitment	In relation to the participants: who are they? what are the inclusion/ exclusion criteria? sampling methods? what are their specific contributions to the case study over time?	Chapter 11	

continued ...

Table 7.2 continued

Case study research component	Key questions	Reading sources in this book	Other useful reading sources
Data collection	What data collection methods and processes will be used? Will they be: solely qualitative? mixed? In what combinations? Will they include, for example:	Chapter 11	Yin (2009) Stake (2006)
	observation/participation? interviews? focus groups? surveys? questionnaires? Will they be undertaken: with individuals or groups? on single or multiple sites? When? consecutively, concurrently? With whom? Over what time range (days, months, years?)	Chapter 4 Chapter 12 Chapter 13	
Data analysis, synthesis and dissemination	How will you: match data collection methods and congruent data analysis methods?	Chapter 1	Yin (2009) Simons (2009) Stake (2006)
	synthesize and integrate multiple data sources? manage discrepancies in results from multiple methods/sources? interpret the overall findings/insights?	Chapter 10	Yin (2009) Simons (2009) Stake (2006)
	present the overall case study? (in narratives, summaries, themes, discourses, etc?) defend the rigour/ trustworthiness of the case study's methods, processes and outcomes? disseminate the findings/ insights/implications?	Chapters 14–16	Yin (2009) Simons (2009) Stake (2006)

papers met the inclusion criteria, according to Whittemore and Knafl's (2005) integrative review method. The results were unsurprising, in that they were similar to other authors' observations about the lack of definitional consensus in case studies (Yin, 2003; Taylor, Kermode and Roberts, 2006). Anthony and Jack (2009, p. 1171) reported that 'confusion exists about the name, nature and use of case study. This methodology, including terminology and concepts, is often invisible in qualitative study titles and abstracts'. The authors noted also, that even though 'a high quality of case study exists in nursing research' (p. 1171), care should be taken to ensure that case studies, as reported in publications, attend to all the details to identify them as such, so that they are acknowledged as contributing to the development of nursing knowledge.

Another example of a systematic review of quantitative and qualitative projects (including case study research) is a project which investigated research evidence in public health decision making processes (Orton, Lloyd-Williams, Taylor-Robinson, O'Flaherty, and Capewell, 2011). The authors reported that to locate eligible sources, they searched 13 bibliographic databases, scanned organizational websites, contacted key informants and scrutinized the bibliographies of the included studies. The 18 selected studies comprised 15 qualitative projects (six of which were case studies) and three surveys (also classified by the authors as qualitative). Selected publications were independently assessed by two reviewers, who 'extracted data and assessed methodological quality'. The data were then 'synthesised as a narrative review' (Orton et al., 2011, p. 1). The authors identified a large number of barriers and facilitative factors within the publications and suggested that 'to more effectively implement research informed public health policy, action is required by decision makers and researchers to address the barriers identified in this systematic review. There is an urgent need for evidence to support the use of research evidence to inform public health decision making to reduce inequalities' (Orton et al., 2011, p. 1).

Unfortunately, the specific contributions of the case study research articles to the overall information about the barriers and facilitators was not possible to separate out in Orton et al.'s (2011) systematic review. However, as all of the reviewed studies were qualitative, the authors' comments may be taken to apply equally to case study research. They concluded that the selected studies 'did not aim for representative samples. Instead, they were based in a diverse range of specific localities where public health decision making takes place. Thus, findings are not generalizable. Clearer descriptions of participants and contexts would have helped interpret the findings from individual studies. The wide variety of study types included in the systematic review also necessitated careful consideration of methods for integrating data and for assessing methodological quality of individual studies' (Orton et al., 2011, p. 8).

In this section, I highlighted the broad choices researchers face when they undertake case study research. I suggested that it is up to you as the researcher to compile your own case study methods into a suitable design according to your specific research focus, aims, objectives and questions, and that there are helpful resources available (e.g., Crowe et al., 2011; Stake, 2006; Yin, 2009). To help you negotiate some of those choices I presented Table 7.2 as an overview of the steps in planning case study research, with key questions to clarify the case study research design. The next section describes some examples of case study research, showing how some researchers in the health sciences have made and applied their case study decisions.

Case study research projects in the health sciences

Database searches for case study research in the health sciences bring up many interesting examples of projects. Because case study research can straddle the 'quantitative/qualitative divide' by employing mixed methods for data collection and analysis, it lends itself equally well to numerically-directed questions about: How much? and How often?, as it does to language-directed questions about: 'What are the effects of this focus of interest? and 'How does this focus of interest present itself over time?' Similarly, the human as experiencing subject does not always have to be centre stage, because areas relating to human patterns and trends in health and illness can be the focus using mixed methods (e.g., Dattilio, Edwards and Fishman, 2010; Habashi and Worley, 2009).

Health-related research interests vary, as shown in examples of case study research in workplace health (Dugdill, 2000; Rothman and Perry, 2004), public health issues, such as anti-alcohol posters in Poland (Gorsky, Krajewski-Siuda, Dutka and Berridge, 2010); the effectiveness of rural telehealth (Singh, Mathiassen, Stachura and Astapova, 2010), ergonomics (Hignett and Wilson, 2004); and the health promotion capacity of sport and recreation organizations (Casey, Payne and Eime, 2009).

Williams, Crooks, Whitfield, Kelley, Richards, DeMiglio and Dykeman (2010) wanted to track the evolution of palliative care in seven provinces in Canada, so they chose a comparative case study approach. The background to their study was that they identified the trends in Canada towards ageing, with consequent increases in chronic diseases, and the flow-on effects of the need for community based care and hospice palliative care (HPC) planning and provision. Therefore, the 'purpose of this study was to analyse the evolution of HPC in seven provinces in Canada so as to inform such planning and provision elsewhere' (p. 1). They were seeking to identify key policy and practice events, as well as barriers and facilitators, to HPC in Canada.

The qualitative comparative case study design included searching grey literature 'to create a preliminary timeline for each that described the evolution of HPC beginning in 1970', and interviewing 42 informants 'to verify the content of each provincial timeline and to discuss barriers and facilitators to the development of HPC' (Williams et al., 2010, p. 1). The research team met to undertake a comparative analysis of the data. Findings pointed to the 'fact that HPC continues to remain at the margins of the healthcare system' (p. 1).

Williams et al. (2010) were able to identify specific barriers and facilitators in establishing HPC in the provinces researched and concluded that 'overall, the evolution of HPC across the case study provinces has been markedly slow, but steady and continuous' (p. 1). They also recognized the effect of demographics on HPC demand in Canada and that the change agents to bring about lasting impact for HPC would be 'concerned citizens, advocacy organizations and local champions' (p. 1).

Williams et al.'s (2010) study shows other researchers that a lot of useful information can be gained by a relatively simple case study design. They connected their research objectives to Gerring's (2007) approach to case study and to qualitative research in general. The researchers used a time span of summer 2006 to summer 2009, to manually track down the grey literature sources through key organizational websites and professional networks in the purposefully selected seven provinces. In that time span they also identified the key informants and interviewed them by phone. The respective rationales for the inclusion of the grey literature and the key informants, plus the analytic techniques, are described in full in the article. The article also describes in full the various barriers and facilitators to HPC in the provinces, and it is immediately apparent to the reader that the two data collection methods over the time span, plus the comparative analysis of the data, were sufficient to reveal many valuable insights in relation to the research objectives.

Another example of a case study is a project undertaken by medical practitioners in Italy to obtain 'comprehensive health outcomes and health services utilization data on stroke patients' (Stuart, Papini, Benvenuti, Nerattinie, Roccato, Macellari, Stanhope, Macko and Weinrich, 2010, p. 271). The research aim was to 'pilot a methodology using administrative data to monitor and improve health outcomes for stroke survivors in Tuscany' (p. 271). The case study used mixed methods. Phase one included 'a series of site visits and interviews with senior health officials and clinicians in AUSLs 10 (Florence district) and 11 (Empoli district) to determine the organization and availability of health services and to identify the availability of relevant data' (Stuart et al., 2010, p. 273). Phase two included 'a retrospective analysis of administrative data 1 year post stroke for all patients in AUSLs 10 and 11 who met study criteria during the calendar year 2002' (Stuart et al., 2010, p. 273).

A working party reviewed the data in Phase three. The authors are silent on the means by which they analysed the interview data, but 'for the statistical significance of differences between AUSLs 10 and 11 for proportions involving the study population (they) used the test for two independent proportions. The t-test was used to test for statistical significance in means between the two groups' (p. 273). The results showed that 'number of inpatient days, number of prescriptions, and prescription costs were significantly higher for patients in AUSL 10 compared with AUSL 11. There was no significant difference between mortality rates' (p. 271). The main recommendation for the future use of the methodology was that administrative data are useful for monitoring processes and outcomes for chronic stroke patients, because it saves money and produces outcomes. However, the outcome measure for the study was mortality rates and the authors recognized that more sensitive outcome measures are important, such as measures of functional impairment.

Stuart et al.'s (2010) project purports in its title to be a case study, but there is no methodological justification for case study in the methods section, rather there is one sentence indicating the use of qualitative and quantitative data. The design is described in phases as discrete data collection methods, which could fit most mixed methods designs. It is difficult to know why the researchers classified their project as a case study as there is no discussion of their methodological choice, so the judgement as to its particular approach rests with readers.

If we take Yin's (2003, pp. 13–14) 'technical definition' of case study, then turn the statements into questions, and ask them of Stuart et al.'s (2010) project, we can make a reasoned judgement. Is Stuart et al.'s (2010) project an empirical inquiry that:

1 investigated a contemporary phenomenon within its real-life context?

2 was used because the boundaries between phenomenon and context were not clearly evident?

3 coped with the technically distinctive situation in which there were many more variables of interest than data points?

4 relied on multiple sources of evidence, with data converged in a triangulating fashion?

5 benefited from the prior development of theoretical propositions to guide data collection and analysis?

From my reading of the technical definition of case study, it is doubtful that Stuart et al.'s (2010) project fits every aspect of Yin's (2003) case study. Stuart et al. (2010) investigated health services and outcomes for stroke survivors, so it was a contemporary phenomenon within its real-life context. To some extent, the boundaries between phenomenon and context were not clearly evident, but the researchers' approach was motivated mainly by their goal to 'develop a methodology that could guide health policy and management decisions, yet be simple and relatively inexpensive to administer. Consequently, (they) wanted to limit the need for multivariate analysis, reduce variation due to case-mix and severity of stroke as much as possible, and use routinely collected data (of mortality rates)' (Stuart et al., 2010, p. 273).

By simplifying the data collection and analysis methods and by using mortality as the outcome measure, the researchers coped with a technically distinctive situation in which there were many more variables of interest than data points, but they relied on minimal sources of evidence. There is no description in the article of the triangulation of data, nor is there evidence that they developed theoretical propositions to guide data collection and analysis, rather their project was motivated by wanting to develop an inexpensive, uncomplicated methodology. Even so, Stuart et al.'s (2010) project still has *some* characteristics of case study as defined by Yin (2003) and other authors (Gerring, 2007; Stake, 2008).

<hr>

Food for thought

Given the loose terminology and lack of definition and consensus as to what constitutes a case study, and the proliferation of projects claiming to be case study research, how will you:

1 decide on what you accept as a case study?

2 decide on whether a project you have in mind is (potentially) a case study?

3 choose a particular case study design?

4 decide on criteria against which to judge a case study's trustworthiness (rigour)?

<hr>

Given the various examples of case study projects and their lack of conformity in design, case study research can be creative in its approach. The particular case study approach you take will be up to you, but you will be accountable for showing that the sequence of methods and processes you use relate directly to exploring the research aims and questions you have posed. To be 'on the safe side' methodologically, you should also be able to claim that your case study approach either reflects or is informed by, published case study approaches (e.g., Gerring, 2007; Yin, 2009; Simons, 2009; Stake, 2006; Woodside, 2010). You need also to consider issues of 'rigour' or trustworthiness in conducting case studies, and appropriate methods of data analysis and interpretation. Read as widely as you can and see how other researchers have organized their case studies and be prepared to critique their methods and designs against published case study approaches.

Chapter summary

The proliferation of case study research has led to considerable variations in the ways disciplines define case study and apply methods and designs. In this chapter, I provided some definitions of case study as research, speculated as to the origins of case study research and identified some common case study research assumptions and key concepts. In the final sections of this chapter, I described some case study research undertaken in the health sciences.

Definitions of case study vary, dependent on whether they are considered as methodology, design or method. Generally considered to be a foundational thinker in case study, Stake's (2008, p. 119) view of case study is that it identifies and explores a specific case as a 'functioning specific' or a 'bounded system'. Yin (2003) agrees with Stake (2000, 2008), that case study is an all-encompassing research strategy, and that definitional consensus has been difficult due to the scope and technical characteristics of case study. While comprehensive definitions of case study are difficult to articulate, it is important not to oversimplify the approach, nor to fail to update definitions in line with contemporary qualitative epistemological assumptions.

It seems that case study as research arose in educational research and evaluation. The success of case study has been propelled by the wave of recognizing qualitative research as a valid paradigm for exploring human interests. For example, Simons (2009) linked the evolution of case study research with the move to qualitative research. When case study was developing as a research approach for evaluating curriculum innovation in the UK and the USA, qualitative research was also gaining ascendancy. Case study research fitted well with evaluative research and the qualitative research paradigm. Stake's writing (1967a, 1967b) in the USA in rethinking evaluation seems to be the catalyst for many other authors to contribute to the discourse on case study as educational research (e.g., MacDonald and Walker, 1975; Simons, 1987).

The key theoretical concepts of case study align, on the whole, with qualitative research assumptions about knowledge. In the same vein, justification of case study mainly parallels responding to critiques that case study does not allow researchers to predict and generalize their findings. Having to justify case study as a valid form of qualitative research has helped to form case study into a methodology, not just a research method or design (Flyvbjerg, 2011). Flyvbjerg's (2011) responses to the misunderstandings about case study not only rely on justifying long-held qualitative research assumptions about knowledge generation and validation, they also rest on his reading of current trends in case study research towards mixed methods.

Case study projects lack conformity in design, so case study research can be creative. Choosing a particular case study approach is up to the researcher(s), but the choice must be justified by showing that the sequence of case study methods and processes relate directly to research aims and questions. Researchers can also be guided by recognized case study approaches (e.g., Gerring, 2007; Yin, 2009; Simons, 2009; Stake, 2006; Woodside, 2010).

Key points

- The popularity of case study research relates to its accessible as an easy-to-apply approach to investigate human interests.

- Writers offering definitions of case study do not necessarily identify their paradigmatic origins and preferences, so it is up to readers to 'read between the lines' to recognize potential difficulties.

- Yin (2003) agrees with Stake (2000, 2008), that case study is an all-encompassing research strategy, and that definitional consensus has been difficult due to the scope and technical characteristics of case study.

- Case study embraces many methods for data collection and analysis, so it sits well as mixed methods research, but for those case studies seeking deep accounts of human experiences over time, case study can sit equally well as a 'stand alone' qualitative research methodology.

- As there are no clear-cut ways of doing case study research, it is up to you as the researcher to set up a practical and systematic approach for gathering, recording, analysing and presenting information.

Critical review questions

1 In what ways is it possible for case study research to inform healthcare practice?

2 To what extent can case study research offer insights into your clients' experiences of health and illness?

References

Anthony, S., & Jack, S. (2009). Qualitative case study methodology in nursing research: An integrative review. *Journal of Advanced Nursing, 65*(6), 1171–1181.

Booth, A., Papanioannou, D., & Sutton, A. (2012). *Systematic approaches to a successful literature review.* London: Sage.

Casey, M.M., Payne, W.R., & Eime, M.E. (2009). Building the health promotion capacity of sport and recreation organisations: A case study of regional sports assemblies. *Managing Leisure, 14,* 112–124.

Charmaz, K. (2006). *Constructing grounded theory: A practical guide through qualitative analysis.* Thousand Oaks: Sage.

Creswell, J.W. (2011). Controversies in mixed methods research. In N.K. Denzin & Y.S. Lincoln (Eds.) *The SAGE handbook of qualitative research,* 4th edn. Los Angeles: Sage, 269–284.

Crowe, S., Cresswell, K., Robertson, A., Huby, G., Avery, A., & Sheikh, A. (2011). The case study approach. *BMC Medical Research Methodology, 11,* 100.

Dattilio, F.M., Edwards, D.J., & Fishman, D.B. (2010). Case studies within a mixed methods paradigm: Toward a resolution of the alienation between researcher and practitioner in psychotherapy research. *Psychotherapy, 47*(4):427–441.

Dugdill, L. (2000). Developing a holistic understanding of workplace health: The case of bank workers. *Ergonomics, 43*(10), 1738–1749.

Flyvbjerg, B. (2011). Case Study. In N.K. Denzin & Y.S. Lincoln (Eds.) *The SAGE handbook of qualitative research,* 4th edn. Los Angeles: Sage, 301–316.

Gerring, J. (2007). *Case study research: Principles and practices.* Cambridge: Cambridge University Press.

Glaser, B.G., & Strauss, A.L. (1967). *The discovery of grounded theory: Strategies for qualitative research.* Chicago: Aldine.

Gorsky, M., Krajewski-Siuda, K., Dutka, W., & Berridge, V. (2010). Anti-alcohol posters in Poland, 1945–1989: Diverse meanings, uncertain effects. *American Journal of Public Health,100,* 2059–2069.

Greenwood, D., & Lowenthal, D. (2005). Case study as a means of researching social work and improving practitioner education. *Journal of Social Work Practice, 19*(2), 181–193.

Habashi, J., & Worley, J. (2009). Child geopolitical agency: A mixed methods case study. *Journal of Mixed Methods Research, 3*(1), 42–64.

Hignett, S., & Wilson, J.R. (2004). The role for qualitative methodology in ergonomics: A case study to explore theoretical issues. *Theoretical Issues in Ergonomics 5*(6), 473–493.

MacDonald, B., & Walker, R. (1975). Case study and the social philosophy of educational research. *Cambridge Journal of Education, 5*(1), 2–12.

Merriam, S.B. (1988) *Qualitative research in education: A qualitative approach.* San Francisco: Jossey Bass

Orton, L., Lloyd-Williams, F., Taylor-Robinson, D., O'Flaherty, M., & Capewell, S. (2011). The use of research evidence in public health decision making processes: Systematic review. *PLoS ONE* 6(7): e21704. doi:10.1371/journal.pone.0021704.

Rothman, E.F., & Perry, M.J. (2004). Intimate partner abuse perpetrated by employees. *Journal of Occupational Health Psychology, 9*(3), 238–246.

Salam, A. (2009). Community and family case study: A community-based educational strategy to promote five star doctors for the 21st century. *South East Asian Journal of Medical Education, 3*(1), 20–24.

Simons, H. (1987). *Getting to know schools in a democracy: The politics and process of evaluation.* Lewes: Falmer Press.

Simons, H. (2009). *Case study research in practice.* Los Angeles: Sage.

Singh, R., Mathiassen, L., Stachura, M.E., & Astapova, E.V. (2010). Sustainable rural tele-health innovation: A public health case study. *HSR: Health Services Research, 45*(4), 985- 1004.

Stake, R.E. (1967a). Toward a technology for the evaluation of educational programs. In R.W. Tyler, R.M. Gagne, & M. Scriven (Eds.) *Perspectives of curriculum evaluation. AERA monograph series on curriculum evaluation. No. 1.* Chicago: Rand & McNally.

Stake, R.E. (1967b). The countenance of educational evaluation. *Teachers College Record, 68*(7): 523–540.

Stake, R.E. (1995) *The art of case study research.* Thousand Oaks, California: Sage.

Stake, R.E. (2000). Case Studies. In N.K. Denzin & Y.S. Lincoln (Eds.) *Handbook of qualitative research* 2nd edn. Thousand Oaks: Sage.

Stake, R.E. (2006). *Multiple case analysis.* New York: Guilford Press.

Stake, R.E. (2008). Qualitative case studies. In N.K. Denzin & Y.S. Lincoln (Eds.) (2008). *Strategies of qualitative inquiry* 3rd edn. Thousand Oaks: Sage, 119–150.

Stuart, M., Papini, D., Benvenuti, F., Nerattinie, E., Roccato, E., Macellari, V., Stanhope, S., Macko, R., & Weinrich, M. (2010). Methodological issues in monitoring health services and outcomes for stroke survivors: A case study. *Disability and Health Journal 3,* 271–281.

Taylor, B.J., Kermode, S., & Roberts, K. (2006). *Research in nursing and healthcare: Evidence for practice,* 3rd edn. Australia: Thomson.

Teddlie, C., & Tashakkori, A. (2011). Mixed methods research. In N.K. Denzin & Y.S. Lincoln (Eds.) *The SAGE handbook of qualitative research,* 4th edn. Los Angeles: Sage, 285–300.

UNESCO. (2011). *Youth X change: Climate change and lifestyle handbook.* Kenya: United Nations Educational, Scientific and Cultural Organization (UNESCO).

Whittemore, R., & Knafl, K. (2005) The integrative review: updated methodology. *Journal of Advanced Nursing, 52*(5), 546–553

Williams, A.M., Crooks, V.A., Whitfield, K., Kelley, M.-L., Richards, J.-L., DeMiglio, L., & Dykeman, S. (2010). Tracking the evolution of hospice care in Canada: A comparative case study analysis of seven provinces. *BMC Health Services Research,* 10,147 http://www.biomedcentral.com/1472-6963/10/147.

Woodside, A.G. (2010). *Case study research: Theory, methods, practice.* UK: Emerald.

Yin, R.K. (1994) *Case study research design and methods.* Thousand Oaks, California: Sage.

Yin, R.K. (2003). *Applications of case study research,* 3rd edn. Thousand Oaks: Sage.

Yin, R.K. (2009). *Case study research: Design and methods* 4th edn. Thousand Oaks: Sage.

Yin, R.K. (2012). *Applications of case study research.* Thousand Oaks: Sage.

8

Feminisms

Bev Taylor

This chapter focuses on feminisms, written intentionally as plural, to denote the multiplicity of feminist approaches to thinking about and researching women's struggles and issues. Feminisms reflect women's interests in their lives within patriarchal cultures and against other various oppressive and hegemonic forces across the world and over time. In this chapter I discuss definitions of feminisms, according to their particular focus on women's lives over time. The origins of feminisms can be traced to the first wave of stirrings of the women's movement at the end of the 19th century in New Zealand and the UK, and it has paralleled key historical events since that time, some of which are traced in this chapter.

Feminisms are mobile methodologies, because they keep on moving with epistemological and ontological trends and adaptations, to encompass the full range of paradigmatic positions and their influences on research. While some feminist researchers keep moving philosophically and take in a wide range of epistemological positions, others choose to work within a chosen paradigm, but they all keep their eyes on certain underlying assumptions about women's lives, viewing them from their various perspectives. Key enduring feminist concepts and the research methods and processes they use to reflect these ideas are discussed in this chapter. To exemplify the methodological variety, I describe a selection of feminist research projects in the health sciences in the last section of this chapter.

Defining feminisms

As with other progressive research methodologies described in this book, it is not possible to settle on one all-encompassing definition of feminism, because the breadth and depth of scholarship and research within the last 100 plus years, has produced many different views and definitions of feminisms. The three waves of feminisms, described in the next section, help readers to locate major moments in feminist thinking. In the first decade of the 21st century, the focus is less on the waves of feminisms (already broken on the shore of feminist history), to a view over the ocean itself, where the breadth and depth of feminisms seems to match more closely the metaphor of waves being whipped up continually by contextual agents and forces within a particular seascape of national, transnational and intersectional possibilities.

It is difficult to locate a precise definition of feminisms in recent published sources, because authors tend to begin from (often unstated) assumptions about the importance of women's lives, experiences and knowledges and go straight into a discussion of ideas and issues from various viewpoints. For example, Hesse-Biber's (2012) edited book *The Handbook of Feminist Research: Theory and Praxis* is a compilation of considered feminist epistemologies, research praxis, and issues and insights in practice and pedagogy, with little or no attention to foundational, 'catch-all' definitions.

Feminisms have gone well beyond the very early years of a dominant ideological position of the equality of women, women's rights and defending the essentialized oppressed woman, to the present era of 'highly diversified, contentious, dynamic, and challenging' approaches and practices (Olesen, 2011, p. 129). Writers prefer to abandon a 'one size fits all' approach to *feminism*, and progress their ideas to encompass wide-ranging *feminisms*, such as feminist empiricism (Hundley, 2012), feminist standpoints (Harding, 2012), postmodern, post-structural, and critical theories (Gannon and Davies, 2012), global feminist ethnography (Bhavani and Talcott, 2012), and intersectionality (Thornton Dill and Kohlman, 2012).

Origins of feminisms

Locating the origins of feminisms depends how far you look back in time and in which direction. If we equate the stirrings of women's reactionary thought with the origins of feminism, it takes us back a long time to the French poet and writer, Christine de Pisan, and her book *The Book of the City of Ladies*. Pisan's (1405, trans. 1982) writing acknowledged women's virtues and nobility of spirit and advocated the need for women's education, while exposing misogyny in the literary establishment of her time. Another early literary catalyst of women's reactionary thought was Mary Wollstonecraft (1792), author of the classic work of early feminist thought, *A Vindication of the Rights of Woman*.

As movements concerned with women's lives and issues, feminisms reflect various transitions in social, cultural, political and economic events and issues, over time, in many parts of the world. Defining and addressing a multiplicity of women's concerns requires many theories to explain the causes of women's lived experiences and the various forms of struggles and oppression they face. Feminist theorists have used the idea of waves, to depict the major shifts in the origins and progression of feminisms. Although there is some disagreement about the timing and exact number of waves, it is generally accepted that there have been three waves of feminisms.

The first wave of feminism refers to events at the end of the 19th century into the beginning of the 20th century, when suffragettes in New Zealand, Australia and the UK, engaged in political action to secure for women the right to vote. 'On 19 September 1893 the governor, Lord Glasgow, signed a new Electoral Act into law. As a result of this landmark legislation, New Zealand became the first self-governing country in the world in which all women had the right to vote in parliamentary elections' (New Zealand History online, 2012, f1). In 1902, Australia was the first country in the world to give women both the right to vote in federal elections and the right to be elected to parliament on a national basis. It was not until 1918, after World War I and considerable political agitation, that women were able to vote in general elections in the UK. In Canada, on 24 May 1918, all female citizens aged 21 and over became eligible to vote in federal elections. In the USA, on 26 August 1920, the 19th Amendment to the Constitution was finally ratified, to allow American women the rights and responsibilities of citizenship, including the right to vote (Cott, 1987).

The first wave of feminisms refers also to the time before, during and after both World Wars, when the heavy losses of fighting men's lives created a need for women to maintain supplies and services in home countries. Women filled their industrial workforce roles well, but they were relegated to home duties and reproductive responsibilities when the troops returned. Consequently, women's issues during the first wave of feminisms included not only their rights to vote, but also ongoing issues related to women's equal status in society, including their rights for equal recognition and benefits in the workforce, their rights to be educated, and a voice in the determination of their reproductive issues, such as contraception and abortion.

During the first wave, women speaking out for women caused such a backlash in the media that 'feminist' became a word of derision and women were afraid to identify as feminists. Cicely Isabel Fairfield, writing with the pen name Rebecca West (1913), expressed the situation courageously and succinctly in *The Clarion*: 'I myself have never been able to find out precisely what feminism is: I only know that people call me a feminist whenever I express sentiments that differentiate me from a doormat, or a prostitute.' As a reaction to the public backlash to feminism between wars, women continued to fight against discrimination. For example, Virginia Woolf wrote *A Room of One's Own* (Woolf, 1989) and *Three Guineas* (Woolf, 1938, 1993).

Second-wave feminism refers to a period of feminist activity beginning in the early 1960s to the late 1980s. Second-wave feminism focused on cultural and political inequalities and identified how women's personal lives were deeply politicized within patriarchal power structures. The second wave included liberal, Marxist, radical and lesbian feminisms. Liberal feminism sought equal rights within the existing social structures, through reasoning and equal educational opportunities for women, to determine their social roles and compete with men on equal terms. Marxist/socialist feminism asserted that ownership of property is the basis of sexism and class division, and that women are oppressed within the family, motherhood, consumerism and class. This approach advocated the freedom to define one's own sexuality, equal sharing of child rearing and domestic roles, and the right to choose, thereby addressing relationships between the economy, family, class and gender.

Marxist/socialist feminist ideas were influential in radical feminism, which withdrew from dominant patriarchal systems to woman-defined systems, thought and culture. Critics who opposed radical feminism questioned the need for a separatist stance, even though they may have agreed that women needed to be free from the biological oppression of motherhood, sexual slavery, and the allocation of womanly work. Lesbian feminists agreed with radical feminists on many levels, and added to those ideas their preferred sexual orientation, by rejecting the dominant heterosexual paradigm and males as sexual partners.

The third wave of contemporary feminism, from the 1980s onwards, includes deconstructive poststructural and postmodern feminisms, reacting to the second-wave thinkers' representations of the 'essential' white, middle-class woman. Feminist poststructuralist thinkers asserted that the division of feminisms into categories was problematic, because the categories were arbitrary and socially produced, and they failed to address issues of power in language, subjectivity, social processes and institutions (Hekman, 1990; Lather, 1991). The debates in this area of feminist thought are lively and controversial, because they take a postmodern epistemological view that 'truth' is partial and illusory. Postmodern feminists urge researchers to question their feminist frames of reference and 'trouble' their own epistemological assumptions, data categories and interpretations (Lather, 2007). The critique of postmodern feminism has been mainly along the lines that it leaves no room for holding true to cherished women's ideals and for standing firm on establishing and maintaining women's reforms, thus giving power to the status quo by failing to address structural power and cultural issues (Ebert, 1996). Other feminisms originating in the third wave are discussed in the next section of this chapter.

Feminisms have evolved according to history and changes in epistemological debates. In the health sciences feminisms have reflected historical changes in disciplinary thought. For example, Kemp and Brandwein (2010) traced the 'intertwined history' of feminisms and social work in the United States. The authors examined the 'ideas, practices, and people that have shaped the complicated organism' of 'feminist social work', from the civic involvement of 19th- and early 20th-century women to 21st-century efforts to craft more global, fluid, and inclusive feminist theories and practices' (Kemp and Brandwein, 2010, p. 341).

In the United States, feminisms and the social work profession shared similar historical trajectories, because they were both 'rooted in the civic involvement of 19th- and early 20th-century women, focused in the interwar years on institution building, were reenergized by the social activism of the 1960s and 1970s, and in the 21st century are struggling to respond adequately to the realities and demands of a highly diverse, fluid, and global world' (p. 341).

In summary, the methodological origins of feminisms are rooted within important historical events, which had as their main objectives the intentions to raise awareness of women's issues related to their fundamental rights as citizens. The right to vote, be educated, have a voice in reproductive issues, and in all political arenas, galvanized the first-wave feminists into action. The second-wave feminists built on the foundations of their predecessors and differentiated the women's movement into liberal, Marxist, radical and lesbian feminisms. The third wave of deconstructive, poststructural and postmodern feminisms, opposed representations of the 'essential' white, middle-class woman and destabilized notions of 'truth' in contemporary feminist research approaches.

Theoretical assumptions and key concepts of feminisms

Given the progression of feminist thought from the first to the third waves and the ongoing rippling surface of the ocean of feminisms, it is not easy to speak of shared assumptions of feminisms, because early ideas have been swept away by successive critiques and adaptations of feminist theories. With no mention of 'waves' as such, Olesen (2011) provides a useful overview of the breadth of feminist qualitative research in the first decade of the 21st century. Olesen's (2011) beginning assumptions are that 'feminisms and qualitative research practices continue to be highly diversified, contentious, dynamic, and challenging', feminist concepts from 'the northern hemisphere are no longer the standard' especially in 'replicating whiteness', and that there is no 'global, homogenous feminism' (p. 129).

While acknowledging the ever-evolving differences in theoretical assumptions about feminisms, Olesen (2011) speculates that

> If there is a dominant theme in feminist qualitative research, it is the issue of knowledges. Whose knowledges? Where and how obtained, by whom, from whom, and for what purposes? It moved feminist research from the lack of or flawed attention to marginalized women, usually non-white, homosexual, or disabled, to recognition of differences among women and within the same groups of women and the recognition that multiple identities and subjectivities are constructed in particular historical and social contexts. It opened discussion of critical epistemological issues, the researcher's characteristics and relationships to research participants. (pp. 129–130)

Having speculated on one possible dominant theme of knowledges in feminist qualitative research, Olesen (2011) goes on to overview the breadth of research from the year 2000, highlighting the key writers in shifting feminist thought. In the vast array of feminisms, Olesen (2011) discusses feminisms as transformative developments, critical trends, continuing issues and enduring concerns. Transformative developments include feminist approaches, such as postcolonial feminist thought (e.g., Kim, 2007); globalization and transnational feminism (e.g., Parrenas, 2008); standpoint theory (e.g., Harding, 2008); and postmodern and poststructural deconstructive theory (e.g., St. Pierre, 2009).

Postcolonial feminist thought

Postcolonial feminist thought emerged from a realization that feminist theories had been generated mainly from a white, industrialized Western perspective, which assumed an essentialized woman, and an inherent 'sameness' of all women and their concerns. That same dominant 'colonized' perspective, although arguably well-intentioned at the time, was the voice of particular-to-context individuals, who were also speaking authoritatively for all other women, regardless of their contexts.

Postcolonial feminisms call for a critique of 'homogenous' feminisms, and require a decolonization process to deconstruct the essentialized concepts of 'woman' and 'women' (Kim, 2007). Postcolonial feminist thought critiques 'constructions of colour', women 'as unified subjectivities located in the category of woman', and whether elite feminist thought silences and speaks for 'subordinates' (Olesen, 2011, p. 130). Also within postcolonial feminist thinking is the idea of 'border work', (e.g., Trinh, 1992), which encourages feminist theorists and researchers to reassess how 'tightly bound … (they) might have become to the specific methodological practices and conceptual definitions of (their) own disciplines' (Hesse-Biber and Piatelli, 2012b, p. 574).

Globalization and transnational feminisms

Globalization feminism takes research interest in the contradictions and tensions in the 'relentless, neoliberal flow of capitalism across national borders' (Olesen, 2011, p. 130), examining issues in dominance of economic forces and women's possibilities for resistance. Transnational feminism 'analyses national and cross-national feminist organizing and action' being careful to avoid imposing 'a Westernised version of feminism' (Olesen, 2011, p. 130).

Feminist standpoint theory

Feminist standpoint theory and research replaces 'the concept of essentialized, universalized woman with the idea of a situated woman with experiences and knowledge specific to her place in her material division of labour and the racial stratification systems' (Olesen, 2011, p. 130). Feminist standpoint research varies as to the interpretation of who is the 'situated woman', according to how she is viewed through various paradigmatic lenses. For example, poststructural standpoint feminists emphasize a critical examination of power relations and postmodernist standpoint feminists argue for using 'powerful analytic tools' to challenge dominant discourses and 'the very rules of the game' (Olesen, 2011, pp. 130–131).

Postmodern and poststructural deconstructive feminisms

Postmodern and poststructural deconstructive theory ushered in the third wave, and it has continued to generate spirited debate among feminists, because these perspectives question the nature of knowledges as grand narratives and thereby potentially unseat some treasured, fundamental feminist ideals and assumptions about women's lives and sources of oppression (Ebert, 1996). Because 'truth' claims are suspect, postmodern/deconstructive feminist researchers focus their investigations on representation and text, and treat as problematic any totalizing claims about power and oppression. For example, Olesen (2011, p. 133) highlights 'sophisticated feminist work in gender and science', which 'discomfort not only male-dominated institutions, such as science, but feminism itself by complicating where and how "women" are controlled, (and) how multiple, shifting identities and selves are produced'.

In summary, although it is a difficult undertaking given the diversity of feminisms, Olesen (2011) has suggested that one overarching concern remains relating to feminist knowledges, now that feminisms have moved away from dominant, homogenous, ethnocentric perspectives of woman and women. She suggests that transformative developments in feminisms include postcolonial feminist thought, globalization and transnational feminisms, feminist standpoint theory, and postmodern and poststructural deconstructive feminisms. Also suggested by Olesen (2011) as transformative developments, but not described in this section, is work by and about specific groups of women, including lesbian research, queer theory, disabled women, women of colour, and problematizing unremitting whiteness.

Feminist research methods and processes

Feminist researchers use methods that best reflect the underlying feminist principles they are supporting and thereby they ensure they generate information relevant to their particular key theoretical assumptions. Particular feminist theories and methods combine synergistically (Hesse-Biber and Piatelli, 2012a, 2012b) in selected methodologies, such as feminist ethnography (Pillow and Mayo, 2012), feminist evaluation research (Brisolara and Seigart, 2012), participatory action research (Lykes and Hershberg, 2012), feminist multiple methods research (Cole and Stewart, 2012), and grounded theory (Clarke, 2012).

Exemplifying feminist ethnography

For example, Pillow and Mayo (2012) began their explication of feminist ethnography by raising questions about the methodology in light of feminist critiques of dominant representations of feminist knowledge. They responded to postcolonial critiques of gender and argued that 'until gender ceases to matter, feminism is necessary, and, correspondingly, feminist research, including feminist ethnography, is necessary' (Pillow and Mayo, 2012, p. 187).

The authors applied as a feminist framework for their project the four stages of doing research: choosing, doing, analysing and writing, and endings, and Reinharz's (1992) three characteristics of feminist research, that it is: 1) focused upon analysing and understanding gender within the context of lived experiences; 2) committed to social change, and 3) committed to challenging thinking about researcher subjectivity and the relationship between the researcher and the researched (Pillow and Mayo, 2012, p. 190).

The remainder of their chapter in Hesse-Biber's (2012) edited book sets out carefully and comprehensively, the *what* and *how* of doing feminist ethnography, congruent with the principles of their chosen feminist framework. For example, in the first step *choosing*, Pillow and Mayo (2012) raise many important issues about *what* to research using a feminist ethnographic approach. They argue for research foci relating to 'women's work', for example, women's 'domestic issues; sexuality; pregnancy; birth; child rearing and mothering; learning styles; communication styles', because it is necessary to address 'the lived realities of women's lives' (p. 193). They add that 'while early feminist theory and ethnography focused on reclaiming women's voices and stories, present-day feminist research focuses on making visible the experiences of women and, at the same time, rethinking these experiences through critical analyses of gendered power relations' (Pillow and Mayo, 2012, p. 193).

In the second step, *doing*, Pillow and Mayo (2012) ask what is 'uniquely different' when undertaking feminist ethnography and what it means 'to have a "feminist" relationship with research subjects [*sic*]' (p. 194). (I have indicated *sic* to mean 'as written' after the word subjects in the direct quote, because it surprises me that the authors would use a word connoting a participant being 'subjected to' feminist research.) They acknowledge the importance of feminist research principles, such as reciprocity, representation and voice, but they concede that there is no one best way of facilitating reflexive researcher–participant relationships and processes. Instead, Pillow and Mayo (2012) suggest that researchers remain mindful of questions about 'how to be a nonexploitative researcher, how to produce research that is useful and empowering to women, and how to make research that is linked with political action' (p. 197).

In *analysing and writing* feminist ethnography, Pillow and Mayo (2012) revisit the published discourses that have troubled established feminist views of data collection and analysis, and of writing up the research. For example, deciding on a narrative voice as researcher is a political issue (Richardson, 1997), deciding how to present the text is a political issue of representation (Visweswaran, 1994), and feminist reflexivity is not so much a matter of showing the trustworthiness or validity of a project as it is a process for continually and critically analysing the nature of the research process throughout the life of the project (Pillow, 2003).

To offer some insights into the conundrums of feminist ethnographic analysis and writing up, Pillow and Mayo (2012) suggest the need for 'sustained engagement'. They cite Lather's (2007) concept of 'naked methodology' laid bare to expose its 'limits of representation', for feminist ethnographers to question 'how research-based knowledge remains possible after so much questioning of the very ground of science' (Lather, 2007, p. viii, in Pillow and Mayo, 2012, p. 199).

In *endings*, Pillow and Mayo (2012) provide an array of possible ways of completing a feminist ethnography, including ongoing relationships and ways of negotiating completion, and suggest that there is no set ending process. They suggest that any ending should not overinflate the researcher's importance and they emphasize the aspects 'that remain key are the researcher's own awareness and reflexivity about power relations in the research setting and the researcher's own acknowledgment of her or his own positionalities in the research and research setting' (Pillow and Mayo, 2012, p. 200).

There are many feminist methods and processes from which to choose, so it is not possible to suggest a prescriptive list. From this overview of Pillow and Mayo's (2012) explication of feminist ethnography, it is possible to note some important principles to which they adhered, which may be of help to you as a researcher seeking to use a feminist approach. Pillow and Mayo (2012) identified feminist ethnography as their methodology, and to ascertain how to put the methodology into action faithfully, they provided an epistemological justification for using ethnography as a feminist approach (i.e., gender issues matter), and the research foci for which it would be most useful (e.g., an area of research interest relating to women's work). They then decided on a method for undertaking the research (the four steps of choosing, doing, analysing and writing, and endings), and feminist principles to guide their processes (e.g. three characteristics of feminist research, Reinharz, 1992). With this theoretical framework in place and with constant attention to the application of the principles and processes of reciprocity, voice, representation and reflexivity, they moved through the four steps of undertaking a coherent and congruent feminist ethnography.

Because there is so much diversity in feminisms, there are many ways of doing feminist research. The challenge for researchers taking a feminist approach is to select wisely from the well-debated alternatives, by reading widely and thinking deeply about questions relating to their potential feminist methodological positioning and their specific research aims, objectives, methods and processes.

Food for thought

Let's assume you would like to use a feminist approach in combination with another methodology, e.g. grounded theory, narrative inquiry, action research, etc.

In relation to your specific health profession, brainstorm some choices you can make about the focus of your research, and your aims, objectives, methods and processes.

Given the diversity of feminist thought, and the particular theoretical assumptions of the methodology with which you will combine a feminist approach, what particular feminist framework and methods will you adopt to inform your project? Why?

Critical trends, continuing issues and enduring concerns

Feminist methods and processes are reflected in critical trends, continuing issues and enduring concerns in feminist thought, as identified by Olesen (2011). She suggests that critical trends in feminist scholarship and research relate to endarkening, decolonizing and indigenizing feminist research, which stresses 'the critical nature of subordinated women's (and men's) knowledge as legitimate foundations for attempts to realize social justice' (Olesen, 2011, p. 134). Writers in this area include Dillard (2008) and Battiste (2008).

Intersectionality is another critical trend in feminisms, denoting 'how social divisions are constructed and intermeshed with one another in specific historical conditions to contribute to the oppression of women not in mainstream, white, heterosexual, middle class, able-bodied America' (Olesen, 2011, p. 134). An example of feminist intersectional inquiry in the health sciences is Bredstrom (2006), in relation to HIV/AIDS research.

Olesen (2011) explains that even though feminist thought is dynamic, there are some feminist issues and enduring concerns which influence feminist research methods and processes. Continuing issues include problematizing the researcher and participant relationship, destabilizing insider–outsider perspectives, and troubling traditional concepts of experience, difference and gender. Enduring concerns relate to issues of 'bias' and objectivity, reflexivity, 'validity' and trustworthiness, participants' voices, deconstructing voice, performance ethnography, ethics in feminist research, and participatory action research.

Being aware of the nature of the critical trends, continuing issues and enduring concerns in feminisms will not automatically indicate the actual methods and processes researchers interested in various areas will select and apply for a particular project. However, there is a very high possibility that in every case, much thought will go into making the *what* and *how* decisions in line with feminist principles, and also into ensuring that these well-considered strategies are embodied throughout before, during and after the project.

Methods do not belong to any one epistemological orientation; they are free to roam across all of the qualitative landscapes, to be taken up as needed. So, when does an interview become a feminist interview? DeVault and Gross (2012, p. 207) confirm that this question is important, because researchers 'who claim the label *feminist* for their methodological projects must be prepared to reply to questions about the meaning and distinctiveness of "feminist" methodology and research'. The authors wrote of two main challenges feminist interview researchers face: firstly, responding to the postcolonial critiques of historical feminism by being cognizant not to reproduce the dominant, homogenized views of women, and secondly, heeding globalization and transnational feminist critiques, to ensure that they explore new, open approaches for interview-based research. DeVault and Gross (2012, p. 215) explained that in 'the conduct of any interview research, feminists attempts to maintain a reflexive awareness that research relations are never simple encounters, innocent of identities and lines of power. Rather, they are always embedded in and shaped by cultural constructions of similarity, difference, and significance'.

In summary, feminist researchers not only emphasize *what* is done in terms of methods, but they are also careful in explicating *how* projects are done. Methods are not prescriptive in feminist projects, so projects may include combinations of all kinds of means undertaken with attention to reflecting feminist principles. Potential methods in qualitative feminist projects may be group work, artwork, performance, storytelling, interviews, participant observation, and so on, depending on the research interests and questions and the particular feminist lens through which the project is viewed. The main process considerations are, again, specific to a particular feminist lens, but they may include providing a trusting, transforming and empowering research focus and setting, and in undertaking research *with*, never *on* women, with mutual respect and sharing.

In the postmodern era of the third-wave feminisms, when possibly the only common feminist focus is on the problematic nature of knowledge generation and validation, continuing issues of the researcher–participant relationship, insider–outsider perspectives, and of troubling experience, difference and gender come to the foreground. 'Bias' and objectivity, reflexivity, 'validity' and trustworthiness, participants' voices, deconstructing voice, performance ethnography, ethics in feminist research, and participatory action research have become enduring concerns. All of these continuing issues and enduring concerns are being debated actively in contemporary feminist literature and they require extensive reading to cover the issues comprehensively.

Even though the selection of feminist methods and processes may differ according to researchers' alignment with underlying assumptions about specific feminisms, it is fairly standard practice in feminist research and scholarly discourse that researchers will review the progression of different feminisms and justify their chosen feminist positioning. Feminist researchers are also guided by key feminist principles, which identify their role relationships with participants and ensure that their research is based on reflexive, woman-centred processes. The following section highlights choices researchers have made in planning and undertaking feminist research projects in the health sciences.

Feminist research projects in the health sciences

Human health issues, as they relate to women, are being discussed, critiqued and researched using feminist lenses in the health and human sciences. For example, fat is still a feminist issue and the debates are re-emerging with renewed vigour in medical sociology and psychiatry (e.g., Chrisler, 2011; Fikkan and Rothblum, 2012; McHugh and Kasardo, 2011; Saguy, 2011). Women's reproductive issues also continue to be feminist issues, including technologies (Gaard, 2010) and gender and childbearing experiences (Carter, 2009). Research in nursing and midwifery apply feminist lenses to women's health and illness experiences and issues (Aranda and Jones, 2010; Glass and Rose, 2008; Goldberg, Ryan and Sawchyn, 2009; Im, 2010; Pannowitz, Glass and Davis, 2009; Ponic, Reid and Frisby, 2010; Scott-Dixon, 2009). Feminist researchers are also active in social work (Abrams and Curran, 2007; Gringeri, Wahab and Anderson-Nathe, 2010), health sociology (Grant and Luxford, 2011; Kuhlmann, 2009; Moore, 2010), psychology (Austin, Rutherford and Pyke, 2006; Fish, 2009; McMullen and Stoppard, 2006), and in issues relating to health disparities (Rogers and Kelly, 2011) and mental health (Muzak, 2009; Kakoti, 2012).

Various researchers in the health sciences have investigated the extent to which feminisms have been used as research approaches in their respective disciplines (Abrams and Curran, 2007; Austin et al., 2006; Gringeri et al., 2010; Im, 2010). For example, Gringeri et al. (2010) were interested in their discovery in the literature, that even though social work was established and has been maintained mainly by women, who have been active in women's issues for 'several generations of feminists', social work 'is curiously and strikingly absent from broader multidisciplinary discussions of feminist research' (p. 390). In the introductory section of the article, Gringeri et al. (2010) overview the feminist research landscape and the third-wave feminisms' progression of thought in relation to power, authority, ethics, reflexivity, praxis, and difference.

Before going into details of how they undertook the literature review, Gringeri et al. (2010) acknowledged their philosophical assumptions as authors, as statements of belief.

> We believe in the existence of feminisms. We also believe quite strongly that feminism is not, nor should it be, solely focused on, for, and/or about female bodies, in part, because what constitutes a female body is not definitive or expansive enough also to address femininities ... we believe that gender is better understood in terms of how it is performed, rather than by ascribing essentialized characteristics on the basis of body sex alone. This is where we diverge from many others who have previously engaged the question of what is feminist research or science. Because we strongly identify with critical and postmodern feminisms that challenge binaries, including the gender binary, we believe that to gain a better understanding of how constructions of gender inform the lived experiences of women, men, and transgendered people, we must also include explorations of the lives of men and transgendered people. (p. 397)

In the method section of the article, the authors describe not only what they did to undertake the literature review, but also how they went about it as a process. The three researchers (two women, one man) worked together by asking if 'such as thing as feminist research exists', then acknowledged 'struggling' with how to answer the question. They described 'peeling back the layers of the onion' and how 'the research process unfolded in a dynamic and iterative way' (p. 396).

They used the Web of Science, a database of 12,000 high impact journals worldwide, to generate a sample of feminist social work studies, and identified high-impact journals social workers read, even if they were not social work journals per se. They also included the journals *Critical Social Work* and *Qualitative Social Work* as sources of published feminist social work research, and searched the broader social science literature, using the keywords feminism and feminist and social work. From the Web of Science journals, the researchers collected citations for all research-based articles containing the keywords feminist or feminism covering the period 2000–2008.

At the conclusion of the detailed search process, the authors examined 50 randomly selected research-based articles 'that claimed feminism within their work' (p. 390). They 'developed a review template to organize and analyze salient data from each article in the sample', which included: 'the article's purpose, treatment of the gender binary, indication of the study's underlying theoretical frame, research methods, data collection strategies, and the degree to which the article incorporated the issues in feminist research identified by Olesen: complexities, approaches to research, and enduring issues in research' (p. 398). The researchers kept in their minds the following questions: What makes the article feminist? How does the article treat binary (essentialized) thinking, particularly in relation to gender? To what degree is the article clearly grounded in theory? (p. 390). They revised the template through several drafts, based on their conversations and insights.

Gringeri et al. (2010) concluded that they

> found a great diversity of topics among the 50 articles in the sample; although 22% dealt with domestic violence in one form or another, the remaining topics represented a broad range, focusing on women of different ages, cultures, racial and class backgrounds, sexual orientations, and geographic locations in relation to issues of health, work, and migration, among others. The articles also dealt with topics such as feminist issues in research and the nexus between a researcher's race or culture and those of the participants. It was surprising that (they) found little diversity in the methods that were used across the sample of articles, suggesting, perhaps, that feminist scholars in social work and related social science disciplines associate qualitative methods with feminist research: only 2 articles were based on quantitative methods, 5 were based on mixed methods, and 43 were based on qualitative methods.

This project is a literature review, therefore, it did not require contact with research participants and an ethics approval process, nevertheless, the research fits the criteria of feminist research, as discussed in this chapter. The hallmarks of Gringeri et al.'s (2010) project that make this research *feminist* are that it: had a focus on feminist research about women's issues; identified and used a feminist framework to organize its research activities; involved a negotiated, iterative process between the research team members; reviewed key contemporary feminist concepts; provided a disclosure of the researchers' feminist positioning; emphasized details about methods and processes equally; reported the findings in light of feminist understandings; and provided a discussion of the implications of the feminist methodology it used. The relatively unusual feature of this project was that it was a feminist project with a male co-researcher, who declared his assumptions equally with the two women co-researchers in this project.

Food for thought
What is your view on Gringeri et al.'s (2010, p. 397) position, that:

> feminism is not, nor should it be, solely focused on, for, and/or about female bodies, in part, because what constitutes a female body is not definitive or expansive enough also to address femininities … (and that) that gender is better understood in terms of how it is performed, rather than by ascribing essentialized characteristics on the basis of body sex alone … (Also) to gain a better understanding of how constructions of gender inform the lived experiences of women, men, and transgendered people, we must also include explorations of the lives of men and transgendered people.

Chapter summary

This chapter focused on feminisms as potential methodologies for qualitative researchers. Precise definitions of feminisms are difficult to locate in recent published sources, because feminisms have gone well beyond the traditional ideas of the first and second waves of feminism. Present-era feminisms include feminist empiricism, feminist standpoints, postmodern and poststructural feminisms, postcolonial feminisms, globalization and transnational feminisms, endarkening, decolonizing and indigenizing feminisms, and intersectionality.

First-wave feminism was characterized by important historical events, which raised awareness of women's issues related to their fundamental rights as citizens, including the right to vote, be educated, have a voice in reproductive issues, and become actively political in all areas of social life. The second-wave feminists differentiated the women's movement into liberal, Marxist, radical and lesbian feminisms. The third wave of poststructural and postmodern feminisms opposed representations of the 'essential' white, middle-class woman and destabilized notions of 'truth' in contemporary feminist research approaches.

Although it is difficult to articulate key concepts in feminisms, an overarching concern relating to feminist knowledges can be identified. Transformative developments in feminisms include postcolonial feminist thought, globalization and transnational feminisms, feminist standpoint theory, and postmodern and poststructural deconstructive feminisms. Also, work by and about specific groups of women, including lesbian research, queer theory, disabled women, women of colour, and problematizing unremitting whiteness.

Because there is so much diversity in feminisms, there are many ways of doing feminist research. Researchers taking a feminist approach select from well-debated alternatives, by reading and thinking about questions relating their potential feminist methodological positioning and their specific research aims, objectives, methods and processes. Methods are selected for undertaking the feminist research and feminist principles are identified to guide the processes. There are many feminist methods and processes from which to choose, but some important principles for selecting them are: recognizing the existence of multiple contemporary feminisms; identifying a feminist methodology for a project, providing an epistemological justification for using a particular feminist approach (i.e., gender issues matter), and the research foci for which it would be most useful (e.g., an area of research interest relating to women's work), before putting the methodology into action faithfully.

The final section of the chapter identified examples of human health issues, which have been discussed, critiqued and researched using feminist lenses in the health and human sciences. Fat is still a feminist issue in disciplines such as medical sociology and psychiatry, and women's reproductive issues, including technologies and gender and childbearing experiences are being researched using feminist methods and processes. Research in nursing and midwifery apply feminist lenses to women's health and illness experiences and issues and feminist researchers are also active in social work, health sociology, psychology, and in issues relating to health disparities and mental health.

A literature review of feminisms in social work was discussed as an example of a feminist approach. Given that feminisms are diverse and continuing to evolve epistemologically, if you are considering using a feminist research approach, you will need to read widely and deeply, to make yourself thoroughly conversant with the philosophies and their applications to research.

Key points

- The word feminisms is written intentionally as plural, to denote the multiplicity of feminist approaches to thinking about and researching women's struggles and issues.

- Originally, feminists cited waves, such as the first wave of feminism, which refers to events at the end of the 19th century into the beginning of the 20th century, when suffragettes in New Zealand, Australia and the UK engaged in political action to secure for women the right to vote.

- The first wave of feminisms refers also to the time before, during and after both World Wars, consequently, women's issues during the first wave of feminisms included not only their rights to vote, but also ongoing issues related to women's equal status in society, including their rights for equal recognition and benefits in the workforce, their rights to be educated, and a voice in the determination of their reproductive issues, such as contraception and abortion.

- Second-wave feminism refers to a period of liberal, Marxist, radical and lesbian feminist activity beginning in the early 1960s to the late 1980s, which focused on cultural and political inequalities and identified how women's personal lives were deeply politicized within patriarchal power structures.

- The third wave of contemporary feminism, from the 1980s onwards, includes deconstructive poststructural and postmodern feminisms, reacting to the second wave thinkers' representations of the 'essential' white, middle-class woman.

- Feminist poststructuralist thinkers assert that the division of feminisms into categories is problematic, because the categories were arbitrary and socially produced, and they fail to address issues of power in language, subjectivity, social processes and institutions (Hekman, 1990; Lather, 1991).

- Transformative feminist developments include postcolonial feminist thought (e.g., Kim, 2007); globalization and transnational feminism (e.g., Parrenas, 2008); standpoint theory (e.g., Harding, 2008); and postmodern and poststructural deconstructive theory (e.g., St. Pierre, 2009).

- The focus now is less on the waves of feminisms (already broken on the shore of feminist history), to a view over the ocean itself, where the breadth and depth of feminisms seems to match more closely the metaphor of waves being whipped up continually by contextual agents and forces within a particular seascape of national, transnational and intersectional possibilities.

- Feminist researchers use methods that best reflect the underlying feminist principles they are supporting and thereby they ensure they generate information relevant to their particular key theoretical assumptions.

- Because there is so much diversity in feminisms, there are many ways of doing feminist research, so the challenge for researchers taking a feminist approach is to select wisely from the well-debated alternatives, by reading widely and thinking deeply about questions relating their potential feminist methodological positioning and their specific research aims, objectives, methods and processes.

- Feminist researchers not only emphasize *what* is done in terms of methods, but they are also careful in explicating *how* projects are done.

- The main process considerations are specific to a particular feminist lens, but they may include providing a trusting, transforming and empowering research focus and setting, and in undertaking research *with*, never *on* women, with mutual respect and sharing.

Critical review questions

1 In what ways is it possible for feminist research to inform healthcare practice?

2 To what extent can feminist research offer insights into your clients' experiences of health and illness?

References

Abrams, L.S., & Curran, L. (2007). Not just a middle-class affliction: crafting a social work research agenda on postpartum depression. *Health and Social Work, 32*(4), 289.

Aranda, K., & Jones, A. (2010). Dignity in health-care: A critical exploration using feminism and theories of recognition. *Nursing Inquiry, 17*(3), 248–256.

Austin, S., Rutherford, A., & Pyke, S. (2006). In our own voice: The impact of feminism on Canadian psychology. *Feminism & Psychology, 16*(3), 243–257.

Battiste, M. (2008). Research ethics for protecting indigenous knowledge and heritage. In N.K. Denzin, Y.S. Lincoln, & L.T. Smith, (Eds.). *Handbook of critical and indigenous methodologies.* Thousand Oaks: Sage, 497–510.

Bhavani, K.-K., & Talcott, M. (2012). Interconnections and configurations: Toward a global feminist ethnography. In S.N. Hesse-Biber *The handbook of feminist research: theory and praxis* 2nd edn. Thousand Oaks: Sage, 135–153.

Bredstrom, A. (2006). Intersectionality: A challenge for feminist HIV/AIDS research? *European Journal of Women's Studies, 13*, 229–243.

Brisolara, S., & Seigart, D. (2012). Feminist evaluation research. In S.N. Hesse-Biber *The handbook of feminist research: Theory and praxis* 2nd edn. Thousand Oaks: Sage, 290–312.

Carter, S.K. (2009). Gender and childbearing experiences: Revisiting O'Brien's dialectics of reproduction. *NWSA Journal. 21*(2), 21.

Chrisler, J.C. (2011). 'Why can't you control yourself?' Fat *should be* a feminist issue. *Sex Roles, 66*(9–10), 608–616.

Clarke, A.E. (2012). Feminism, grounded theory, and situational analysis revisited. In S.N. Hesse-Biber *The handbook of feminist research: Theory and praxis* 2nd edn. Thousand Oaks: Sage, 388–412.

Cole, E.R., & Stewart, A.J. (2012). Narratives and numbers: Feminist multiple methods research. In S.N. Hesse-Biber *The handbook of feminist research: Theory and praxis* 2nd edn. Thousand Oaks: Sage, 368–387.

Cott, N.F. (1987). *The grounding of modern feminism.* New Haven, CN: Yale University Press.

DeVault, M.L., & Gross, G. (2012). Feminist qualitative interviewing. In S.N. Hesse-Biber *Handbook of feminist research: Theory and praxis.* 2nd edn. Thousand Oaks: Sage, 206–236.

Dillard, C.B. (2008). When the ground is black, the ground is fertile. In N.K. Denzin, Y.S. Lincoln, & L.T. Smith, (Eds.). *Handbook of critical and indigenous methodologies.* Thousand Oaks: Sage, 277–292.

Ebert, T. (1996). *Ludic feminism and after: Postmodernism, desire and labor in late capitalism.* Ann Arbor: University of Michigan Press.

Fikkan, J.L., & Rothblum, E.D. (2012). Is fat a feminist issue? Exploring the gendered nature of weight bias. *Sex Roles, 66*, 575–592.

Fish, J. (2009). Our health, our say: towards a feminist perspective of lesbian health. *Feminism & Psychology, 19*(4), 437–453.

Gaard, G. (2010). Reproductive technology, or reproductive justice? An ecofeminist, environmental justice perspective on the rhetoric of choice. *Ethics & the Environment, 15*, 103.

Gannon, S., & Davies, B. (2012). Postmodern, post-structural, and critical theories. In S.N. Hesse-Biber *The handbook of feminist research: Theory and praxis* 2nd edn. Thousand Oaks: Sage, 65–91.

Glass, N., & Rose, J. (2008). The importance of emancipatory research to contemporary nursing practice, *Contemporary Nurse, 29*(1), 8.

Goldberg, L., Ryan, A., & Sawchyn, J. (2009) Feminist and queer phenomenology: a framework for perinatal nursing practice, research, and education for advancing lesbian health. *Health Care Women International* 30(6): 536–549.

Grant, J., & Luxford, Y. (2011). 'Culture it's a big term isn't it'? An analysis of child and family health nurses' understandings of culture and intercultural communication. *Health Sociology Review, 20*(1), 16.

Gringeri, C.E., Wahab, S., & Anderson-Nathe, B. (2010). What makes it feminist?: Mapping the landscape of feminist social work research. *Affilia: Journal of Women and Social Work, 25*(4), 390–405.

Harding, S. (2008). *Sciences from below: Feminisms, postcolonialities, and modernities.* Durham, NC: Duke University Press.

Harding, S. (2012). Feminist standpoints. In S.N. Hesse-Biber *The handbook of feminist research: Theory and praxis* 2nd edn. Thousand Oaks: Sage, 46–64.

Hekman, S. (1990). *Gender and knowledge: Elements of a post-modern feminism.* Boston: Northeastern University Press.

Hesse-Biber, S.N. (2012). *Handbook of feminist research: Theory and praxis.* 2nd edn. Thousand Oaks: Sage.

Hesse-Biber, S.N., & Piatelli, D. (2012a). The synergistic practice of theory and method. In S.N. Hesse-Biber *The handbook of feminist research: Theory and praxis* 2nd edn. Thousand Oaks: Sage, 176–186.

Hesse-Biber, S.N., & Piatelli, D. (2012b). The feminist practice of holistic reflexivity. In S.N. Hesse-Biber *The handbook of feminist research: Theory and praxis* 2nd edn. Thousand Oaks: Sage, 557–582.

Hundley, C.E. (2012). Feminist empiricism. In S.N. Hesse-Biber *The handbook of feminist research: Theory and praxis* 2nd edn. Thousand Oaks: Sage, 28–45.

Im, E.-O. (2010). Current trends in feminist nursing research. *Nursing Outlook, 58,* 87–96.

Kakoti, S.A. (2012). Arab American women, mental health, and feminism. *Affilia: Journal of Women and Social Work, 27*(1), 60–70.

Kemp, S. & Brandwein, R. (2010). Feminisms and social work in the United States: An intertwined history. *Affilia: Journal of Women and Social Work, 25*(4), 341–364.

Kim, H.S. (2007). The politics of border crossings: Black, postcolonial, and transnational feminist perspectives. In S.N. Hesse-Biber. *Handbook of feminist research: Theory and praxis.* Thousand Oaks, Sage, 107–122.

Kuhlmann, E. (2009). From women's health to gender mainstreaming and back again: Linking feminist agendas and new governance in healthcare. *Current Sociology, 57*(2), 135–154.

Lather, P. (1991). *Getting smart: Feminist research and pedagogy within the postmodern.* New York: Routledge.

Lather, P. (2007). *Getting lost: Feminist efforts towards a double(d) science.* Albany: State University of New York Press.

Lykes, M.B., & Hershberg, R.M. (2012). Participatory action research and feminisms: Social inequalities and transformative praxis. In S.N. Hesse-Biber *The handbook of feminist research: Theory and praxis* 2nd edn. Thousand Oaks: Sage, 331–367.

McHugh, M.C., & Kasardo, A.E. (2011). Anti-fat prejudice: The role of psychology in explication, education and eradication. *Sex Roles, 66*(9–10), 617–627.

McMullen, L.M., & Stoppard, J.M. (2006). Women and depression: A case study of the influence of feminism in Canadian psychology. *Feminism & Psychology, 16*(3), 273–288.

Moore, S.E.H. (2010) Is the healthy body gendered? Toward a feminist critique of the new paradigm of health. *Body Society* 16(2): 95–118.

Muzak, J. (2009). Trauma, feminism, and addiction: cultural and clinical lessons from Susan Gordon Lydon's take the long way home: Memoirs of a survivor. *Traumatology, 15*(4), 24–34.

New Zealand History online (2012). New Zealand Women and the vote: Suffrage and beyond 'brief history – women and the vote', URL: http://www.nzhistory.net.nz/politics/womens-suffrage/brief-history, (Ministry for Culture and Heritage), updated 16 January 2012.

Olesen, V. (2011). Feminist qualitative research in the millennium's first decade: Developments, challenges, prospects. In N.K. Denzin, Y.S. Lincoln, & L.T. Smith, (Eds.) *The SAGE handbook of qualitative research*, 4th edn. Thousand Oaks: Sage, 129–146.

Pannowitz, H.K., Glass, N., & Davis, K. (2009). Resisting gender-bias: Insights from Western Australian middle-level women nurses. *Contemporary Nurse, 33*(2), 103–109.

Parrenas, R.S. (2008). *The force of domesticity: Filipina migrants and globalization*. New York: New York University Press.

Pillow, W.S. (2003). Confession, catharsis or cure: The use of reflexivity as methodological power in qualitative research. *International Journal of Qualitative Studies in Education, 16*(2), 175–196.

Pillow, W.S., & Mayo, C. (2012). Feminist ethnography: Histories, challenges and possibilities. In S.N. Hesse-Biber *The handbook of feminist research: Theory and praxis* 2nd edn. Thousand Oaks: Sage, 187–205.

Pisan, C. (1982 trans.). *The book of the city of ladies*, New York: Persea Books.

Ponic, P., Reid, C., & Frisby, W. (2010). Cultivating the power of partnerships in feminist participatory action research in women's health. *Nursing Inquiry, 17*, 324–335.

Reinharz, S. (1992). *Feminist methods in social research*. New York: Oxford University Press.

Richardson, L. (1997). *Fields of play (constructing an academic life)*. New Brunswick, NJ: Rutgers University Press.

Rogers, J., & Kelly, U.A. (2011). Feminist intersectionality: Bringing social justice to health disparities research. *Nursing Ethics, 18*(3), 397–407.

Saguy, A. (2011). Why fat is a feminist issue. *Sex Roles, 66*(9–10), 600–607.

Scott-Dixon, K. (2009). Public health, private parts: a feminist public-health approach to trans issues. *Hypatia, 24*(3), 33–55.

St. Pierre, E.A. (2009). Afterword: Decentering voice in qualitative inquiry. In Y. Jackson & L.A. Mazzei (Eds.) *Voice in qualitative inquiry: Challenging conventional, interpretive, and critical concepts in qualitative research*. New York: Routledge, 221–236.

Thornton Dill, B., & Kohlman, M.H. (2012). Intersectionality: A transformative paradigm in feminist theory and social justice. In S.N. Hesse-Biber *The handbook of feminist research: Theory and praxis* 2nd edn. Thousand Oaks: Sage, 154–174.

Trinh, T.M.. (1992). *Framer framed*. New York: Routledge.

Visweswaran, K. (1994). *Fictions of feminist ethnography*. Minneapolis: University of Minnesota Press.

West, R, (1913) Mr Chesterton in hysterics. A study in prejudice. *Clarion* 14 November 1913, p.5.

Woolf, V. (1938, 1993). *Three guineas*. Harmondsworth: Penguin.

Woolf, V. (1989). *A room of one's own*. New York: Harcourt Brace.

Wollstonecraft, M.A. (1792). *Vindication of the rights of woman: An authoritative text backgrounds criticism*. C.H. Poston (Ed.) (1975). New York: Norton.

9

Action research

Karen Francis

Chapter overview

Action research is a popular methodology adopted by health and educational researchers interested in practice innovation. In this chapter action research will be defined and the theoretical assumptions that underpin this approach delineated. The origins of the methodology will be described, followed by an overview of the process of conceptualizing and undertaking a study using this approach.

Definition

Action research consists of a family of research methodologies that have an action intent, that is the research undertaken seeks to answer a question that results in affirmative action (Cassell and Johnson, 2006; Koshy, Koshy, and Waterman, 2011; McMurray, Pace, and Scott, 2004). These approaches are informed by critical social theory advanced by Habermas who argued that people are oppressed if they do not understand the systems of domination and their associated dependence that are artefacts of western society. Habermas contended that if individuals were aware of these structures they would be positioned with the knowledge to challenge oppression and/or act or be emancipated to change the status quo (Kemmis and McTaggart, 2008; McCarthy, 1989).

As a research methodology, action research is the catalyst for researchers to collaborate and ask questions arising from their social worlds that require resolution (Fay, 1975). Action research is a collaborative and systematic endeavour inspired by concern and interest to facilitate change that is mutually acceptable to those involved in the project (Kemmis and McTaggart, 2008). Kemmis and McTaggart, educational action researchers, conclude that action research is 'a form of collective self-reflective enquiry undertaken by participants in social situations in order to improve the rationality and justice of their own social or educational practices' (Kemmis and McTaggart, 1988). Koshy et al. (2011) offer that 'action research creates knowledge based on enquiries conducted within specific and often practical situations' (p. 4).

Theoretical assumptions of action research

Theoretical assumptions are the beliefs that underpin the methodology. For action research these include:

- An intent for action that leads to change
- Social process
- Participatory
- Practical
- Critical
- Context specific
- Reflexive.

Action research is a social process that leads to change through a collaborative and transformative set of actions. The research is a reflexive process that occurs in a specific context and has a practical application (Kemmis and McTaggart, 2008).

Origins of action research

Kurt Lewin (1890–1947) pioneered action research methodology (Cassell and Johnson, 2006). He was a Prussian psychologist who emigrated to the USA in 1933 to escape Nazi persecution. As a psychologist he was interested in human behaviour. Lewin gained notoriety for the research he undertook that was focused on social issues (Koshy et al., 2011). He coined the term 'action research' to describe a process of inquiry for understanding social management or social engineering (Kemmis and McTaggart, 2008). Investment in engagement with action research leads to social action that is acceptable and/or rewarding for those involved (Corbett, Francis, and Chapman, 2007). Lewin proffered that action research provides a way of generating knowledge about a social system while providing a method for changing it (Infed, 2012). Patton explains that action research 'aims at solving specific problems within a program, organization or community' (2002). He went on to cite Whyte who explained that:

> Action research explicitly and purposely becomes part of the change process by engaging the people in the program or organization in studying their own problems in order to solve those problems.
>
> (Patton, 2002)

The action research approach adopted by Lewin was followed by Corey and others in the USA to investigate questions of concern related to education (Koshy et al., 2011).

Action research has been used widely in education and health research including nursing since the 1980s. This methodology does not treat those who are the focus of the research as passive subjects of the research, but seeks to empower them to act on their own behalf as active participants in change (Kemmis and McTaggart, 2008). Kemmis and McTaggart (2008) proffer that action research should be considered a social process and as such, power relationships are of importance and need to be managed at the commencement of the project. Resolving unequal relationships can be achieved if participants are considered and valued as co-researchers and their contributions acknowledged and celebrated by all members of the team. In recent years the term 'appreciate inquiry' has been used to describe an approach to action research that has been adopted by organizations interested in capitalizing on what is done well rather than what is bad (Cassell and Johnson, 2006). This approach is underpinned by a belief that the solutions sought already exist. Adopting an affirmative action process firstly confirms the strengths of organization and through this process empowers them, the group, to consider what could be, and what will be (Hall and Hammond, 2012).

Action research methods

Action research is a cyclical process that is participatory, collaborative and reflexive in nature. Action research studies are often developed from a need to explain a concern that is shared by a group and begins with a concrete problem being posed (Mills and FitzGerald, 2008a). The initial identification of the concern may be by a third party such as a researcher or by senior administrators (Cassell and Johnson, 2006). The group which is formed from those willing to be involved, may include external researchers who are willing to be involved and to meet with the group to consider the issues, clarify and prioritize these (Kemmis and McTaggart 2008). Kemmis and McTaggart (2008) caution that the role of facilitator must be in keeping with the methodology, that is, the facilitator is not just concerned with the technical skills of project management but has a vested interest in the group and that their motivation aligns with that of the research group. The facilitator and the group decide on a process for investigating the issues and formulate an action plan that is cyclical in nature (Koshy et al., 2011) but, as highlighted by Kemmis and McTaggart (2008), is flexible. The action plan involves a series of activities:

> problem identification, diagnosis, planning, intervention and evaluation of the results of action in order to learn and to plan subsequent intervention that are repeated until the desired outcomes are reached.
> (Cassell and Johnson, 2006, p. 814)

A review of achievements for each action set is undertaken at the conclusion of each cycle of activity and forward planning for the next series of actions occurs until the group is satisfied that the goals initially agreed on, are met. A study undertaken by Mills and FitzGerald (2008a), looking at the changing role of practice nurses, originally sought to report on the techniques used to develop a new model of service delivery. The project intent changed however when it was identified by the nurse participants that they were encountering obstacles in changing their scope of practice to accommodate their new knowledge and skills (Mills and FitzGerald, 2008b). The focus of the study became an empowering process that led to the participants developing methods to overcome the barriers that were limiting the implementation of the new model of care.

Koshy et al. (2011) suggest that the aim of action research is to learn through action that results in professional and/or personal growth. Action research is participatory and the process of doing the research evolves through a self-reflective spiral of activity (see Figure 9.1).

Participating in an action research study facilitates individual and group reflection. Taylor et al. (2008) found in an action research study they facilitated with palliative care nurses that the reflective aspects of the approach supported the nurses to review their practice to isolate opportunities for practice modification that would better meet the needs of their patients. Projects adopting an action research methodology within healthcare settings provide

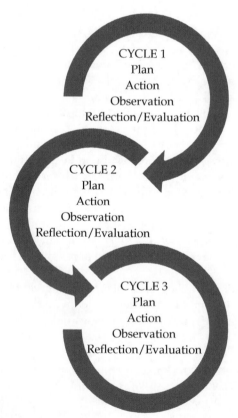

Figure 9.1 Action research cycle

an opportunity for critical review of practices, processes and systems as they impact on service delivery and ultimately patient outcomes. Indeed, Dick (2004) emphasized that action research is by its very nature about systems and system change. He submitted that the process facilitates openness to change and proactivity (Dick, 2004).

Action research is a politically motivated research methodology. The intent is always action, which can lead to theorizing and the development of innovative practice (Kemmis and McTaggart, 1988).

The action research cycle

Action research typically uses a cyclical model of action to achieve the agreed aims of the project (see Figure 9.1). Each cycle or action set involves four basic steps: planning, action, observation and reflection. Each step scaffolds the next and each cycle articulates with the next until the project is completed.

- *Planning*: A plan is developed that will inform action to improve an action (practice) that is already happening. It should be forward looking. It recognizes that to some degree all social action is unpredictable and therefore risky. The plan needs to be flexible to be able to adapt to unforeseen effects or constraints. The plan should empower participants to act more appropriately and more effectively.

- *Action*: This is deliberate and controlled. It is a careful and thoughtful variation on existing practice. It is critically informed. It uses action as a platform for future development and later action. Action is flexible and open to change in the light of changing circumstances. An essential difference that sets action research apart is that actions are observed.

- *Observation*: In action research this process is planned, it looks forward, providing the basis for reflection. Observation is responsive, open-minded and open-eyed (Kemmis and McTaggart, 1988). Researchers observe the action process; the effects of the action, both intended and unintended; the circumstances of, and the constraints on action; how circumstances and constraints change planned action; and any other issues that may arise.

- *Reflection/Evaluation*: This phase of the cycle involves reviewing the process and making sense of the decisions made and outcomes achieved, the problems encountered and the implications for the project considered. Group discussions provide the basis for revising the research plan and identifying the way forward, the next cycle of activity (Koshy et al., 2011).

Action research is a dynamic process that is integrative rather than a rigid model for directing a research process (Kemmis and McTaggart, 1988). As pointed out by Mills and FitzGerald (2008a), the research begins with the isolation of a tangible problem in context (place and space) that requires investigation either by an individual, a group, or an organization.

157

A group of people interested in solving the problem, and someone designated to facilitate and manage the process, constitute the action group. The research facilitator or facilitators (if more than one) may be the person/s who initially identified the problem such as a researcher or a team member of a workplace or community group nominated to take on this role (Kemmis and McTaggart, 2008; Streubert, 2011). If the facilitator is external to the group then it is important that they acknowledge their motivations for being involved, and their underlying beliefs particularly as they relate to the research (etic perspectives). The etic beliefs held by the facilitator and any other external members of the group may be different to that of the groups (emic perspective). These differences if voiced can add depth to the project provided there is collective understanding of the value of each perspective (Streubert, 2011). The integrity of the research is reliant on the group's collective thinking and the collaborative negotiation processes that feature throughout the life of the project.

Data analysis

The analysis of data in action research projects occurs throughout the lifetime of the study. Data generated in each cycle of activity are analysed and reflected on. This process then informs the next cycle of activity. Determining the type of data required is informed by the research question/s that the group believes require answering. A number of action researchers have used mixed methods such as survey data when large amounts of information from an organization are needed, focus and individual groups to elicit information from a user, employee and consumer perspectives on a targeted issue. For some researchers the data are generated from the action group through focus group meetings and reflections. In some ways action research data generation is eclectic as process is driven by need. The following examples are included as the projects have adopted a diversity of data generation and analysis approaches that have met the research groups' needs.

Mahone et al. (2011) reported that they utilized group processes to discuss implementing a shared decision making (SDM) model in an intervention to improve therapeutic medication use among people with a serious mental illness. An action group was formed which met monthly to discuss options for achieving this objective. The discussion was recorded and transcribed using a content analysis approach (Mahone et al., 2011). Each individual transcript was reviewed and themes identified that captured the ideas generated. All transcripts (each meeting) were subsequently compared and themes categorized and ranked according to the most frequent responses. This information was shared with the group who used the information to inform service delivery (Mahone et al., 2011).

A study undertaken to identify the usefulness of participatory action research methodology to empower youth to contribute to health service delivery utilized a survey as a means of data generation (Dold and Chapman, 2012). The survey data included demographic information (age, gender, role) and qualitative responses to a set of five questions. Responses to each question were analysed using a thematic approach.

A systematic review to identify best practice featured as one of several data generation techniques adopted in an action research study to develop an intervention for bereaved fathers (Aho, Astedt-Kurki, Tarkka, and Kaunonen, 2011). The systematic review utilized predetermined selection criteria to select studies that informed the development of the intervention for the identified group (Aho et al., 2011).

Concluding the study

All research projects, including action research projects, are time limited. Timeframes are generally developed at the commencement of all research studies, although recognizing and managing for contingencies is an important part of the planning process. Action researchers engage in a dynamic collaborative problem solving process that leads to negotiated change. The intent of action research is to support and emancipate through active involvement in the process.

Case study

Twenty-four nurses employed at a rurally located small general hospital work on a 32-bed medical/surgical ward. The majority of patients admitted to the ward are elderly, aged from 65 to 92 years, with varying levels of mobility. Preventing falls is an advocated risk management strategy by the hospital. In the past month, the ward has reported nine separate incidences of patients falling. The Nurse Unit Manager is concerned and decides that something must be done to address this problem. She wants to report to senior management that an intervention is being implemented that will reduce falls risk by 50 per cent in the next 12-month period, by 75 per cent in 24 months and 99 per cent in 36 months. You are appointed to lead the groups by the Nurse Unit Manager.

Limitations

Action research has been criticized because it is context specific, problem focused and often involves small numbers of people. The 'grass roots' nature of this approach impacts on the generalizability of findings.

Conclusion

In this chapter action research has been described. The theoretical assumptions underpinning the approach have been explained and the process of doing research using this process depicted. Limitations have been highlighted and a case example provided to guide conceptualization of an action research study.

Karen Francis

Key points

- Action research consists of a family of research methodologies that have an action intent, that is, the research undertaken seeks to answer a question that results in affirmative action.

- As a research methodology, action research is the catalyst for researchers to collaborate and ask questions arising from their social worlds that require resolution.

- Action research seeks to empower participants to act on their own behalf as active participants in change.

- The action plan involves a series of activities: problem identification, diagnosis, planning, intervention and evaluation of the results of action, in order to learn and to plan subsequent intervention that are repeated until the desired outcomes are reached.

- A review of achievements for each action set is undertaken at the conclusion of each cycle of activity and forward planning for the next series of actions occurs until the group is satisfied that the goals initially agreed on, are met.

- Each cycle or action set involves four basic steps: planning, action, observation and reflection. Each step scaffolds the next and each cycle articulates with the next until the project is completed.

Critical review questions

1 Develop a plan for establishing a research group to address this clinical problem.

2 What strategies would you adopt to ensure that the group remains focused, develops an appropriate plan and implements an agreed intervention?

3 Identify measures that the group will need to consider to measure outcomes arising from the interventions implemented.

References

Aho, A.L., Astedt-Kurki, P., Tarkka, M., & Kaunonen, M. (2011). Development and implementation of a bereavement follow-up intervention for grieving fathers: an action research. *Journal of Clinical Nursing, 20*, 408–419.
Cassell, C., & Johnson, P. (2006). Action research: Explaining the diversity. [Discussion paper]. *Human Relations, 59*(6), 783–814.
Corbett, A.M., Francis, K., & Chapman, Y. (2007). Feminist-informed participatory action research: A methodology of choice for examining critical nursing issues. *International Journal of Nursing Practice, 13*(2), 81–88.
Dick, B. (2004). Action research, themes and trends. *Action Research, 2*(4), 425–444.

Dold, C.J., & Chapman, R.A. (2012). Hearing a voice: Results of a participatory action research study. *Journal of Child and Family Studies, 21*, 512–519. doi: 10.1007/s10826-011-9505-9.

Fay, B. (1975). *Social theory and political practice*. London: Allen & Unwin.

Hall, J., & Hammond, S. (2012). What is appreciative inquiry? Retrieved 19 November 2012 from http://www.thinbook.com/docs/doc-whatisai.pdf

Infed. (2012). Kurt Lewin: Groups, experiential learning and action research. Retrieved 1 May 2012 from http://www.infed.org/thinkers/et-lewin.htm.

Kemmis, S., & McTaggart, R. (1988). *The action research planner*. Geelong: Deakin University Press.

Kemmis, S., & McTaggart, R. (2008). Participatory action research, communicative action and the public sphere. In N.K. Denzin & Y.S. Lincoln (Eds.), *Strategies of qualitative inquiry*. (3rd edn, pp. 271–330). Los Angeles: Sage.

Koshy, E., Koshy, V., & Waterman, H. (2011). *Action research in healthcare*. London: Sage.

Mahone, I.H., Farrell, S.P., Hinton, I., Johnson, R., Moody, D., Rifkin, K., & Barker, M. (2011). Participatory action research in public mental health and a School of Nursing: Qualitative findings from an academic community partnership. *Journal of Participatory Medicine, 3.*

McCarthy, T. (1989). *The critical theory of Jurgen Habermas*. Cambridge, UK: Polity Press.

McMurray, A.J., Pace, R.W., & Scott, D. (2004). *Research: A common sense approach*. Southbank, Victoria: Thomson.

Mills, J., & FitzGerald, M. (2008a). The changing role of practice nurses in Australia: An action research study. *Australian Journal of Advanced Nursing, 26*(1), 16–20.

Mills, J. and Fitzgerald, M. (2008b). Renegotiating roles as part of developing collaborative practice: Australian nurses in general practice and cervical screening. *Journal of Multidisciplinary Health Care* 1: 35–43.

Patton, M.Q. (2002). *Qualitative research and evaluation methods* (3rd edn). Thousand Oaks: Sage.

Streubert, H.J. (2011). Action research method. In H.J. Streubert & D. Rinaldi Carpenter (Eds.), *Qualitaive research in nursing, advancing the humanistic imperative* (5th edn). Philadelphia: Wolters Kluwer/Lippincott Williams & Wilkins.

Taylor, B.J., Bewley, J., Bulmer, B., Fayers, L., Hickey, A., Hill, L., & Stirling, K. (2008). Getting it right under pressure: Action research and reflection in palliative nursing. *International Journal of Palliative Nursing, 14*(7), 326–331.

10

Mixed methods research

Bev Taylor

Mixed methods research (MMR) might seem like an unlikely inclusion in this book on qualitative methodologies, methods and processes, but it is included because not only does MMR combine methods and processes commonly used in quantitative and qualitative research approaches, it is also now claimed to be a research methodology. MMR has developed considerably from being simply the mixing of methods to gaining methodological status. Indeed, MMR has become so popular in the last three decades that some researchers regard it as the 'third paradigm' in research (Plano Clark and Wang, 2010; Ploeg et al., 2010; Tashakkori and Teddlie, 2010; Thogersen-Ntoumani, Fox, and Ntoumanis, 2005), following on third in line after the quantitative and qualitative paradigms. For some researchers, MMR is 'the best of both worlds', but even though it has become established, not all researchers accept it unconditionally, nor do they necessarily embrace MMR wholeheartedly as the third major research approach.

In this chapter, we explore some definitions of MMR and examine the underlying theoretical assumptions in mixing quantitative and qualitative research methods. Many of the epistemological assumptions of MMR can be traced to its origins, so we review the history and evolution of MMR, discuss the claim that MMR is based conceptually in pragmatism, and locate the main MMR approaches that have been developed. The chapter concludes with critiques of MMR and examples of health science projects using MMR approaches.

Definitions of MMR

MMR has 'taken on a life of its own' since the late 1980s, so definitions of MMR have changed and grown with its popularity. The best approach to disentangling the array of MMR definitional possibilities is to rely on Creswell and Plano Clark's (2011) summary of the shifts in defining MMR according to authors' particular foci. For example, Creswell and Plano Clark (2011, p. 2) cite an early definition of MMR by Greene, Caracelli and Graham (1989), who emphasized mixing methods and 'the disentanglement of methods and philosophy'. Greene et al. (1989) defined mixed methods designs as those that include at least one quantitative method (designed to collect numbers) and one qualitative method (designed to collect words), where neither type of method is inherently linked to any particular inquiry paradigm (p. 256).

In Greene et al.'s definition, we see methods as 'free agents', able to collect information devoid of methodological foundations and intentions. While qualitative researchers in the later 1980s may have agreed that research methods did not have to serve a particular paradigm exclusively, the surge of qualitative research approaches from a decade previously were underscored with interpretive and critical philosophies that addressed epistemological issues. Consequently, some qualitative researchers expressed their reservations about the non-methodological mixing of methods in early versions of MMR (Giddings, 2006; Giddings and Grant, 2007; Holmes, 2006).

MMR definitions continued to change in response to critiques of MMR and through its increasing maturity. Creswell and Plano Clarke (2011) explain that within a decade, the simple definition of MMR as the mixing of methods was adapted to combining 'qualitative and quantitative approaches in the methodology of a study' (Tashakkori and Teddlie, 1998, p. ix), then to definitions reflecting its emergence as a methodological approach 'with its own worldview, vocabulary, and techniques' (Tashakkori and Teddlie, 2003, p. x).

In view of the burgeoning array of MMR approaches and definitions, Johnson, Onwuegbuzie and Turner (2007) suggested 'a composite understanding based on 19 different definitions provided by 21 highly published mixed methods researchers' (Creswell and Plano Clarke (2011, p. 3). Johnson et al. (2007) came up with the composite definition, that

Mixed methods research is the type of research in which a researcher or team of researchers combines elements of qualitative and quantitative research approaches (e.g., use of qualitative and quantitative viewpoints, data collection, analysis, inference techniques) for the purposes of breadth and depth of understanding and corroboration (p. 123).

By 2011, Creswell and Plano Clarke were keen to put forward a definition of 'core characteristics of mixed methods research' (p. 5). In six bullet points, Creswell and Plano Clarke (2011, p. 5) asserted that in:

mixed methods, the researcher
- collects and analyses persuasively and rigorously both qualitative and quantitative data (based on research questions);
- mixes (or integrates or links) the two forms of data concurrently by combining them (or merging them), sequentially by having one build on the other, or embedding one within the other;
- gives priority to one or both forms of data (in terms of what the research emphasizes);

- uses these procedures in a single study or in multiple phases of a program of study;
- frames these procedures within philosophical worldviews and theoretical lenses; and
- combines the procedures into specific research designs that direct the plan for conducting the study.

Creswell and Plano Clarke's (2011) comprehensive bullet point definition is more like a summary of MMR than it is a definition. Thus, we see that since the late 1980s MMR researchers have responded to the critiques against mixing methods with longer, more comprehensive definitions that have reflected the exponential growth of MMR. More recent definitions of MMR indicate its development into a research approach which mixes every aspect of research at all levels. Now we have a definitional sense of MMR, we will retrace its origins to understand its evolution as a research approach.

Origins and evolution of MMR

The history of MMR differs according to the people describing the events. For example, Teddlie and Johnson (2009a,b) trace the history of MMR within the history of methodological thought. The thoughts of philosophers from antiquity, the Middle Ages and the Scientific Revolution and its aftermath occupy the first three stages (Teddlie and Johnson, 2009a). The emergence of the social and behavioural sciences in the 19th and early 20th centuries occurred in Stage 4, during which logical positivism became the dominant philosophical and research paradigm. At Stage 5, the 'traditional period from 1900 to World War II', Teddlie and Johnson (2009) attest to the critiques of logical positivism, the development of qualitative research methods, and the use of mixed methods during this transitional period. This account of MMR history differs from other accounts, such as those given by Creswell and Plano Clark (2011, p. 21), who describe the turn-of-the-20th-century events as only 'key antecedents to what would later be more systematic attempts to forge mixed methods into a complete research design and to create a distinct approach to research'.

From its genesis in Stage 5, Teddlie and Johnson (2009) trace the history of MMR through three more stages. In Stage 6, the 'postpositivist era from the end of World War II to 1970', early grounded theorists (Glaser and Strauss, 1967) were advocates for multi-methods and mixed methods research. During Stage 7, 'diversification of and advances in methodologies in the human sciences – 1970 to 1990', constructivism emerged and paradigmatic positions were debated. In this period, Teddlie and Johnson (2009, p. 62) also note the increasing 'sophistication and popularity of qualitative methods', the use of triangulation as validity measures, and the continued emergence and development of MMR.

According to Teddlie and Johnson (2009), Stage 8 in the history of methodological thought was from 1990 to the present time. Stage 8 is the period of the 'institutionalization of mixed methods as a distinct methodological orientation', in which dialogues have been set up between qualitative and quantitative communities, and there has been a proliferation of MMR books, articles and research throughout the human (and health) sciences. As noted earlier, Teddlie and Johnson's (2009) account of the origins of MMR is inclusive of early trends from Stage 5, where qualitative and quantitative methods were first mixed. Johnson and Gray (2010) take a similar approach to tracking the history of MMR, by contextualizing it within the history of ideas within philosophy. Unsurprisingly, because Johnson is a co-author on both publications (Johnson and Gray, 2010; Teddlie and Johnson 2009), they are in agreement that 'MM-like thinking' (Johnson and Gray, 2010, p. 69) has been in existence for some time.

Creswell and Plano Clark (2011) consider that from the early 1990s MMR emerged for a number of reasons. Essentially, their position is that MMR was a necessary next step, because complex research questions require complex 'answers beyond simple numbers in a quantitative sense or words in a qualitative sense' (Creswell and Plano Clark, 2011, p. 21). Also, in their opinion, qualitative research had evolved into 'a legitimate form of inquiry' to the point where 'quantitative researchers recognize(d) that qualitative data can play an important role in quantitative research' (p. 21). Qualitative researchers also recognized that participants' accounts were not generalizable and therefore, multiple forms of evidence were necessary.

As a qualitative researcher, who will most probably be branded a purist, I need to confess to some irritability when I read Creswell and Plano Clark's (2011) words. On the face of it, the words as written fuel my suspicion that, for some researchers, MMR may be a way of legitimizing and extending the potential of qualitative research. Like Giddings and Grant (2007) before me, I am concerned that MMR may be a Trojan horse, being used to carry quantitative soldiers into the heart of qualitative territory and unseat its basic epistemological assumptions from within. While complex research questions do require complex answers, numbers alone in quantitative research are not necessarily simple; neither are words alone in qualitative research necessarily simple. Complex methods and processes to accommodate complex research questions are characteristic of both approaches, so that numbers or words alone, not mixed of necessity, can be totally sufficient for complex research questions and aims. This is not to say that MMR approaches are not also able to answer complex questions, but they should be seen as an option, not an imperative.

Also, I am wary of the suggestion that qualitative research *needed to evolve* into 'a legitimate form of inquiry' *as judged by some (mostly) quantitative researchers*, before it could 'play an important role in quantitative research' (Creswell and Plano Clark, 2011, p. 21). This view, as written, reflects the dominant attitude of some researchers that qualitative research was, and may still be, substandard, and needs to prove its legitimacy before it can be of practical use to quantitative researchers. The so-called 'paradigmatic battles' between quantitative and qualitative research approaches were then, and still are, real points of epistemological differences, if we base our 're-search' for new and extended knowledge on philosophical assumptions about the way knowledge is generated and validated. Simply brushing away these epistemological differences in the name of progress and pragmatism does not change the fact that the basic epistemological views are very different. Attempts to neutralize epistemological differences in MMR may be a means of suppressing the debate, thereby ultimately appropriating and subjugating qualitative research all over again to the ever-dominant quantitative paradigm.

Lastly, any qualitative researcher who wants to generalize findings as an end point to their inquiry has missed the point that qualitative knowledge about human experiences is relative, subjective and context-boundable and, therefore, generalizability is neither possible nor desirable and no amount of multiple forms of evidence will make it so. The intention to generalize is connected to fundamental positivistic assumptions about knowledge through quantifiable means. Quantifying qualitative data for the purpose of generalization rests on another fundamental assumption, that data (and epistemologies) integrate as one set of data moves into another and loses their identity in the transition. The question needs to be asked continually of both data shifts in MMR: Is this integration or subjugation?

Even so, in terms of its continued evolution, Creswell (2011) is optimistic that in the next decade MMR will become firmly established. He predicts that 'there will be a gradual acceptance of pragmatism as the primary philosophical orientation associated with MMR'; 'a generic set of MMR designs will emerge over time and be popularized in textbooks'; 'analysis issues will become more important'; MMR will 'continue to be adopted throughout the social and behavioral [sic] sciences'; and MMR will 'continue to pave the way for human sciences research to be more inclusive (eclectic) and research question oriented' (Creswell, 2011, p. 296).

Food for thought

In an attempt to secure MMR as the third research paradigm, it is possible that some MMR researchers created novelty from what had already been in existence since the emergence of qualitative research approaches at the turn of the 20th century. If that is the case, it is worth considering that it is highly likely that the earliest emergence of MMR in Teddlie and Johnson's (2009) Stage 5 may have been a means of controlling and 'legitimizing' qualitative methods, which were emerging at that time.

Is it possible that mixing methods, as advocated in Stages 5 and 6, was a way of keeping qualitative methods and methodologies 'in check', so they could be controlled and 'legitimized' against quantitative standards? If yes, how? If no, why not?

If you argue yes, that MMR was possibly a controlling and legitimizing strategy at that time, does it then follow that, many decades hence, the continued popularity and ultimate dominance of MMR may one day lead to a demise of specific qualitative methodologies and a renewed and even stronger era of quantitative research dominance?

Theoretical assumptions of MMR

Proponents of MMR approaches assume that a variety of research methods can be mixed and that this mixing can be defended methodologically, most notably by the philosophy of pragmatism (Creswell, 2011; Creswell and Plano Clark, 2011; Tashakkori and Teddlie, 2010). From my reading of MMR literature (Greene et al., 1989), MMR did not begin its evolution with pre-stated philosophical assumptions that would tie it methodologically to particular epistemological ideas. Rather, MMR began simply as mixing methods to strengthen evidence and subsequent critiques about the lack of a philosophical underpinning and the ad hoc mixing of paradigmatic assumptions (Giddings, 2006; Giddings and Grant, 2007; Holmes, 2006) led to a post hoc search for a suitable methodological basis (Tashakkori and Teddlie, 1998; Johnson and Onwuegbuzie, 2004; Greene, 2008). Given the practical advantages of mixing research methods, the suggestion is that MMR lends itself well to pragmatism.

Pragmatism

At its simplest level, pragmatism means acting according to a practical imperative. The earliest applications of pragmatism to MMR were based simply on the practical need to begin with the research question(s), rather than starting with a particular methodological stance. For example, Tashakkori and Teddlie (1998, p. 20) wrote of the 'dictatorship of the research question' and Johnson and Onwuegbuzie (2004, p. 17) suggested that researchers should 'choose the combination or mixture of methods and procedures that works best for answering (their) research questions'. While these suggestions had a practical imperative for getting on with managing the work of research projects, more cautious views have been presented (Biesta, 2011; Gorard and Taylor, 2004; Greene, 2008). For example, Biesta (2011, p. 96) calls for 'a better and more precise understanding of what pragmatism entails (and) to engage in more detail with the question of how ideas from pragmatism might be relevant for mixed methods research'.

For some MMR researchers, pragmatism emphasizes the expediency of mixing methods. For example, Tashakkori and Teddlie (2010) describe the practical benefits of MMR, as:

- methodological eclecticism (freedom to combine the best methods for answering the research questions) (p. 8);

- paradigmatic pluralism (a variety of paradigms can serve as underlying philosophies) (p. 9);

- an emphasis on diversity at all levels of the research enterprise (p. 9);

- an emphasis on continua rather than a set of dichotomies (p. 10);

- an iterative, cyclical approach to research (p. 10);

- a focus on the research question (or research problem) in determining the methods employed within any given study (p. 10);

- a set of basic 'signature' research designs and analytical processes (p. 10);

- a tendency towards balance and compromise that is implicit within the 'third methodological community' (p. 11); and

- a reliance on visual representations (e.g., figures, diagrams) and a common notational system (p. 11).

However, all the espoused practical and methodological benefits of MMR are not necessarily explained by pragmatism. Biesta (2011, p. 96) reviewed pragmatism and the philosophical foundations of MMR by differentiating between what he termed *'everyday* pragmatism' as a practical justification for mixing methods and *'philosophical* pragmatism', which is 'a set of philosophical tools that can be used to address problems'. After systematically identifying key principles of Dewey's philosophical pragmatism (e.g., Dewey 1933), Biesta (2011) argued that pragmatism does not provide a comprehensive methodology on which to rest all of MMR's epistemological assumptions. Biesta (2011) came to that conclusion by systematically outlining the fundamentals of Dewey's pragmatism as knowing as a way of doing. According to Biesta (2011) the consequences of Dewey's pragmatism as a form of transactional constructivism are that it

> holds that knowledge is at the very same time constructed *and* real ... (and) given that knowledge concerns the relationship between (our) actions and (their) consequences, knowledge will ever offer us only *possibilitie*s but not certainty ... Sometimes what is possible in one situation turns out also to be possible in another situation; but in other situations, the transactional determinants of the situation are different, so what is possible in one case is no longer possible in another case.
>
> (Biesta, 2011, p. 111)

A major consequence of this transactional, constructivist view is that only 'warranted assertions' can be made from inquiry and there can be no absolute 'truth'. Also, the ultimately transactional, subjectivist position of pragmatism leads to the construction of 'an *intersubjective* world out of our individual, subjective worlds' (Biesta, 2011, p. 112), thereby calling into question the possibility of objective knowing and 'truth'. Therefore, whereas pragmatism may suit MMR (QUAN) on a design level, it is at odds with QUAN on a methodological level. Biesta (2011, p. 114) concluded that 'although pragmatism is unable to provide *the* philosophical foundation for mixed methods research, it has some important things to offer, particularly in helping mixed methods researchers to ask better and more precise questions about the philosophical implications and justifications of their designs'. Therefore, Biesta (2011) suggested that pragmatism can be regarded as a 'philosophical companion' (p. 97), rather than an underlying philosophical position to justify all of the aspects MMR. Given that Creswell (2011, p. 296) is of the opinion that 'there will be a gradual acceptance of pragmatism as the primary philosophical orientation associated with MMR', it will be interesting to watch how the methodological debate plays out over time between MMR researchers.

MMR designs

Since its inception in the late 1980s, MMR research designs have proliferated in accord with the freedom to mix methods according to the requirements of the research aims and questions. Consequently, there is a 'dizzying' array of MMR design possibilities. For example, even though few studies use these notational systems when publishing their projects (Creswell, 2007; Tashakkori and Teddlie, 2010), it is possible to differentiate MMR designs according to weighting of the importance and the timing of the methods. For example, MMR projects can be described according to a dominant-less dominant, sequential design (QUAN to qual; quan to QUAL; QUAL to quan; qual to QUAN); or an equal weighting, sequential design (QUAL to QUAN; QUAN to QUAL). Undertaken simultaneously, concurrent designs that are dominant-less dominant can be 'nested' (QUAL plus QUAN; QUAN plus qual), or they can be equal weighting and 'fully integrated' (QUAL and QUAN) concurrent designs (Creswell, 2003; Miller and Fredericks, 2006).

However, Creswell and Plano Clark (2011) dispel any illusion that MMR designs are relatively few or simple. To assist would-be mixed methods researchers to make reasoned choices about their MMR designs, Creswell and Plano Clark (2011) suggest that a good beginning point is to realize that there are *fixed MMR designs*, which have been planned ahead in a research plan, and *emergent MMR designs*, which are added on as deemed necessary as the project progresses. Also, MMR designs can take a *typology-based approach*, where pre-existing useful designs are adopted, or they can take *dynamic approaches*, that consider and interrelate 'multiple components of research design rather than placing emphasis on selecting an appropriate design from an existing typology' (Creswell and Plano Clark, 2011, p. 59). According to Creswell and Plano Clark (2011, pp. 69–70), the six major typology-based MMR designs are the:

- convergent parallel design
- explanatory sequential design
- exploratory sequential design
- embedded design
- transformative design
- multiphase design.

Also known as the convergent design, the *convergent parallel design* uses concurrent timing to implement equally 'the quantitative and qualitative strands during the same phase of the research process, prioritizes the methods equally, and keeps the strands independent during analysis and then mixes the results during the overall interpretation' (Creswell and Plano Clark, 2011, pp. 70–71).

Also known as the explanatory design, *the explanatory sequential design* has two interactive phases. The first phase is explanatory, because it prioritizes QUAN (quantitative data collection and analysis), and follows up in the second phase with qual (qualitative data collection and analysis), to help explain the first phase.

Also known as the exploratory design, the *exploratory sequential design* begins with QUAL (qualitative data collection and analysis), and follows up in the second phase with quan (quantitative data collection and analysis), to test or generalize the findings from the first phase.

In the *embedded design* the 'researcher collects and analyzes both quantitative and qualitative data within a traditional both quantitative and qualitative design' (Creswell and Plano Clark, 2011, p. 71). The design may include a supplemented qual strand within a QUAN design, or a supplemented quan strand within a QUAL design, depending on the needs of the evolving project.

In the *transformative design*, the methodological considerations of projects with transformative intentions, methods and processes are fundamental to the project, and the methods are mixed to achieve the research aims and questions. Examples of research methodologies with transformative intentions are action research, feminist and critical ethnographic approaches. In the *multiphase design*, concurrent and sequential strands are created, as the project evolves over time and the aims of the project are being achieved, for example, in evaluation research.

There are many published MMR typology-based designs from which to choose that have been evolved within a range of disciplines (Creswell and Plano Clark, 2011, pp. 56–59). The practical suggestions given by Creswell and Plano Clark (2011) for making well-reasoned decisions about the selection of a particular MMR design are to:

- match the design to the research problem, purpose and questions (p. 60);

- be explicit about the reasons for mixing methods (p. 61);

- determine the level of interaction between the quantitative and qualitative strands (p. 64);

- determine the priority of the quantitative and qualitative strands (p. 65);

- determine the timing of the quantitative and qualitative strands (p. 65); and

- determine where and how to mix the quantitative and qualitative strands (p. 66).

As the other factors have already been mentioned in this chapter, the last point needs elaboration. In relation to determining where and how to mix the quantitative and qualitative strands, MMR researchers need to consider the possible points of integration for the data strands. For example, there are four possible 'points of interface' where data can be mixed: at interpretation, data analysis, data collection and design. It is interesting that Creswell and Plano Clark (2011) describe the research process in reverse when suggesting points of interface for mixing quantitative and qualitative strands.

Critiques of MMR

A review of the literature over the last two decades confirms support for MMR, but as it grows, some cautionary notes have been sounded. Some qualitative researchers are calling for a closer inspection of the claims for epistemological integration and balance, by pointing out methodological differences between QUAL and QUAN (Giddings, 2006; Giddings and Grant, 2007) and the risk of the qualitative research tradition being subsumed by the persistently dominant quantitative research tradition. Giddings and Grant (2007) argue that MMR

> has been captured by a pragmatic postpositivism ... which secures mixed methods within the broader positivist project to know the world in particular ways. The effect of this capture is to reinstall the marginalization of other forms of knowing. Moreover, the resultant narrowing of focus means more circumscribed fields of values at play, questions being asked, forms of data being collected, modes of analysis being undertaken, and possible outcomes being generated (p. 52).

As a qualitative researcher, I have for a long time been wary about, but somewhat unable to articulate comprehensively, my concerns about MMR. Preparing this chapter has helped me to see that, for me, it is not so much an either/or choice, that is, to accept or reject MMR. I come from a background of being enthusiastic to learn about and debate the various epistemological standpoints of qualitative methodologies. Even taking on board the admonitions from critics along the way that I, as a qualitative researcher, may have misappropriated philosophical principles to approaches, such as grounded theory (Glaser, 1992) or phenomenology (Crotty, 1996), I at all times tried to bend my mind to the philosophical nuances and apply them as best I could to qualitative projects I undertook or supervised.

Then, along came MMR, initially mixing methods with no concern for methodological congruence, and later, defending its practical benefits with pragmatism. In both locations, my standpoint has been somewhat bemused and wary. I realize that I have an underlying concern, that having worked hard to gain a foothold in the philosophical cliff of knowledge generation and validation, qualitative researchers may be abandoning their relativistic viewpoints about knowledge and grasping on to MMR, which is being put forward as a firmer hold on 'truth' and 'true' knowledge. If this is the case, we as qualitative researchers may have forgotten that knowledge about human experience is as uncertain as a cliff face, and we accept that is how it is – uncertain, tenuous, 'safe' enough only for this moment, but in no way is knowledge about human experience secure, solid and immutable.

If we accept that foundational differences in quantitative and qualitative research lie in the nature of 'truth' and how to generate 'true' knowledge, it then follows that the means of validating knowledge differs from both standpoints. Traditionally, quantitative researchers have appealed to means for demonstrating rigour and qualitative researchers have attempted to achieve trustworthiness criteria in their respective projects. The claims of MMR to be able to integrate MMR data have been addressed through various means. For example, traditionally the approach has been to discuss validity from a QUAL and QUAN perspective, but to not mix them (Tashakkori and Teddlie, 1998), to extend the idea of construct validity to cover all phases of the MMR (Leech et al., 2010), to link inferences in evaluation standards with validity (Teddlie and Tashakkori, 2009), to develop nine forms of legitimation (Onwuegbuzie and Johnson, 2006) and to review validity concerns as related to types of designs (Campbell, 1986; Creswell, Plano Clark, and Garrett, 2008).

A willingness to take on any or all of these approaches to knowledge validation in MMR projects will rest on a number of consensual factors, such as agreement with the practical expediencies of MMR, agreement to reject or suspend philosophical foundations for *doing* research of any type, and/or a belief in the paramount importance of answering the research questions by whatever mixed means necessary. The proliferation of MMR in general, and in the health sciences in particular, suggests that these criticisms of MMR have possibly not been considered at all, they have been addressed completely at various levels, or there are other possible reasons falling in between these polar options. Regardless, I agree with Creswell (2011) that MMR is here to stay, although I have reservations about what this trend might ultimately mean for qualitative research, if it becomes *always accompanied* by quantitative methods.

MMR projects in the health sciences

The emergence of MMR has mirrored the emergence of evidence based practice (EBP) in the health sciences, so these two movements have been highly influential in determining what counts as evidence and how projects need to be designed to answer complex health-related research questions. The highest levels of evidence in EBP are quantitative in nature and design. Consequently, qualitative researchers seeking research funding have increasingly joined forces with quantitative researchers to develop MMR designs.

MMR has been successful in the health sciences for many reasons, an important one being that it allows for large-scale projects to be undertaken, which incorporate researchers' expertise in mixing methods in a variety of MMR designs (Carter, Callaghan, Khalil and Morres, 2012; van Staa, 2011). For example, writing on behalf of a research team, van Staa (2011) reported on the 'added value' of using MMR in a project 'unraveling triadic communication in hospital consultations with adolescents with chronic conditions'. The objective of the project was to 'integrate findings of a mixed methods research (MMR) into adolescents' preferences and competencies for communication during consultations, in order to demonstrate the added value of MMR for health communication research' (van Staa, 2011, p. 455). The sequential design MMR involved adolescents (12–19 years) with various chronic conditions, who were being cared for in a university hospital. The MMR methods comprised: '(1) 31 face-to-face interviews; (2) Q-methodology; (3) 39 observations of outpatient consultations; (4) three focus groups with 27 healthcare providers; (5) webbased questionnaire in 960 adolescents' (p. 455). Following the data analyses, the researcher concluded that

> Adolescents had different preferences regarding health communication, but all wished to be involved as partners. Yet, their actual participation during consultations was low. They often acted as bystanders rather than main characters because their participation was neither requested nor encouraged. Parents filled the gap, to healthcare providers' frustration. The questionnaire confirmed the discrepancy between self-efficacy and self-reported independent behavior during consultations ... Triadic communication was all but multi-party-talk and adolescents did not act and were not considered as main partners.

van Staa (2011) reiterated that the research team acknowledged that 'MMR was of pivotal importance' for understanding the participants' experiences and they recommended that adolescents needed to be more actively encouraged by healthcare providers to 'take the lead in communication by initiating independent visits and changing the parents' roles' (p. 455).

MMR has been interpreted and applied in a variety of ways in the health sciences. For example, researchers have applied mixed methods to pretest the Pressure Ulcer Quality of Life (PU-QOL) instrument (Gorecki, Lamping, Nixon, Brown and Cano, 2012), while others have systematically reviewed quantitative and qualitative research articles on various topics, such as: medication administration technologies and patient safety (Wulff, Cummings, Marck and Yurtseven, 2011); investigating community-based health and health promotion for homeless people (Coles, Themessl-Huber and Freeman, 2012); and exploring the quality of nursing documentation and approaches to its evaluation (Wang, Hailey and Yu, 2011).

Even though MMR has gained incredible success, it is not without issues in health science research. In addition to the MMR methodological issues discussed already in this chapter, health science researchers have written about various research process problems. For example, Curry, O'Cathain, Plano Clark, Aroni, Fetters and Berg (2012) explored the role of group dynamics in mixed methods health sciences research teams. Curry et al. (2012, p. 5) conceptualized

> mixed methods research teams as 'representational groups,' in which members bring both their organizational and professional groups (e.g., organizational affiliations, methodological expertise) and their identity groups, such as gender or race, to the work of research. Although

diversity and complementarity are intrinsic to mixed methods teams, these qualities also present particular challenges. Such challenges include (a) dealing with differences, (b) trusting the 'other,' (c) creating a meaningful group, (d) handling essential conflicts and tensions, and (e) enacting effective leadership roles.

These group dynamic issues are hardly surprising, because experts in their preferred methods have developed a great deal of knowledge and skill over time, which may not be easily 'essentialized' for the benefit of other team members. Also, working in a research team is exacting enough even when the methods are homogenous to a particular paradigm, so it may be understandably even more difficult when working in teams with different paradigmatic backgrounds. While there is a general consensus that MMR is a good and worthwhile research pursuit, it can bring up many methodological and process issues, which need to be unpacked and sorted through carefully, in order for the MMR team to work cohesively to attain the best possible research outcomes.

Chapter summary

Mixed methods research (MMR) is included in this book on qualitative methodologies, methods and processes because MMR combines methods commonly used in quantitative and qualitative research approaches, and it is also a research methodology. MMR has developed from being simply the mixing of methods, to gaining methodological status, and being heralded by some researchers as the 'third paradigm' in research (Plano Clark and Wang, 2010; Ploeg et al., 2010; Tashakkori and Teddlie, 2010; Thogersen-Ntoumani, Fox, and Ntoumanis, 2005). While it may be 'the best of both worlds' for some researchers, MMR is not necessarily embraced wholeheartedly by all researchers in all respects.

In this chapter, we explored some definitions of MMR, examined the underlying theoretical assumptions in mixing quantitative and qualitative research methods, reviewed the history and evolution of MMR, discussed pragmatism, and identified the main MMR designs. The chapter concluded with critiques of MMR and some examples of health science projects using MMR approaches.

Key points

- MMR definitions have changed in response to critiques of MMR, from the mixing of methods to a methodological approach.

- Johnson et al.'s (2007) composite definition of MMR is that it 'is the type of research in which a researcher or team of researchers combines elements of qualitative and quantitative research approaches (e.g., use of qualitative and quantitative viewpoints, data collection, analysis, inference techniques) for the purposes of breadth and depth of understanding and corroboration' (p. 123).

- Perspectives differ about the history of MMR, from being situated within the history of methodological thought, to emerging in the late 1980s.

- Proponents of MMR approaches assume that a variety of research methods can be mixed and that this mixing can be defended methodologically, most notably by the philosophy of pragmatism.

- Biesta (2011) has argued that pragmatism does not provide a comprehensive methodology on which to rest all of MMR's epistemological assumptions, thus he has suggested that pragmatism can be regarded as a 'philosophical companion' (p. 97), rather than an underlying philosophical position to justify all of the aspects MMR.

- According to Creswell and Plano Clark (2011, pp. 69–70), the six major typology-based MMR designs are the: convergent parallel design; explanatory sequential design; exploratory sequential design; embedded design; transformative design; and multiphase design.

- MMR projects can be described according to a dominant-less dominant, sequential design (QUAN to qual; quan to QUAL; QUAL to quan; qual to QUAN); or an equal weighting, sequential design (QUAL to QUAN; QUAN to QUAL).

- Undertaken simultaneously, concurrent designs that are dominant-less dominant can be 'nested' (QUAL plus QUAN; QUAN plus qual), or they can be equal weighting and 'fully integrated' (QUAL and QUAN) concurrent designs (Creswell, 2003; Miller and Fredericks, 2006).

- To assist would-be mixed methods researchers to make reasoned choices about their MMR designs, Creswell and Plano Clark (2011) suggest that a good beginning point is to realize that there are *fixed MMR designs,* which have been planned ahead in a research plan, and *emergent MMR designs,* which are added on as deemed necessary as the project progresses. Also, MMR designs can take a *typology-based approach*, where pre-existing useful designs are adopted, or they can take *dynamic approaches,* that consider and interrelate 'multiple components of research design rather than placing emphasis on selecting an appropriate design from an existing typology' (Creswell and Plano Clark, 2011, p. 59).

- The practical suggestions given by Creswell and Plano Clark (2011) for making well-reasoned decisions about the selection of a particular MMR design are to: match the design to the research problem, purpose and questions (p. 60); be explicit about the reasons for mixing methods (p. 61); determine the level of interaction between the quantitative and qualitative strands (p. 64); determine the priority of the quantitative and qualitative strands (p. 65); determine the timing of the quantitative and qualitative strands (p. 65); and determine where and how to mix the quantitative and qualitative strands (p. 66).

- Although the literature over the last two decades confirms support for MMR, some cautionary notes have been sounded for a closer inspection of the claims for epistemological integration and balance, by pointing out methodological differences between QUAL and QUAN (Giddings, 2006; Giddings and Grant, 2007; Holmes, 2006) and the risk of the qualitative research tradition being subsumed by the persistently dominant quantitative research tradition.

- MMR has been successful in the health sciences for allowing for large-scale projects to be undertaken, which incorporate researchers' expertise in mixing methods in a variety of MMR designs, and for its potential to be interpreted and applied in a variety of ways.

Critical review questions

1 In what ways is it possible for mixed methods research to inform healthcare practice?

2 To what extent can mixed methods research offer insights into your clients' experiences of health and illness?

References

Biesta, G. (2011). Pragmatism and the philosophical foundations of mixed methods research. In A. Tashakkori & C. Teddlie *Handbook of Mixed Methods in Social & Behavioral Research*. Thousand Oaks: Sage, 95–117.

Campbell, D.T. (1986). Relabeling internal and external validity for applied social scientists. *New Directions for Program Evaluation, 1986*(31), 67–77.

Carter, T., Callaghan, P., Khalil, E., & Morres, I. (2012). The effectiveness of a preferred intensity exercise programme on the mental health outcomes of young people with depression: A sequential mixed methods evaluation. *BMC Public Health, 12*, 187–193.

Coles, E., Themessl-Huber, M., & Freeman, R. (2012). Investigating community-based health and health promotion for homeless people: a mixed methods review. *Health Education Research, 27*(4), 624–644.

Creswell, J.W. (2003). *Research design: Qualitative, quantitative, and mixed methods approaches set* (2nd edn). Thousand Oaks: Sage.

Creswell, J.W. (2007). *Qualitative inquiry and research design: Choosing among five traditions* (2nd Ed). Thousand Oaks: Sage.

Creswell, J.W. (2011). Controversies in mixed methods research. In N.K. Denzin & Y.S. Lincoln. *The Handbook of Qualitative Research*. Los Angeles: Sage, 269–283.

Creswell, J.W., & Plano Clark, V. (2011). *Designing and conducting research methods* (2nd edn). Los Angeles: Sage.

Creswell, J.W., Plano Clark, V., & Garrett, A.L. (2008). Methodological issues in conducting mixed methods research designs. *Advances in mixed methods research: theories and applications*. Los Angeles: Sage, 66–84.

Crotty, M. (1996). *Phenomenology and nursing research*. Melbourne: Churchill Livingstone.

Curry, L.A., O'Cathain, A., Plano Clark, V.L., Aroni, R., Fetters, M., & Berg, D. (2012) The role of group dynamics in mixed methods health sciences research teams. *Journal of Mixed Methods Research, 6*(1), 5–20.

Dewey, J. (1933). How we think: A restatement of the relation of reflective thinking to the educative process. In J.A. Boydston (Ed.), *The later works (1925–1953)* (Vol. 8, pp. 105–352) Carbondale and Edwardsville: Southern Illinois University Press.

Giddings, L. (2006). Mixed-methods research. *Journal of Research in Nursing, 11*(3), 195–203.

Giddings, L., & Grant, B. (2007). A trojan horse for positivism?: a critique of mixed methods research. *Advances in Nursing Science, 30*(1), 52–60.

Glaser, B.G. (1992). *Emergence vs forcing: Basics of grounded theory analysis*. Mill Valley: Sociology Press.

Glaser, B.G., & Strauss, A.L. (1967). *The discovery of grounded theory: Strategies for qualitative research*. Chicago: Aldine.

Gorard, S. & Taylor, C. (2004). *Combining methods in educational and social research*. Buckingham, UK: Open University Press.

Gorecki, C., Lamping, D.L., Nixon, J., Brown, J.M., & Cano, S. (2012). Applying mixed methods to pretest the Pressure Ulcer Quality of Life (PU-QOL) instrument. *Quality of Life Research, 21*, 441–451.

Greene, J.C. (2008). Is mixed methods social inquiry a distinctive methodology? *Journal of Mixed Methods Research, 2*(1), 7–22.

Greene, J.C., Caracelli, V.J., & Graham, W.F. (1989). Toward a conceptual framework for mixed-methods evaluation designs. *Educational Evaluation and Policy Analysis, 11*, 255–274.

Holmes, C.A. (2006). Mixed (up) methods, methodology and interpretive frameworks. Paper presented at the Mixed Methods Conference, Cambridge, UK.

Johnson, B., & Gray, R. (2010) A history of philosophical and theoretical issues for mixed methods research. In A. Tashakkori & C. Teddlie. *Handbook of Mixed Methods in Social & Behavioral Research*. Thousand Oaks: Sage, 69–94.

Johnson, R.B., & Onwuegbuzie, A.J. (2004). Mixed methods research: A paradigm whose time has come. *Educational Researcher, 33*, 14–26.

Johnson, R.B., Onwuegbuzie, A.J. & Turner, L.A. (2007). Toward a definition of mixed methods research. *Journal of Mixed Methods Research, 1*, 112–133.

Leech, N.L., Dellinger, A.B., Brannagan, K.B., & Tanaka, H. (2010). Evaluating mixed research studies: A mixed methods approach. *Journal of Mixed Methods Research, 4*(1), 1731.

Miller, S.J., & Fredericks, M. (2006). Mixed methods and evaluation research: Trends and issues. *Qualitative Health Research, 16*(4), 567–579.

Onwuegbuzie, A.J., & Johnson, R.B. (2006). The validity issue in mixed research. *Research in the Schools, 13*(1), 48–63.

Plano Clark, V., & Wang, S. (2010). Adapting mixed methods research to multicultural counseling. *Handbook of multicultural counseling*, 427–438.

Ploeg, J., Skelly, J., Rowan, M., Edwards, N., Davies, B., Grinspun, D., & Downey, A. (2010). The role of nursing best practice champions in diffusing practice guidelines: a mixed methods study. *Worldviews on Evidence Based Nursing. 7*(4): 238–251.

Tashakkori, A., & Teddlie, C. (1998). *Mixed methodology: combining qualitative and quantitative approaches*. Thousand Oaks: Sage.

Tashakkori, A., & Teddlie, C. (2003). *Handbook of Mixed Methods in Social & Behavioral Research*. Thousand Oaks: Sage.

Tashakkori, A., & Teddlie, C. (2010). *Handbook of Mixed Methods in Social & Behavioral Research*. Thousand Oaks: Sage.

Teddlie, C., & Johnson, R.B. (2009a). Methodological thought before the 20th century. In A. Tashakkori & C. Teddlie. *Foundations of mixed methods research: Integrating quantitative and qualitative approaches in the social and behavioral sciences.* Thousand Oaks: Sage, 40–61.

Teddlie, C., & Johnson, R.B. (2009b). Methodological thought since the 20th century. In A. Tashakkori & C. Teddlie. *Foundations of mixed methods research: Integrating quantitative and qualitative approaches in the social and behavioral sciences.* Thousand Oaks: Sage, 62–82.

Thogersen-Ntoumani, C., Fox, K.R., & Ntoumanis, N. (2005). Relationships between exercise and three components of mental well-being in corporate employees. *Psychology of Sport and Exercise, 6,* 609–627.

van Staa, AL. (2011). Unraveling triadic communication in hospital consultations with adolescents with chronic conditions: The added value of mixed methods research. *Patient Education and Counseling, 82,* 455–464.

Wang, N., Hailey, D., & Yu, P. (2011). Quality of nursing documentation and approaches to its evaluation: a mixed-method systematic review. *Journal of Advanced Nursing, 67*(9), 1858–1875.

Wulff, K., Cummings, G.G., Marck, P., & Yurtseven, O. (2011). Medication administration technologies and patient safety: a mixed-method systematic review. *Journal of Advanced Nursing, 67*(10), 2080–2095.

Part II

Methods and processes

Welcome to Part II of this book. Part I was designed to refresh your memory of some fundamental ideas relating to qualitative research, by defining methodologies, methods and processes. Although we assume you already know about research in general, Part I began with foundational concepts, such as world views guiding approaches to research, including quantitative, qualitative and mixed methods research, before reviewing postmodern influences on paradigmatic shifts in research inquiry. The methodologies featured in Part I were grounded theory, historical research, ethnography, phenomenology, narrative inquiry, case study research, feminisms and action research. Mixed methods were also described.

Overview of Part II

Part II features qualitative research methods and processes. Methods are *what* researchers do to collect and analyse data, and processes are *how* they go about doing them. Part II takes as its starting point, the idea that methods and processes are 'free agents', able to roam across a variety of qualitative methodologies, because they do not 'belong' to a specific theoretical tradition. On the whole though, the methods and processes qualitative researchers use in collecting and analysing data depend on their choice of methodology. The research methods and processes merge into a meshwork of what researchers are doing and how they are doing it, according to the methodological assumptions of the specific approach and in accord with the research aims, objectives and questions.

The data collection and analysis methods and processes featured in Part II are for interviewing (Chapter 12), group work (Chapter 13), narrative analysis (Chapter 14), discourse analysis (Chapter 15) and other creative approaches (Chapter 16). Part II concludes with Chapter 17, which describes the uptake of qualitative research in clinical settings to improve evidence-based practice.

Revising the process of developing a research project

Bev Taylor

Chapter overview

This chapter revises the process of developing a research proposal, in relation to a project's title, background, aims, objectives, questions, methodology, ethical considerations, participant recruitment and sampling, and data collection and analysis. Proposal development is also discussed in relation to a project's limitations, timeframes, resources and funding. The chapter concludes with a discussion of trustworthiness issues and offers suggestion for writing up a project.

A successful qualitative research project often reflects the due care researchers take in thinking the research through initially, developing a thorough research plan, considering trustworthiness issues and in disseminating the insights and implications. The following section revises these aspects of developing a research project, so you can judge for yourself the extent to which you attend to the details of good project development.

Developing and writing a qualitative research proposal

A qualitative research proposal is a written account of your plan for the research project, which presents an argument for why the project is necessary, the choice of methods and processes to facilitate it, and a guide for action over the time of the project. Although the proposal is written sequentially, in some qualitative projects, certain aspects of the research proposal are written in broad terms because the plan may evolve with time and participation.

Initially, the planning may be highly flexible and open to interpretation, with you and your colleagues meeting to 'flesh out' some ideas around a mutually agreed topic, or focused on the published criteria of a call for research funding. Developmental ideas may begin with spontaneous suggestions and sketchy strategies, which are then refined to fit the specific requirements of a manageable project within personnel, cost and time constraints. When the initial ideas firm up, the plan helps you, the researcher, to design and organize the project carefully from the title of the research to research report dissemination details.

It is important to identify the audience for whom the proposal is aimed, as these people have the power to approve or reject your proposal. Funding and ethics committees will have different emphases, but they are generally concerned that your project is worthwhile and that it is of high quality. Funding panels want to know that your research is worth funding against a competitive field, that it has a realistic budget and it will make a significant contribution to knowledge and practice. Human ethics committees will be most concerned with all of the ramifications of the risks and benefits of the project to participants.

Before you write, you need to have in mind the fundamentals of the proposed project. You need a research focus, either stated as a research problem or described in exploratory terms. You will have read and reviewed some literature, unless you are working using a qualitative approach in which this may not be appropriate. You will have identified the basic sequence of events in your research plan, although some of these ideas may firm up as you write and revise drafts of the proposal. After drafts of the initial planning comes the writing of a formal research proposal, to communicate clearly and concisely every step that you can reasonably foresee in your research project.

The overall headings structure of a research proposal is fairly standard, but variations may occur in specific guidelines according to context, for example, from a university, clinical area, funding body or human ethics committee. Become very conversant with the application forms and guidelines organizations provide and ensure you follow them 'to the letter'. The panel members of these organizations have most probably been selected for their eye for detail and their insistence on doing things correctly, so don't try to be too innovative and creative in the way you write your research proposal.

The proposal should develop a logical flow of ideas and should be laid out in the specified order. If you are using a standard set of guidelines written for quantitative research designs, use the headings supplied, but explain briefly the qualitative research equivalents within the respective sections, for example, why hypotheses are not applicable, why and how sampling methods differ, that you are describing strategies for enhancing trustworthiness, not means for measuring rigour, and so on. Allow plenty of time to prepare your proposal, because it may take longer than you expect to develop a proposal and get all of the necessary approvals.

To revise the essentials of how to prepare a qualitative proposal, in sections where the writing is not self-evident, I offer an example of a proposal, but always be mindful that there are lots of variations in the ways proposals can be written. The example is of a proposal I submitted to a Human Research Ethics Committee (HREC), in which there was only one member of my healthcare profession (nursing) with qualitative expertise deciding on the merits of the proposal. Other HREC members occupied roles required for Australian HREC composition, but they did not necessarily have expertise in qualitative research. Therefore, it was important to be clear about the focus and methodology of the project, as it would have to be clear and acceptable to predominantly quantitative interests at the HREC meeting.

Research proposal preliminaries

The research proposal usually begins with the title page, an abstract or summary and researchers' details. This structure varies according to the reasons for which the proposal is being developed and written, however, if not otherwise specified, it is a good idea to include preliminary pages prior to the body of the proposal.

The title page

The title page of the proposal should clearly convey the research focus within the title, by using key words. Although the title is usually no longer than 20 words, some agencies require both long and short titles, while others do not specify a word limit. It is advisable to indicate the qualitative methodology within the title, so this can be placed after a well-placed semicolon. As well as the title of the proposal, the title page of the research proposal usually indicates the date of submission, plus the authors' names, positions and qualifications. If the proposal is being submitted for ethics, funding, or other outside approvals, the authors' postal and email addresses are given, as well as telephone and fax contact numbers.

The abstract

The abstract is a brief summary of the proposal, which gives the reader an overview of the project and includes the major themes or threads of the project. Primarily, it should focus on the project's aims, objectives, methods, processes and outcomes. It should be concise and written within a specified word limit. For example:

> Nurses and midwives work in busy healthcare settings, facing work constraints and issues on a daily basis, which challenge their value systems and impede their best efforts to deliver quality care. This project aims to facilitate action research and reflective processes for experienced Registered Nurses and Midwives, in order to: raise their critical awareness of practice problems they face every day; work systematically through problem solving processes, to uncover constraints against effective nursing and midwifery care; and improve the quality of care given by nurses and midwives, in light of the identified constraints and possibilities. Over a 16-week period, the RNs' and RMs' action research groups will meet weekly, for one hour, on a negotiated day and time and in a mutually agreed venue within the hospital, to discuss clinical problems they raise in their journal writing and in group discussion. In the first two weeks the participants will be oriented to action research and reflective practice principles and discuss how to work together as a group. Action research

cycles will then be undertaken. Group discussion will identify thematic concerns (practice issues) and the most practical and useful plan of action. Thematic analysis of journal experiences and participant observation will be managed by individual and group critical reflection. The action plan will be revised until it improves identified aspects of clinical practice.

The researchers' details

This section usually indicates the researchers' names, positions, and qualifications. It requires that one person be first named as the person responsible and for contact in relation to the project. Sometimes, the researchers' curricula vitae (CVs) are included so that panel members evaluating the proposal can judge whether the applicants have the necessary expertise to carry out the project successfully. The CVs include qualifications, relevant experience, a list of publications, any other research projects undertaken and any previous research grants awarded to members of the research team. The particular details to be highlighted in the attached CVs are usually clarified by the grant funding body, so ensure you follow their requests carefully.

The body of the research proposal

Because qualitative proposals are often scrutinized by academic departments, health agency organizations, funding bodies and ethics committees that are often composed of people with backgrounds in quantitative research, qualitative proposals must conform to some extent with these people's expectations of what constitutes a 'proper' research proposal. Even though qualitative research has moved a long way into the postmodern era, too much creativity at this stage of the research may result in obstruction to the proposed research at the outset. Therefore, it is important that the body of qualitative proposals is written carefully, clearly and with a sound rationale for all of the proposed steps in the project.

Title

Be clear about what it is you want to know and why you want to know it, to give the research a title. For example, the project title can be simply:

Improving Nursing and Midwifery Practice with Action Research and Reflection

Background

Sometimes a background statement precedes the literature review, to set the context for how the ideas for the proposed research project came into being. It basically answers the question: What are the researchers' interests in doing this project? For example:

When I visited rural hospitals in the local region recently to discuss my previous research and my research role in the School of Nursing and Midwifery, nurses and midwives requested opportunities to engage with me in action research and reflection.

The background section includes a literature review or the results of a systematic review of literature, to overview the knowledge gained to date in the area of a research interest. The research studies chosen should relate to the research questions you are trying to answer. The literature review summarizes and critiques the previous relevant research findings and identifies the gaps and weaknesses in what has been researched to date. Primarily, the literature review convinces the target audience that your research is important and timely.

Literature reviews are notoriously easy to critique, but difficult to write. The best way to write better literature reviews is to keep on practising writing them and to continue to collect hints in how to do them more effectively (Garrard, 2010). Remember, there may not be much research-based literature in a highly unusual area of interest, as is the case with qualitative projects that try to push the boundaries of what can be known about phenomena. In this case, the literature can be linked indirectly to the main ideas in the research. Allied, nonspecific articles may inform the research interest and add to the argument of why your project is necessary. Also, some approaches such as grounded theory may claim that their inductive style suggests that literature not be amassed at this stage. This is a good enough stance if it can be substantiated. However, be aware that some people reading the proposal may assume that the failure to present a literature review is a 'cop out' and they may assume you are actually not aware of literature in the area.

Some helpful questions to keep in mind, to ensure a thorough literature review are:

- What is the purpose of the literature review? In other words, what is the relationship between the literature review and the research questions?

- Who has written in the area? What social/occupational roles do they occupy?

- What has been written in the area? What key propositions have been made and do they fall into key areas? What has been seen as problematic and what solutions/strategies/actions have been proposed and/or tested in relation to the area of concern?

- How have other scholars received this material? Has this material been subsumed into existing paradigms? Has it challenged existing theories or does it reinforce present ideas?

- What research projects have been carried out in this area? What methods have been employed and were they appropriate for the research questions investigated?

- What are the major findings of the research projects?

- Are research findings across various studies consistent, conflicting or both?

- What debates have there been about the content (substantive) and approach (methodological) components of these projects?

- What have been the main issues in the debates?

- What important issues appear to be overlooked, and constitute gaps, silences and omissions?

- What are the common threads in the research issues, debates, findings and themes?

- How can these common threads guide an evaluation of the knowledge that has been gathered to date, and how they can be informative for further inquiry?

The literature review or systematic review of the research focus needs to be adjusted to the requirements of the particular proposal. For example, funding bodies will specify strict word limits and the formatting in their form will probably cut off extra words. This means that you will need to get to the heart of the issue as quickly as you can, keeping in mind that citations need to be as recent and relevant as possible. An example of an excerpt of a brief literature review incorporated into an ethics submission is:

> Nurses and midwives work in busy healthcare settings, facing work constraints and issues on a daily basis, which challenge their value systems and impede their best efforts to deliver quality care (Freshwater, Taylor and Sherwood, 2008). Added to this, their fast-paced workdays preclude possibilities for them to engage in research, or to practice reflectively. Given the imperative for healthcare practitioners to apply best evidence to their practice and to engage in reflective practice, nurses and midwives can benefit greatly from being facilitated in action research and reflection, by experienced researchers, who come to them in their immediate work contexts, to assist them in collaborative research. The research methodology has been used successfully in previous projects (for example, Rowley and Taylor, 2011; Taylor, Edwards, Holroyd, Unwin and Rowley, 2005; Taylor, Bulmer, Hill, Luxford, McFarlane and Stirling, 2002), leading to improved nursing practice. Given the infinite possibilities for clinical challenges and the potential of participatory research approaches to assist, this project is timely and important.

The references may be included in the proposal immediately after the literature review, or may appear in an appendix attached to the proposal. You will find the references for this literature review at the end of this chapter.

Research aims and objectives

Aims are overall research intentions and objectives are specific subsets of the intentions. Objectives are the specific research intentions, which you write in answering the question: In order to do what? For example:

> This project aims to facilitate action research and reflective processes for experienced Registered Nurses and Midwives, in order to:
>
> - raise their critical awareness of practice problems they face every day;
> - work systematically through problem solving processes, to uncover constraints against effective nursing and midwifery care; and
> - improve the quality of care given by nurses and midwives, in light of the identified constraints and possibilities.

Significance

At this point, a statement may be made about the potential significance of the project. The statements of significance inform readers why this research is worthwhile, because of the successful outcomes you are anticipating. For example:

> The project is significant because it has the potential to improve healthcare by facilitating an action research and reflection process, on site, with registered nurses and midwives. Experiencing the use of action research and reflective practice in this project will give the nurses and midwives the 'research tools' they require to undertake their own collaborative research projects in the future. Therefore, the project will not only serve as a medium for immediate improved practice, but also serve a lifelong educative process for nurses and midwives for ongoing cycles of future practice improvements.

Research questions

Specific questions related to the research objectives may be posed at this point, which indicate the problem focus you are taking in the research. Questions of this nature may not be appropriate in all qualitative proposals, because some creative approaches may use participatory processes in which the project evolves, as participants work collaboratively to raise questions as the research moves through phases and group processes. If you are unsure of your research questions, look at the project objectives and adjust these statements to questions. For example:

- What are the practice problems nurses and midwives face every day?
- What constraints weigh against effective nursing and midwifery care?
- How can nurses and midwives improve the quality of the care they give, in light of the identified practice constraints and possibilities?

Methodology

In qualitative research, methodology usually refers to the theoretical assumptions underpinning the choice of research methods and processes. The term can become confused with its use in quantitative research, which uses methodology to mean the research design. In qualitative research, the equivalent to a research design is a research plan, although some researchers may not bother with making that distinction.

As we discovered in Part One of this book, there are many philosophical traditions that lend their epistemological assumptions to qualitative research inquiry. The originating philosophies all have something different to say about how knowledge is generated and validated, so they create new and adapted knowledge by looking through their particular paradigmatic lenses. To do this, they use the methods and processes that are most likely to gather the type of data they need. Therefore, the epistemological assumptions of particular methodologies directly influence the selection of research methods and processes. Qualitative researchers tend to identify with a methodological position and give a rationale in the research proposal for why the theoretical ideas fit with the aims and objectives of their project. For example:

> The methodology of choice for this project was action research and reflection. In any healthcare profession involving complex practices involving knowledge, skills and human connection, there are many opportunities for using reflection and action research as a collaborative research approach. Nursing has used reflective processes for some time to improve practice (Thorpe and Barsky 2001; Stickley and Freshwater 2002; Johns, 1999), clinical supervision (Todd and Freshwater 1999; Heath and Freshwater 2000; Gilbert 2001), education (Freshwater 1999a, 1999b; C. Johns 2000; Platzer et al. 2000a) and research (Freshwater 2001; Taylor 2001). Midwifery is also a rich source of reflection and midwives have been encouraged to use reflective processes to inform and improve their practice (Taylor 2002a, 2002b).
>
> Kurt Lewin (1946) first used the term 'action research' when in the mid-1940s he used a group research process for community projects in post-war America. Action research goes to the site of the concern or practice and works with the people there as co-researchers, to generate solutions to the problems with which they are keen to deal. Action research involves a four-stage process of collectively planning, acting, observing and reflecting (Dick 1995; Stringer 1996). Each phase leads to another cycle of action, in which the plan is revised, and further acting, observing and reflecting is undertaken systematically, to work towards solutions to problems of a technical, practical or emancipatory nature (Kemmis and McTaggart 1988; Taylor 2000). Cycles of action research lead to further foci and co-researchers can keep an action research approach to their work for as long as they choose, to find solutions to their practice problems.

Reflective processes and action research combine well to create an effective collaborative qualitative research approach for identifying and transforming clinical issues, because reflection is part of the action research method of planning, assessing, observing and reflecting. Reflection is drawn out especially in this combined approach of collaborative research, because this distinction gives more importance to the role of reflective processes in helping practitioners to make sense of their practice and to bring sustained improvements to it.

Ethics

Human research cannot proceed without ethical clearance. In all human research it is necessary to provide a full account of ethical considerations to be given to participants, including informed consent to ensure their privacy and anonymity, and the assurance that they can choose to withdraw from the research at any time, without penalty. Full ethical clearance will need to be sought from participating institutions. It is usual to submit a full research plan, including ethical statements, a plain language statement and a consent form for each category of participants.

Organizations will have ethical approval forms to complete, which are often accompanied by detailed guidelines. Follow the guidelines and complete the form carefully, ensuring you respond to all the necessary sections. If you have had previous experience with ethics committees you probably know already that it is not easy to get an approval on the first attempt. An ethics submission you thought was very clear can attract a lot of comments and questions, all of which need to be clarified for the committee members. Ethical assurances may include, but are not limited to, these sorts of statements:

The group sharing process will involve participants talking confidentially with the other group members about de-identified practice incidents, in which events did not happen as participants might have ideally chosen. Sometimes, the 'space' to speak honestly and be heard supportively in a safe group environment, may cause clinicians to experience emotional catharsis in the form of laughter, or sometimes, tears. In the case of tears being shed, there will be respectful silence and, as facilitator, I will model to the other members how to thoughtfully manage the situation. The plans to minimise the risks associated with emotional catharsis, as shown possibly by tearfulness are to: acknowledge the potential sign of emotional discomfort; check to see if the assumption of discomfort is correct (the participant might explain that the tears mean joy, relief, pride, etc.); and offer 'time out' and privacy. If it eventuates that the tearfulness represents deeper emotional concerns, in a private place away from the group, I will offer my emotional support as an experienced facilitator and counsellor. If my emotional support is insufficient, I will advise the participant of professional, no-cost counselling services within the community, for example (contact details of local counselling services). In the unlikely event of unforeseeable extreme emotional discomfort (i.e., there have been no such cases in previous, similar projects) requiring professional counselling, I will remind the participant of their right to withdraw from the project, should they choose, with no coercion. In such a case of wanting to withdraw from the project, I will suggest professional counselling, and offer to maintain regular phone or in-person contact re their ongoing emotional welfare, but only if they wish it to be so.

Any distress, embarrassment or other harm that might be caused when the data is reported, will be prevented by: participants being fully aware of the aims and objectives of the project; identifying participants by pseudonyms only, only sharing de-identified practice stories and reflections in the group; participants assisting in writing, checking and approving all drafts of reports and publications; and by reporting de-identified results only in publications and conference presentations.

Pseudonyms will be used in place of participants' names in publications. As action research is a medium for teaching co-researchers how to write for publication and they are named on publications according to their contribution, complete privacy will not be possible. Therefore, every attempt will be made to hide their identities within the text of the publication and to conceal any other identifiable person, or organisation connected to the project, by using broad terms, e.g., 'the hospital, 'the participant', 'the patient'. Also, before submission to journals, participants will read all drafts of publications to ensure that they, and all other associated details, have been de-identified sufficiently.

Data collected will be stored in accordance with X University regulations, kept on university premises, in a locked filing cabinet for five years. The researcher only will have access to the information.

Sampling and participant recruitment

Sampling procedures for qualitative and quantitative projects differ, because decisions about who will be involved as research participants are based on different assumptions about knowledge generation and validation. Unless the project is part of a mixed methods design, it will be rare (I dare not claim impossible) for you to see a qualitative project intentionally seeking a representative sample drawn from a research population. Strict, specific sampling criteria apply for quantitative projects, to ensure a representative 'catch' of all the people comprising a specific population, in order to make generalizable claims at the completion of the project.

Qualitative researchers assume knowledge is dynamic and context dependent, therefore, it is not generalizable to all or most cases (people, human situations). Qualitative researchers do not attempt stringent sampling procedures, because they are interested in purposively gaining localized, personal accounts from people who have experienced a particular phenomenon and are willing to speak about it. If more participants are needed in the sample the people already in the project are invited to suggest other people who may be interested, so in this way the sample 'snowballs' until the numbers are sufficient. A purposive and snowballing sampling approach in qualitative projects immediately attracts claims of bias from quantitative researchers, who insist on objective approaches to prevent researchers and participants prejudicially contaminating a sample.

Having gained a sense of who might be the best participant group to inform the research questions, recruitment methods and processes will include determining the specific inclusion and exclusion criteria, such as gender, age range and other relevant factors. The proposal also describes the means by which participants will be invited into the project. For example,

> Purposive sampling will be used to target intentionally experienced female and male RNs and RMs, in an age range of 25 to 65 years, who are interested in using action research and reflecting in their practice, in order to improve it. I will send copies of the Explanatory Statement to the RNs' and RMs' managers in hospitals, who will distribute them to the nurses' and midwives' ward settings. Interested RNs and RMs will respond to me via email or phone contact, as indicated on the Explanatory Statement. If recruitment is slow or delayed, I will seek permission from the Director of Nursing to go to the hospital and speak to nurses and midwives at their respective clinical meetings, to explain the project and the benefits and (low) risks of their involvement.

It may be necessary to provide a rationale for the sampling methods and the number of participants, especially if the proposal is likely to be judged against empirico-analytical criteria, where large numbers are required for statistical significance. The extent to which you will need to produce a strongly referenced rationale to HREC or funding body members will depend on the likelihood of it being needed. It may be worthwhile checking on the composition of certain committees judging research proposals to see if they are open to and aware of the epistemological assumptions of qualitative research. For example, in justifying purposive sampling you may write something like:

> This research approach is interested in accessing participants who have experience in the research interest. A purposive sampling method is appropriate, because participants will be sought intentionally for their ability to inform the research from accounts of their personal experiences.

You may decide that it is wise to give a sound set of reasons for what may be construed by some audiences as a 'small sample size'.

> Up to 10 nurses and midwives will be invited to participate in the action research and reflection groups. The number of participants is appropriate,

because successful group processes rely on active participation and no more than 10 participants will enhance opportunities for participants' contributions to the group. Also, in qualitative research generally, the focus is on the richness and quality of the research process and the data collected, not on high participant numbers and the quantity of data.

Data collection

Data are the collections of information gained from using methods and processes to gather them in. Data collection choices depend on the type and amount of information you need. There are so many data collection methods and processes from which to choose, so rather than rush and make an ad hoc grab at them, spend some time in thoughtfully selecting the best ones for your project. For an overview of the possibilities, look at the rest of the chapters in Part II of this book. A good way to organize your thinking about the best data collection methods and processes, is to work through certain questions systematically and thoroughly. For example:

- What are the project's aims and objectives?
- What are the research questions?
- What is the methodological positioning of this project?
- What methods and processes fit with the methodology and give me the best possible chance of answering the research questions?

The best choices about methods and processes you make are those that are congruent with every aspect of the overall project. For example:

Over a 16-week period, the RNs' and RMs' action research groups will meet weekly with me, for one hour, on a negotiated day and time and in a mutually agreed venue within the hospital, to discuss clinical problems they raise in their journal writing and in group discussion. The data collection activities embedded in the group processes are:

In the first two meetings I will orient the participants to action research and reflective practice principles. We will also discuss how they will work together as a group (e.g., the need for confidentiality and trust in the group, freedom to speak honestly without animosity, and the need to feel free to name and challenge any behaviour within the group, which is not in keeping with the mutually agreed collaborative processes).

RNs and RMs will be given opportunities to write de-identified journal reflections of practice experiences. As is the case with all nursing and midwifery care, the details of patients' care will be completely confidential. No patient names will be used in group discussion, in journal writing or as transcribed data for the project report and publication.

The participants' practice reflections will be shared verbally in the group meetings.

The researcher will guide the group in a collective thematic analysis approach, to critically analyse the content of all the shared practice stories and identify common themes and issues in their nursing or midwifery practice.

A theme common to all of the reflections will be identified as the thematic concern (issue) as an action research focus for the respective group.

Action cycles of planning, assessing, observing and reflecting will generate an action plan for addressing and amending the identified thematic concern.

The action plan will be instituted in nursing or midwifery practice settings as part of the clinician's reflective practice and the results of the changed approach to the thematic concern will be noted, through continued planning, acting, observing and reflecting.

The action plan will undergo revision until it achieves some positive changes in successfully managing the identified thematic concern, to the group's satisfaction.

The research results will be disseminated collaboratively. The researcher will guide participants in how to prepare publications and conference presentations.

Data analysis

The proposal must set out clearly the methods for sorting (analysing) and making sense of (interpreting) the data, so the people judging the merits of the proposal can consider whether your plans for this phase are reasonable in relation to the intentions of the project. For example:

Data analysis will be undertaken collectively in meetings with group participants. The data, in the form of summarized practice stories and reflections, will be gathered by the researcher as meeting notes during meetings. Meeting notes will be verified for accuracy by participants at the beginning of each meeting. Corrections to meeting notes (data) will be made by the researcher, as specified by participants, and presented for participants' verification at the next meeting.

Thematic analysis of journal experiences will be managed by individual and group critical reflection. Group discussion will also be used to identify thematic concerns (practice issues) and the most practical and useful plan of action. Descriptions of participant observation will be analysed by a manual thematic analysis method (Taylor, Kermode and Roberts, 2006). In each action research cycle the findings will be pooled and discussed and the appropriate action will be planned and taken. Successive observation of the effects will follow, before further reflection leads to further action and analysis.

Limitations

At the end of the research plan, acknowledge any weaknesses of the approach that you have chosen. Proposal readers are chosen to be panel members because of their expertise, so they will most likely spot flaws in your plan. Remember though, that you are acknowledging the extent to which your research proposal fits the assumptions of qualitative research. In writing a qualitative research plan you were not intending to develop an objective design, which would be judged against quantitative criteria. Your research plan needs to reflect the central assumptions of your chosen methodology. Consequently, the methods and processes need to be congruent with those epistemological ideas. All too often, qualitative researchers fall into the trap of listing as limitations, the aspects of the project which do not 'measure up' to quantitative expectations, such as sampling deficits, which are in fact sampling *differences*. Be sure then, that what you are identifying as a limitation is a weakness in the application of the chosen qualitative methodology, which you realize could have been stronger in your plan, given other, more ideal circumstances.

Timeframes

The proposal needs to show that you have considered realistic timeframes and that you have planned for the necessary resources to carry out the project effectively. Time management of every research phase and activity will ensure you have allowed enough time to complete the project within the prescribed period. The research proposal will assure the funding body or your authorizing organization that you know what you are going to do, and when. An example of a short timeframe might be as illustrated in Table 11.1.

Table 11.1 An example of a short timeframe

Timing	Activity
Month 1	Finalize ethics approval
Month 2	Recruit participants Begin reflective and action research methods and processes
Month 3	Continue and document action cycles of planning, acting, observing and reflecting
Months 4–5	Facilitate tuition and practice in preparing for professional presentations and publications
Month 6	Submit the journal article(s) and organize presentations

Resources and funding

A good research proposal shows that the physical and human resources have been considered to carry out the project satisfactorily. A section on the background of the researcher, the physical resources and the budget required to run the project will be required by granting agencies and universities.

In the budget section, indicate the costs for all of the materials, personnel and equipment that you will require to carry out the project to a successful completion. The major cost components are direct costs, that is, costs that are specific to the project, and indirect costs or infrastructure costs that are incurred by the institution as a result of supporting your project.

Direct costs are usually salary costs and costs for equipment, materials and procedures. Salary costs are for research personnel, such as secretaries, research assistants and the researcher. They should also include salary costs of clinicians who may be acting as data collectors. Salary costs include a component for on-costs such as annual leave and payroll tax, so check with your financial services personnel, who can advise you as to the appropriate costs to itemize in the budget. There may also be costs for work by non-salaried personnel such as typing, consulting, data entry, and data transcription services. Costs for equipment include any instruments, computer software, equipment such as video cameras or tape recorders, and purchase or rental of computers. Materials include stationery, videocassettes, audiocassettes, postage, report preparation and dissemination. Procedure costs include printing, photocopying and laboratory analysis of data. There may also be other incidental costs such as travel and accommodation.

Indirect costs are 'infrastructure costs', such as the use of the telephone, fax, office, computing time, and so on. Proposals for grants from outside a sponsoring institution will normally include an infrastructure component in the budget. Infrastructure costs are usually calculated by a formula devised by the institution and you should use this formula to calculate any such costs.

If you are applying for a research grant to assist you in completing your project, you will need to give careful consideration to the costs involved. Most granting bodies provide a form for you to complete, outlining costs for the research personnel (research assistants, desktop publishers, clerical assistance and so on); equipment (computer data analysis system, audiotapes and so on); travel at x cents per kilometre; and other costs, such as photocopying, mailing and so on. The grant application guidelines will make it clear what the funding body will or will not fund, so be sure to read the information carefully. Funding bodies want to know about each item of research expenditure in your budget, to know that the money is justified and that you will use it prudently. You need to be as clear as possible in writing this section. For example:

Justification of the budget
Although I will be responsible for the conduct and evaluation of the project, I will need the help of an experienced research assistant (RA), who is also a registered nurse with at least an honours degree. Duties will include assistance in arranging access and consent and helping in the conduct and evaluation of cycles. Two hundred and forty hours of work are needed to assist me in these duties over the action research period (seven hours per week for 34 weeks). The HEW Level 5/1 reflects the level of qualification and experience of a RA with established clinical

competence and a high degree of confidentiality, capable of working with minimal supervision in a sensitive area of research.

The transcription assistant costs reflect the lengthy and tedious process of transcribing audiotapes. It takes three hours to transcribe a one-hour tape, and it must be done by a proficient and reliable person to maintain the integrity of the data. The number of tapes is an estimate for the data-gathering period. High-quality audiotapes are required for safe recording and storing of interview data for analysis.

Dissemination

Dissemination of qualitative research insights and implications is through the usual channels of publications and presentations. Publications include refereed journal articles, books, monographs and theses documents. Presentations can be given at professional conferences, seminars, research workshops, in-service meetings and so on. The proposal should contain a plan for the dissemination of findings, to show that you are aware that the research will be meaningless if the results are not shared with the people who may benefit from them. For example:

> The researcher will teach RNs and RMs how to plan for verbal presentations to peers, and to write for publication in refereed professional journals. A potential target for national presentation is the annual clinical practice conference. Local venues for speaking about the research may also include nurses' seminars at local hospitals and various nurse interest groups in the region. National refereed journals, which could be targeted for publication, include 'Contemporary Nurse' and the 'Australian Journal of Advanced Nursing Practice'. International refereed journals for which the project is suitable include 'The International Journal of Nursing Practice' and 'The International Journal of Nursing'. Articles will be written by a combination of group members, depending on who is interested and willing to expend time and energy in getting quality articles ready for publication. In all presentations and articles each member of the group will receive acknowledgment, although they may not necessarily be listed as contributors if they have not taken a share of the workload for the verbal presentation or written article.

Final elements of a research proposal

The final pages of a research proposal contain supporting materials that relates to the material in the body of the proposal. Principally, these materials are a full reference list and any appendices containing additional material not central to the proposal, but providing additional information and examples.

References

The list of references comes at the end of the proposal, usually before the appendices. Follow the referencing system recommended by the funding body or institution. If you have a choice, use a user-friendly referencing system such as the author–date system (Harvard), because entries can be added, deleted, or changed with a minimum of disruption to the rest of the document. In addition, the reader is able to tell immediately who the author is and when the reference was published. Other systems, such as the footnote (Oxford) system require an adjustment of all following reference numbers whenever a reference is inserted or removed.

Appendices are included if it is necessary to provide extra material. Use appendices judiciously to avoid filling the proposal with unnecessary detail and interrupting the flow of the main text. Include only material that supports or expands on the information in the body of the text, such as participants' explanatory statements, consent forms and letters of support. Start each appendix on a new page and name them alphabetically, i.e. Appendix A, Appendix B and so on.

Trustworthiness issues

Trustworthiness is an alternative term for 'rigour', which is 'strictness in judgement and conduct, which must be used to ensure that the successive steps in a project have been set out clearly and undertaken with scrupulous attention to detail, so that the results/findings/insights can be trusted' (Taylor et al., 2006, p. 400). Achieving trustworthiness criteria ensures research consumers that the project is transparent and it can be investigated for evidence of the worthiness of knowledge claims reflected in methodological accuracy.

Qualitative research is rigorous, but it usually uses words other than reliability and validity, because it is based on different epistemological assumptions, having thrown off quantitative epistemological assumptions of measures for 'truth'. Qualitative researchers' concerns about 'rigour' began with Guba and Lincoln (1981), who suggested renaming of validity and reliability categories into trustworthiness, to reflect the people-oriented nature of qualitative research. Various means of determining 'rigour' in qualitative research have been suggested (Sandelowski 1986; Denzin 1989). There is not one accepted test of 'rigour' in qualitative research, because there is not singular way of doing qualitative research. In the postmodern era, the 'translation' of criteria extends to less structured thinking and the concept of goodness (Emden and Sandelowski, 1998; 1999). This means that qualitative researchers use the most appropriate means of assessing 'rigour', which reflect the methodological assumptions of the project.

In contrast to less-structured postmodern criteria, Denzin (1989) suggested a cross-checking data system of data, investigator, theory and methodological triangulation to converge data sources and thereby create stronger conclusions that could be claimed as 'truth'. Triangulation has become more popular in contemporary times, where postmodern relativism pulls against the increasingly structured design influences of mixed methods research.

Data triangulation uses multiple data sources, such as interviewing many participants about the same topic in a study. Investigator triangulation uses many individuals to collect and analyse a single set of data. Theory triangulation uses many theoretical perspectives to interpret data. Methodological triangulation uses multiple methods such as interviews, document analysis and observation (Taylor et al., 2006, p. 403).

An approach to trustworthiness which falls in between highly structured and detailed triangulation methods and the extreme relativism of postmodern influences has been suggested for some time by Sandelowski (1986), who suggested the criteria of credibility, fittingness, auditability and confirmability.

Credibility means the extent to which participants and readers of the research recognize the lived experiences described in the research as similar to their own. If there is recognition of the phenomenon just from reading about it in the transcripts or research reports, credibility is achieved. Fittingness refers to the extent to which a project's findings fit into other contexts outside the study setting. The term is also used to mean the extent to which the readers of the research find it has meaning and relevance for their own experiences. Auditability is the production of a decision trail, which can be scrutinized by other researchers to determine the extent to which the project has achieved consistency in its methods and processes. A high degree of auditability would allow another researcher to use a similar approach and possibly arrive at similar or comparable conclusions. Confirmability of a project is achieved when credibility, auditability and fittingness can be demonstrated. This relies on the confirmation of participants, whose subjectivity is valued as instructive in assessing the extent to which the project achieves neutrality from the researcher's stated biases (Taylor et al., 2006, pp. 402–403).

Trustworthiness criteria (however named) differ for judging the worth of qualitative research projects, because projects are based on differing epistemological assumptions. This means that the best set of criteria for judging any one project are those that are congruent with (fit with) the assumptions of a specific methodology. Basically, the questions to ask of a project retrospectively to judge its worth are:

- What were the research aims, objectives and questions?
- What was the chosen methodology?
- To what extent did the chosen research methods and processes reflect the project's methodological assumptions about knowledge generation?
- How successful were the chosen methods and processes in fulfilling the aims and objectives and in answering the research questions?
- Did the research insights come directly from the information sources, such as participants' accounts, documents, observations, and so on?
- Were the research insights checked and validated directly with the information sources?
- Were the claims for new or amended knowledge appropriate for the methodology?
- Were the knowledge claims expressed in the language of the methodology?

You will be able to locate specific trustworthiness (validity) criteria for particular methodologies by going to the literature sources and searching for them according to the type of methodology. For example, there are published criteria for grounded theory (Strauss and Corbin, 1998; Charmaz, 2008), historical research (Kincheloe, 2001), ethnography (Fetterman, 2010), phenomenology (Armour, Rivaux and Bell, 2009), narrative inquiry (Dodge, Ospina and Foldy, 2005), case study research (Yin, 2009, 2012), feminisms (Pillow and Mayo, 2012) and action research (Minkler and Wallerstein, 2011).

Suggestions for writing up a project

Having completed the project, it is time to write a report. The specific requirements of research reports vary as to type, so they are written in various documentary forms, such as research theses, research books, monographs and journal articles. A research report is written in the past tense, because it is an account of research events as they unfolded within a project. Locate and follow carefully the specific requirements for writing a research report in the form of a thesis, book, monograph or journal article, as the guidelines will give information about the writing style, referencing, word length, essential inclusions and so on.

Regardless of the type of research report, the best sequence for a research report is the same as for a research proposal, because it ensures you account for each and every aspect of the research, as projected. Rather than rework the research proposal example in this chapter to past tense throughout, the approach I will take in this section is to raise certain questions you can use to check that you have attended to the fundamental requirements of writing a good research report.

Research report preliminaries

- Have you included a title page, an abstract or summary and researchers' details?
- Have you indicated the authors' names, qualifications, postal and email addresses and telephone and fax contact numbers?
- Does the title page of the proposal clearly convey the research focus within the title, by using key words?
- Is the qualitative methodology within the title?
- Does the abstract focus on the project's aims, objectives, methods, processes and outcomes? Is the abstract concise and within a specified word limit?

The body of the research report

- Does the background statement contextualize why the research project came into being?

- Is the literature review an amalgam of the original literature plus that which has come to light since the project began?
- Does the literature review summarize and critique the previous relevant research findings and identify the gaps and weaknesses in what has been researched to date?
- Do the research aims and objectives convey the specific research intentions?
- Is there a clear, appropriate claim for the successful outcomes (significance) of the project?
- What were the research questions?
- Are the methodological assumptions described?
- How did the methodology relate to this project?
- From which committees was ethical approval gained for the project?
- Are the ethical issues and ramifications described fully?
- Is the sampling technique explained?
- Are the participant recruitment methods and processes discussed?
- Are the data collection methods and processes described and congruent with every aspect of the overall project?
- Are the data analysis methods and processes described and congruent with the methodology of choice?
- Whose writing informed the choice of analysis?
- What were the steps in the analysis?
- Who did the analysis; that is, was it done by an individual or by a group?
- How did the individual/group go about doing the analysis?
- How were the data organized when they reached analysed form?
- Are the research insights (interpretations, results, findings) described in detail?
- What were the sub-themes/collective themes/competing discourses?
- Does the report reflect faithfully the roles and contributions of all the people in the research to data analysis and interpretation?
- Who made the interpretations?
- How were the interpretations made?
- What interpretations were made?
- How were the interpretations validated?
- Are excerpts of actual dialogue between researchers/co-researchers/participants quoted as sources of data validation?

- Are suggestions/recommendations offered for readers in practice, education, administration and research?

- Are the project's limitations acknowledged in relation to the chosen methodology?

- Have the trustworthiness issues and strategies been discussed in relation to the chosen methodology?

- Does the report demonstrate that the final discussion and conclusions are congruent with the overall plan, methods and processes of the research?

Final elements of a research proposal

- Are the references complete and in the required referencing style?

- Are the required appendices included?

The questions listed in this section are indicative of questions you may ask of yourself as a writer of a research report. Other questions and requirements may arise, dependent on your overall research plan and how it played out over the course of the project. A good way to learn how to write comprehensive research reports is to read as many of them as you can, in their various forms. You will soon start to see that research reports have a particular style and tone and that various inclusions are essential. As this is the first means of disseminating the overall research results, a well-written research report will begin to communicate the details of your project and possibly influence readers' thinking and practices, if the research insights and implications resonate with them.

Conclusion

In this chapter I revised the process of developing a research proposal, in relation to a project's title, background, aims, objectives, questions, methodology, ethical considerations, participant sampling and recruitment, and data collection and analysis. Proposal development was also discussed in relation to a project's limitations, timeframes, resources and funding. The chapter concluded with a discussion of trustworthiness issues, and offered suggestion for writing up a project.

Key points

- Methods and processes are 'free agents', able to roam across a variety of qualitative methodologies, because they do not 'belong' to a specific theoretical tradition.

- The methods and processes qualitative researchers use in collecting and analysing data depend on their choice of methodology.

- The research methods and processes merge into a meshwork of what researchers are doing and how they are doing it, according to the methodological assumptions of the specific approach and in accord with the research aims, objectives and questions.

- A successful qualitative research project often reflects the due care researchers take in thinking the research through initially, developing a thorough research plan, considering trustworthiness issues and in disseminating the insights and implications.

- A qualitative research proposal is a written account of a plan for the project, which presents an argument for why the project is necessary, the choice of methods and processes to facilitate it, and a guide for action over the time of the project.

- Developmental ideas may begin with spontaneous suggestions and sketchy strategies, which are then refined to fit the specific requirements of a manageable project within personnel, cost and time constraints.

- When the initial ideas firm up, the plan helps the researcher to design and organize the project carefully from the title of the research to research report dissemination details.

- The audience for whom the proposal is aimed must be identified, as these people have the power to approve or reject the proposal.

- The research proposal preliminaries usually include the title page, an abstract or summary and researchers' details.

- The body of qualitative proposals describe the research aims, objectives, questions, significance, data collection and analysis methods and processes, limitations and trustworthiness issues.

- The final elements of a research proposal are the references and appendices.

- A research report is written in the past tense as an account of past research events.

- Specific requirements for writing a research report differ according to whether it is a thesis, book, monograph or journal article.

- Regardless of the type of research report, the best sequence for a research report is the same as for a research proposal, because it ensures a comprehensive account of the research, as projected.

Critical review questions

1 Why is it important to ensure that each and every aspect of a qualitative research proposal is covered?

2 To what extent is it possible to follow *exactly* every projected aspect of a qualitative research proposal?

References

Armour, M., Rivaux, S.L., & Bell, H. (2009). Using context to build rigor: Application to two hermeneutic phenomenological studies. *Qualitative Social Work*, 8(1), 101–122.

Charmaz, K. (2008). Reconstructing grounded theory. In P. Alasuutari, L. Bickman & J.B. Brannen (Eds.) *The SAGE handbook of social research methods*. Thousand Oaks: Sage.

Denzin, N.K. (1989). *The research act*. New York: McGraw Hill.

Dick, R. (1995). A beginner's guide to action research. *ARCS Newsletter*, 1(1), 5–9.

Dodge, J., Ospina, S.M., & Foldy, E.G. (2005). Integrating rigor and relevance in public administration scholarship: The contribution of narrative inquiry. *Public Administration Review*, 65(3), 286–300.

Emden, C., & Sandelowski, M. (1998). The good, the bad and the relative: Conceptions of goodness in qualitative research: Part one. *International Journal of Nursing Practice*, 4(4), 206–612.

Emden, C., & Sandelowski, M. (1999). The good, the bad and the relative: Conceptions of goodness in qualitative research: part two. *International Journal of Nursing Practice*, 5(1), 2–7.

Fetterman, D.M. (2010). *Ethnography: Step by step*. Thousand Oaks: Sage.

Freshwater, D. (1999a). Clinical supervision, reflective practice and guided discovery: Clinical supervision. *British Journal of Nursing*, 8(20), 1383–1389.

Freshwater, D. (1999b). Communicating with self through caring: the student nurse's experience of reflective practice. *International Journal of Human Caring*, 3(3), 28–33.

Freshwater, D. (2001). Critical reflexivity: A politically and ethically engaged method for nursing, *NT Research*, 6(1), 526–537.

Freshwater, D., Taylor, B., & Sherwood, D. (2008). *International textbook of reflective practice in nursing*. United Kingdom: Blackwell.

Garrard, J. (2010). *Health sciences literature review made easy: The matrix method* 3rd edn. Sudbury, MA: Jones & Bartlett.

Gilbert, T. (2001). Reflective practice and supervision: Meticulous rituals of the confessional. *Journal of Advanced Nursing*, 36(2), 199–205.

Guba, E., & Lincoln, Y. (1981). *Effective evaluation*. San Francisco: Jossey-Bass.

Heath, H., & Freshwater, D. (2000). Clinical supervision as an emancipatory process: Avoiding inappropriate intent. *Journal of Advanced Nursing*, 32(5), 1298–1306.

Johns, C. (1999). Reflection as empowerment? *Nursing Inquiry*, 6(4), 241–249.

Johns, C. (2000). Working with Alice: A reflection. *Complementary Therapies in Nursing and Midwifery*, 6, 199–303.

Kemmis, S., & McTaggart, R. (Eds.) (1988). *The action research planner*, 3rd edn. Geelong: Deakin University Press.

Kincheloe, J.L. (2001). Describing the bricolage: Conceptualizing a new rigor in qualitative research. Qualitative Inquiry, 7(6), 679–692.

Lewin, K. (1946). Action research and minority issues. *Journal of Social Issues*, 2, 34–46.

Minkler, M., & Wallerstein, N. (2011). *Community-based participatory research for health: From process to outcomes*. San Francisco: Jossey-Bass.

Pillow, W.S., & Mayo, C. (2012). Feminist ethnography: Histories, challenges and possibilities. In S.N. Hesse-Biber. *The handbook of feminist research: Theory and praxis* 2nd edn. Thousand Oaks: Sage, 187–205.

Platzer, H., Blake, D., & Ashford, D. (2000a). Barriers to learning from reflection: A study of the use of groupwork with post-registration nurses. *Journal of Advanced Nursing*, 31(5), 1001–1008.

Rowley, J., & Taylor, B. (2011). Dying in a rural residential aged care facility: An action research and reflection project to improve end-of-life care to residents with a non-malignant disease. *International Journal of Nursing Practice; 17*, 591–598.

Sandelowski, M. (1986). The problem of rigour in qualitative research. *Advances in Nursing Science, 8*(3), 27–37.

Stickley, T., & Freshwater, D. (2002). The art of loving and the therapeutic relationship. *Nursing Inquiry, 9*(4), 250–256.

Strauss, A.L., & Corbin, J.M. (1998). *Basics of qualitative research: Techniques and procedures for developing grounded theory.* Thousand Oaks: Sage.

Stringer, E.T. (1996). *Action research: A handbook for practitioners.* Thousand Oaks: Sage.

Taylor B.J., (2000) *Reflective practice: A guide for nurses and midwives.* St Leonards: Allen and Unwin.

Taylor, B.J., (2001) Identifying and transforming dysfunctional nurse–nurse relationships through reflective practice and action research. *International Journal of Nursing Practice, 7*(6), 406–413.

Taylor, B.J. (2002a). Technical reflection for improving nursing and midwifery procedures using critical thinking in evidence based practice. *Contemporary Nurse, 13*(2–3), 281–287.

Taylor, B.J. (2002b). Becoming a reflective nurse or midwife: Using complementary therapies while practising holistically. *Complementary Therapies in Nursing and Midwifery, 8*(4), 62–68.

Taylor, B.J., Bulmer, B., Hill, L., Luxford, C., McFarlane, J., & Stirling, K. (2002) Exploring idealism in palliative nursing care through reflective practice and action research. *International Journal of Palliative Nursing 8*(7): 324–330

Taylor, B.J., Edwards, P., Holroyd, B., Unwin, A., & Rowley. J. (2005). Assertiveness in nursing practice: An action research and reflection project. *Contemporary Nurse, 20*(2), 324–347.

Taylor, B.J., Kermode, S., & Roberts, K. (2006). *Research in nursing and healthcare: Evidence for practice*, 3rd edn, Thomson, Australia.

Thorpe, K., & Barsky, J. (2001). Healing through self-reflection. *Journal of Advanced Nursing, 35*(5), 760–768.

Todd, G., & Freshwater, D. (1999). Reflective practice and guided discovery: Clinical supervision, *British Journal of Nursing, 8*(20), 1383–1389.

Yin, R.K. (2009). *Case study research: Design and methods.* 4th edn. Thousand Oaks: Sage.

Yin, R.K. (2012). *Applications of case study research.* Thousand Oaks: Sage.

12

Interviewing and analysis

Bev Taylor

When qualitative researchers consider their projects they usually begin with some general ideas of the research aims, questions and significance. After the *what* and *why* ideas have taken some shape, *how* questions usually arise, leading to decisions about methods and processes. Given that qualitative researchers are interested in people's individual and collective experiences, interviews are often used to gather participants' experiential accounts as data.

Interviews are versatile, serving as effective information collection methods across the whole range of qualitative research methodologies, from grounded theory to projects influenced by poststructural and postmodern thinking. Consequently, there is a wide range of texts (e.g., Bourgeault, Dingwall and de Vries, 2010; Denzin and Lincoln, 2011; Gubrium, Holstein, Marvasti and McKinney, 2012; Hesse-Biber and Leavy, 2011) available for gathering and analysing interview data, much of which 'dives in at different places', to focus on various aspects of interviewing.

In order to contextualize the various descriptions of qualitative interview, this chapter begins by outlining some fundamental ideas, such as the types of interviews, according to their different degrees of structure, depth, approximation and sensitivity. Undertaking interviews with research participants also varies according to the nature of the projects for which they are selected. Consequently, some interviews are named according to specific methodologies, for example, narrative interviewing, feminist interviewing, and so on. To demonstrate the methodological versatility of qualitative research interviews, this chapter explores various methodological adaptations in methods and processes for undertaking interviews. Interview analyses also vary according to the knowledge assumptions of the various methodologies in which they are used, therefore, the chapter concludes with examples of analytic strategies.

Types of interviews

This book assumes that you have already made progress in your research studies and projects, but given the proliferation of literature on interviewing, you may benefit from a review of some ideas about types of interviews, described according to contemporary thinking. Interviews have typically been described in various ways, according to features relating to their structure, depth, and interviewer–interviewee approximation. More recently, the degree of project and participant sensitivity in interviewing, and specific methodological considerations relating to interviewing, are also receiving attention.

Interview structure

In general, the degree of interview structure varies from highly structured to relatively unstructured, with various gradations of structure in between. Unsurprisingly, the degree of structure relates to the underlying intentions for collecting interview information and the epistemological assumptions of the chosen research methodology.

Structured interviews are conducted with a list a predetermined questions, asked by trained interviewers, who use a standardized approach and formal tone. The uniformity in approach to structured interviews often, but not always, reflects the epistemological assumptions of positivistic and post-positivistic approaches that value knowledge gained through objective, standardized and controlled means. Although structured interviews reflect an intention to gather information uniformly to prevent bias from contaminants such as subjectivity and spontaneity, structured interviews are 'making a comeback' to qualitative research within some 21st-century quasi-qualitative, qualitative and mixed methods research approaches.

Quasi-qualitative approaches are essentially quantitative research approaches deigning to be qualitative, by virtue of a descriptive design. There is evidence of conceptual slippage in what constitutes qualitative, when researchers label as qualitative, data gained in surveys and questionnaires, which have descriptive elements. Likert scales and open-ended items attached to questions in a structured interview guide do not gather rich qualitative data. Structured, open-ended survey questions gather data which can be analysed into rudimentary themes and organized into percentages of incidences. Other valid and reliable instruments used in quantitative descriptive designs may also collect language-based data, but these data do not, in themselves, constitute qualitative research. On the whole, structured interviews are suitable for quasi-qualitative approaches, because they use a list of multiple, closed and/or open-ended questions, which could just as effectively be posed in a survey or questionnaire. If the intention is to ask as many people as possible about focused areas of interest, the question needs to be asked: Why bother with interviews at all, when surveys and questionnaires may be less work intensive, less expensive, and more amenable to quantification?

Categorical distinctions blur in the postmodern era. Where we may have reasonably argued that structured interviews 'belong' in quantitative and quasi-qualitative projects, researchers working within established qualitative methodologies may choose relatively structured interviewing methods and processes, based on their attention to rigour within their preferred methodology. For example, the feminisms are generally considered to lie within the qualitative research paradigm, but they are plural because they constitute many types, ranging from relatively objective to highly abstract approaches (Olesen, 2011). Feminists working within the empirical paradigm, asking research questions that require quantitative methods to find objective answers, may choose to use structured interviews for gathering and analysing data.

Mixed methods research can use any degree of structure in the interview component. Given the alignment of methods most often used to gather information from different epistemological standpoints, however, the choice is open to mixed methods researchers to use structured interviews, especially if the project has a large sample, multi-site, multi-national design. In large-size projects, structured interviews may give mixed methods researchers some confidence that questions have been asked with some degree of uniformity, and with a sharpened focus on the research aims and objectives, so comparisons can be made between data sets (Creswell, 2011; Morse, 2012; Tashakkori and Teddlie, 1998, 2010).

Semi-structured interviews have some guiding questions, but not too many, when the intention is to draw out participants' descriptions of their lived experiences using relatively informal processes. The underlying epistemological assumption in seeking participants' lived accounts from semi-structured interviews is that the information gathered constitutes valid and valuable knowledge, relative to participants' unique contexts of time, place and personal experiences.

The guiding questions in semi-structured interviews reiterate the project's focus and invite participants to give a spontaneous, relatively uninterrupted 'free flow of consciousness'. If participants diverge too far from a research interest, researchers can use short communicative deflections, such as: 'You were saying before ...' If participants are hesitant to speak, or they are having difficulty in maintaining a steady flow of ideas, researchers may use prompts, such as: 'You mentioned before ... can you tell me more about that please?' and so on. If participants are clear about the research focus and their part in it, they usually respond with generous, focused accounts to semi-structured interview questions.

Unstructured interviews give an invitation to speak on a topic, followed with silence or little more than the hint of a focus, when the informal interviewing process intends to open up what emerges from a well of individual or collective life stories. Unstructured interview methods and processes are often, but not always, based on postmodern epistemological assumptions that people are the owners and authors of their own experiences and personal knowledge. Based on these relativistic epistemological assumptions, researchers are relatively silent in unstructured interviews, using nothing more than the nod of a head and other non-verbal cues to encourage participants to continue their accounts. Although there is no prescription for their use in qualitative research, unstructured interviews are used in projects where participants' experiential knowledge is valued as paramount to the research focus (Gubrium et al., 2012).

Interview depth

Interestingly, when classifying interviews according to depth, there is little or no mention of increasing degrees of depth. To engage in depth discussions infers that some interviews can be superficial or shallow, and even if these distinctions are honest in some cases, these qualifiers suggest that shorter, briefer, depth-lacking interviews are of no real value. The literature speaks mainly of in-depth interviews, inferring, but not necessarily owning the possibility, that other forms of interviews are 'less than deep'.

Linguistic conventions aside, interviews move qualitative researchers into an ocean of knowledge, 'fishing' for information at various depths. Extending the metaphor of an ocean of knowledge made accessible through qualitative interviews, there are three possible types of interview based on depth: 1) overview interviews, consistent with the shallows; 2) intermediate interviews, with the depth of reefs and shoals; and 3) in-depth interviews, with the potential of the deep ocean.

Overview depth interviews seek varying breadths of information, but the methods and processes skim across the surface of a topic, sometimes floating in ideas, and sometimes sitting in the shallows to note the ideas that swirl past. Overview interviews can be used to gather demographic information as an alternative to a short answer survey, or when initial interviews are being used to ascertain the participants' fit with inclusion criteria.

Intermediate depth interviews seek varying breadths of information with some degrees of detail and immersion, as they wade out and begin to leave safe, overview interview depths. Intermediate interviews are characteristic of projects seeking participants' experiential accounts, but not at depths that require them to respond beyond their basic recollections.

In-depth interviews go beyond the shallows and reefs, to dive deeply in participants' experiential accounts, to discover hitherto unreflected knowledge, with the potential for rich insights and research implications. The depth gained in in-depth interviews is not by the number of questions, but by participants' thoughtful attention to an invitation, posed informally and with open-endedness, to encourage them to feel free to reveal as much as they can about an area of interest.

Interview approximation

Interview structure and depth differences have traditionally been used to distinguish the various types of formal and informal interviews, but in this highly technological era, approximation is another consideration. Approximation, in relation to interviews, refers to the proximity of the interviewer to the interviewee, such as face to face, or by phone, email, Skype, and so on. Depending on the size and scope of projects, some interviews may be conducted in close approximation face to face, or they may be by distance, by various technological means.

Face-to-face interviews are preferable when it is advisable or convenient for interviewer and participant to be present in the same room. Face-to-face interviews are possibly the most personal and immediate approximation for interviewing, but they may not always be possible, due to constraints relating to a project's size, scope and consequent costs. Sometimes, face-to-face interviews may not be convenient for participants, especially if they are ageing, or if they have disabilities and other personal constraints and preferences, which weigh against them being face to face with a researcher. Whereas it might be reasonable to think that all projects with sensitive content *should* use face-to-face interviews, there are health research examples where interviews were conducted comprehensively and with a high degree of ethical safety, by non-face-to-face approximation (Holt, 2010; McCoyd and Kerson, 2006).

Telephone interviews are a possibility when it is not possible, preferable or necessary to be in the same room for face-to-face interviews. Telephone interviews are generally hands free and on speaker for ease of audiotaping. Not to be confused with telephone interview surveys, which fall arguably into a quasi-qualitative category (e.g., Genovese, 2004), qualitative interviews by telephone are influenced by the methods and processes of face-to-face interviewing, while acknowledging the constraints of the technology (Harris, Kelly, Hunt, Plant, Kelley, Richardson and Sitzia, 2008; Holt, 2010).

The advantages and disadvantages of phone interviews are exemplified well in a study by Harris et al. (2008). As part of a larger study, Harris et al. (2008) undertook telephone interviews with 'elite' Directors of Nursing Services (DNSs), who worked within acute National Health Service (NHS) Trusts in two health regions in Southern England. The DNSs were considered an elite group, because they were executives, and as such, they were deemed to possess authority, knowledge and power by virtue of their role positions. The researchers' reasons for accessing the DNSs for telephone interviews included the relatively low number of participants, who were separated by relatively large distances, and an interview schedule with relatively few questions not geared towards in-depth responses.

After discussing issues related to getting past the DNSs gatekeepers (secretaries, personal assistants, and so on), who usually protect the interests of vulnerable or 'hard to reach' research participants, Harris et al. (2008, p. 243) identified the issue of 'being stripped of the face-to-face interpersonal skills normally used to negotiate difficult situations during interviews – such as facial expressions and gestures to encourage dialogue and assessing the interviewee's response to probe their views further'. Even though they found the telephone interviews 'allowed a franker, more confiding relationship to be rapidly established between two strangers', as researchers they had to adjust rapidly to non-visual cues, such as tone of voice, 'working quickly to establish a dialogue in a short time' (p. 243). They also identified the need for assertiveness, tact and empathy in communication skills, especially in relation to allowing for silence for participants to think and respond.

Harris et al. (2008, p. 244) suggested that the 'emotional demands associated with the conduct of these telephone interviews was found to be significant and a range of interview styles were required from being fairly hard-nosed about the process, which may be likened to people selling over the telephone, to having to draw on all possible interpersonal skills'. The benefits of telephone interviewing identified by Harris et al. (2008) included the collection of more DNSs' perspectives than they originally imagined, plus they were able to access more participants for high quality data, with fewer costs associated with research personnel, time and travel.

Email interviews use computer-mediated recruitment to access participants for sharing their experiences in relation to research foci (Hamilton and Bowers, 2006; Hunt and McHale, 2007; James and Busher, 2006; McCoyd and Kerson 2006). Varying degrees of success have been documented and insights have been gained as to the advantages and disadvantages of email interviews. For example, McCoyd and Kerson (2006, p. 389) used 'computer-mediated recruitment and email intensive interviewing' in a study of 'the decision-making and bereavement process of women, who terminated desired pregnancies after diagnosis of a fetal anomaly'. The researchers' intentions were to include 'isolated, geographically dispersed and/or stigmatized groups who are often overlooked or ignored' in their study, but they experienced ethical and methodological issues related to computerized communication for interviewing.

The study used grounded theory analysis methods, which revealed 'the tremendous grief that these women experience in the face of societal silencing'. Email recruitment was chosen when face-to-face and telephone interview recruitment netted poor response rates, so a recruitment letter was posted on a listserv connected with a website called TOPS (Termination of Pregnancy Support). The researchers noted that participants 'recruited through the Listserv letter spontaneously requested email interviews (likely because they received support from one another via emails and a listserv at TOPS)' (p. 390). Approvals and modifications were made to address ethical imperatives, and 'email interviews were used for those who requested them – the majority of the study group' (p. 390). The same interview guide was used for the three interview formats, allowing for a comparison of approaches. Of the three types of interviews – face to face, telephone and email – the researchers claimed that 'email interviews tend to be more complete, to include more self-reflection by respondents, and to be seemingly more candid' (p. 390). These insights show that email interviews can be informal, relatively unstructured and in-depth, even if they focus on sensitive issues at a distance.

McCoyd and Kerson (2006) identified ethical and methodological issues associated with email interviews. Given the sensitive nature of the research, ethical issues were concerns about confidentiality and informed consent. The researchers were keenly aware of the need to de-identify the data and to keep the data secure online. Participants were given full details regarding the project and their participation in it, and electronic signatures and statements of consent were used instead of paper-based forms. Researchers were also highly attentive to cues that participants may have been experiencing emotional stress and discomfort, and they had detailed plans in place to deal with *emotional assessment and referral*. The specific details in view of the potential ethical issues are listed within their research article (McCoyd and Kerson, 2006).

The methodological issues with email interviews related mainly to sampling, concerns to which they responded to their social work and medical colleagues using qualitative sampling rationales and arguments.

There are many advantages to email interviewing including inclusiveness of geographically disadvantaged participants with relative ease of access cheaply and quickly, resulting in larger sample sizes, large amounts of in-depth data and pre-written data for analysis. Even so, email interviewing needs to be undertaken cautiously. Researchers warn that email interview 'users must take account of a number of sensitive issues, and there are a number of serious disadvantages that limit its use to specific areas. The e-mail interview cannot be used simply as a cheap alternative to face-to-face interviews in all circumstances' (Hunt and McHale, 2007). There are also methodological issues 'affecting the credibility and trustworthiness of the research design of the studies, and issues around the authenticity of participants' voices and how (they are) affected by power and control in the interview process' (James and Busher, 2006). Hamilton and Bowers (2006, p. 281) have also identified and addressed multiple 'issues of appropriateness, adequacy, representativeness, sample bias, data fraud, flexibility and consistency in interviewing, timing, elimination of the need for transcription, oral versus written communication, reliability and validity, and ethical concerns' relating to Internet recruitment and email interviewing.

Interview sensitivity

The types of qualitative interviews can be differentiated according to their sensitivity, from relatively low to extremely high sensitivity, depending on the research focus, the nature of participants, and researcher–participant processes. Qualitative researchers are often interested in deep accounts of participants' lived experiences, so interviews may be classified as sensitive, depending on the research focus, the nature of the participants, and the researcher–participant relationship.

Sensitive research foci involve projects seeking to explore areas not often disclosed and discussed publicly, which may have ethical and legal implications, such as drug-taking habits, domestic violence, and sexual preferences and health. Projects of a sensitive nature undertaken by health researchers include reproductive issues (McCoyd and Kerson, 2006), sexual activities (Walby, 2010), sexual health (Bischofberger and Vischer, 2010; Perry, Thurston and Green, 2004) and sexual assault (Campbell, Adams, Wasco, Ahrens and Sefl, 2009, 2010).

For example, Campbell et al. (2009) undertook face-to-face interviews with adult rape survivors. The researchers wanted to guide the development of interviewer training programmes, so they 'asked survivors what interviewers should know about rape and how they should interact with participants'. The 92 survivors in the study suggested that 'interviewer training needs to emphasize diversity so that researchers are capable of working effectively with individuals with different life circumstances' and 'interviewers need to show warmth and compassion and allow (participants) to exercise choice and control during the interview process' (Campbell et al., 2009, p. 595). In another article relating to the same research, Campbell et al. (2010) analysed the narrative data from the interviews and found that 'the overwhelming majority of survivors found the interview to be a helpful, supportive, and insightful experience' in which 'feminist interviewing principles were noticed and appreciated by the participants and contributed to (participants') overall positive participation outcomes' (p. 60).

Sensitive research participants are those people deemed vulnerable, if they fit within definitions and categories pre-determined by various national and global health research committees. Vulnerable research participant categories vary from country to country, but they are generally agreed to be people who have sensitivities according to: age, such as children and ageing people; condition, such as debilitated and frail people; ethnicity, such as indigenous people and diverse migrant groups; and disadvantage, such as low socio-economic groups, homeless people and minority groups.

For example, Sands, Bourjolly and Roer-Strier (2007) explored cultural barriers between a white non-Muslim female interviewer and an African American Muslim interviewee. This social work research was an opportunity to critically examine a qualitative research interview in terms of 'cultural barriers, warming up, crossing the racial barrier, connecting as social workers, connecting as women, connecting as students, and crossing the tape recorder barrier' (p. 353). In another project, Bischofberger and Vischer (2010) highlighted the challenges they faced when conducting qualitative interviews on HIV prevention and care in a multilingual, transcultural setting with sub-Saharan migrants. Other examples of using interviews in transcultural and culturally sensitive qualitative projects are Winchatz (2006), Birks, Chapman and Francis (2007), and Lagesen (2010).

Researcher–participant sensitivities are associated with projects in which there are relatively high ethical risks when the methodology encourages abstract, dynamic and intersubjective research processes, often reflected in the intentional blurring of traditional researcher–participant roles. In these projects, close relationships and highly participatory processes, attempt to lessen or eradicate researcher–participant power imbalances and participants become co-researchers (DeVault and Gross, 2012). In other interview situations the researchers may already know the participants (McConnell-Henry, James, Chapman and Francis, 2009).

Methodological interviews

Lastly, in this discussion of types of interviews, we arrive at interviews categorized according to their particular methodological assumptions and influences. Extending the definition of methodology in this instance to mean *both* the theoretical assumptions underlying the choice of methods and processes *and* the basics of research design, types of methodological interviews include focus group interviews, case study research, feminist interviews, narrative interviews, ethnographic interviews, and so on. As the methodological distinctions for interviews are associated with congruent analysis methods, these types of interviews are described in the next section.

Conducting and analysing interviews

By way of introduction, this section begins with some thoughts on the various representations of interviews, before reviewing some fundamental considerations when planning to do interviews within qualitative research. Following on from these preliminary contextual discussions, this section moves on to elaborate on some important methodological differences in undertaking and analysing interviews.

Thoughts on representations

Interviews have become so popular in qualitative and mixed methods research that they have been identified as interview research (Gubrium et al., 2012). While interview research is handy keyword in a title for a research text, and a 'catch all' strategy to underscore the technical and epistemological 'complexity of the craft', it seems that interviews have the potential to outstrip epistemological (methodological) 'boundaries'. Rather than be regarded as methods and processes for collecting and analysing information in a wide range of qualitative projects, interviews and interviewing have the potential to become a research approach in and of themselves. The question remains for qualitative researchers: Are we speaking of interview research, or research in which interviews are integral methods and processes?

Taking the view that interviews are not a research approach per se, but the means by which qualitative research projects can be assisted to achieve their purposes, discussions of various representations of interviews continue. For example, as methods and processes, interviews are represented in relation to their methodological congruency, the nature of inquiry developed, and the positioning of researcher and participant in communicative roles within them.

The methods and processes for conducting and analysing interviews depend on their type and the way they function to collect and make sense of information in light of methodological assumptions. When methodological congruency is the underlying principle, interviews can be undertaken and analysed in a thoughtful, intentional manner and not just 'dropped into' a project haphazardly, in the hope of 'catching' comprehensive data.

Roulston's (2010) advice is given to novice interviewers, but it is useful for any researcher who intends to make the best use of interviews. She suggests that the quality of a project and of interviews can be enhanced by

six conceptions of interviewing (she labels) as: neo-positivist, romantic, constructionist, postmodern, transformative and decolonizing. These include:

- What are the theoretical assumptions underlying this conception of interviewing?
- What kinds of research questions are made possible from this perspective?
- What methodological issues are highlighted in the literature in qualitative inquiry with respect to this conception?
- What are criticisms of this conception of interviewing and/or research?
- What kinds of approaches have researchers documented to establish the 'quality' of research using interviews from this conceptualization? (p. 204)

The neo-positivist, romantic, constructionist, postmodern, transformative and decolonizing classifications Roulston (2010) uses fit within broader typologies, such as quantitative (neo-positivist); qualitative interpretive (romantic, constructionist); qualitative critical (transformative); and poststructural, postmodern (decolonizing, postmodern) approaches to research. Specific methodologies can be located within these research approaches, but they do not necessarily stay in stable theoretical positions, so they can be represented as mobile methodologies (Taylor, Kermode and Roberts, 2006).

The mobile nature of some qualitative methodologies necessitates considerable flexibility of thought, when qualitative researchers using interviews are seeking earnestly to reflect the central assumptions of a particular methodology located at a particular point on a paradigmatic continuum. For example, ethnography is a mobile methodology, which can be located along the entire paradigmatic continuum, taking on at one time or concurrently, interpretive, critical, poststructural and postmodern forms. Therefore, a researcher's choices relating to interview methods and processes will differ according to the theoretical assumptions of the type of ethnography chosen, determined beforehand by the intentions of the project, and guided thereafter by the questions to ask and *how* to ask them. If methodological congruency is valued, only then will an ethnographic researcher not only be clear about *how to be* within a culture, but also have clarity about how make sense of participants' interview responses. The discussion of this example is extended later in this section.

Added to considerations of methodological congruency when selecting and enacting interview methods and processes, is a core consideration of the nature of inquiry developed within interviews. Brinkmann (2007) discusses the idea that successful qualitative interviews are not so much geared towards gathering 'mere opinions about a given topic', rather they are discursive methods. The author argues a very simple point, that 'by probing their respondents' experiences and opinions (the *doxa*), interview researchers are often engaged in what seems like a time-consuming kind of opinion polling for which quantitative instruments such as questionnaires often appear to be much more efficient' (p. 1117).

Brinkmann (2007) argues that doxastic interviews are limited in their knowledge generating potential, and that the Socratic dialogical form of

Food for thought

- When deciding on the type of interview, to what extent do I consider the:
  - project's aims, objectives, research questions and potential significance?
  - structure, depth, and interviewer–interviewee approximation?
  - degree of project and participant sensitivity?
  - specific methodological considerations?
  - overall congruency of the project's methodology, methods and processes?
  - practical constraints, such as the availability and location of participants and their personal characteristics and preferences?
  - specific project constraints, such as timelines and funding?
- When getting ready to interview, to what extent do I consider practical necessities, such as:
  - gaining entry to the 'field'?
  - accessing participants?
  - recruiting participants?
  - ensuring participants' full ethical rights?
  - preparing documents and equipment?
  - negotiating a time and place?
  - preparing myself technically and emotionally?
- When undertaking an interview, do I:
  - greet the participant?
  - offer sincere preliminary courtesies?
  - allow time to get 'settled in' together?
  - have in mind a particular communicative process, such as a dialogical, conversational style?
  - begin the interview with an appropriate invitation, opening focus or question?
  - keep in mind a particular communicative process?
  - maintain the natural flow of the interview with appropriate silence, nonverbal encouragement, and occasional communicative encouragement?
  - remain aware of, and manage, potential risks, such as participant's emotional catharsis, physical tiredness, and so on?
  - monitor the practicalities, such as the timing, and 'coverage' of the question(s)?
  - sense completion?
  - explore ongoing plans for the participant's participation?
  - complete the interview with sincere gratitude?

interviewing 'addresses not opinions but knowledge (*episteme*)', so that 'both parties are engaged in dialectically examining a topic, with the aim of gaining knowledge in a normative–epistemic sense' (p. 1116). While qualitative researchers may agree instantaneously with Brinkmann that Socratic interviewing methods and processes are preferable, and they are to some extent the norm, due attention must be paid to interview questions in terms of the what, why, where, when, how and by whom choices for interviews to be successful in knowledge generation.

Ezzy (2010) discusses yet another aspect of interviewing – the emotional dimension. In his argument that interviewing involves 'embodied emotional performance', Ezzy makes apparent a phenomenon within the interviewing process, which can remain invisible and unarticulated, yet it is highly influential in qualitative interviewing processes. Drawing on Benjamin's (1988) psychoanalytic theory of the emotional dimensions or structures of interaction, Ezzy (2010) argues that 'the emotional framing of interviews plays a major role in shaping the content of interviews', making the interview experience into 'either conquest or communion' (p. 163). Essentially, the features of interpersonal communication, including those attitudes, behaviours and ways of being engaged in when interviewing, attain either a conquest or communion outcome.

Eloquently encapsulating the differences between communion and conquest, Ezzy (2010, p. 164) explains

> At the heart of Benjamin's account of knowing as communion is the experience of mutual recognition. This cannot be achieved through seeking obedience or repressing the Other … This contact is a moment of recognition of simultaneous sameness and difference. It requires a recognition that the subject is both independent of the Other and that this independence is dependent on the Other recognizing the subject … this seeming contradiction is a paradox that is never resolved but rather lived out as a constant tension. Mutual recognition is a product of a self-confidence that is also emotionally open to, or dependent on, the Other. Good interviewing, like good romance, engages with precisely the tension between self-confidence and emotional dependence. To ask questions, and to listen to the answers, requires a simultaneous sense of one's own sense of self as an interviewer independent of the interviewee and an openness to, a dependence on, what the interviewee has to say because without this the relationship is impossible. Good interviews are not dominated by either the voice of the interviewer or the agendas of the interviewee. Rather, they feel like communion, where the tension between the research question and the experience of the interviewee is explored.

Ezzy (2010, p. 164) makes the point that 'masculine metaphors of conquest: probing, directing, questioning, active listening' are typically used to direct, control and shape interviews, identifying interviewing as a form of conquest. He argues that 'reflexive awareness of, and engagement with, the emotional, embodied, and performed dimensions of the interview' (Ezzy, 2010, p. 163) allow qualitative researchers to engage in communion with participants, whereby mutual respect, trust and openness lead to deeper, richer insights for researchers and participants alike.

In summary, interviews have become so popular and integral to qualitative research that they have been identified as interview research, implying that they have taken on a research approach status. Various representations of interview methods and processes proliferate, such as those attempting to reflect methodological congruency and others concerned with the nature of the knowledge generating and communicative potential of the interviewing process. While these thoughts on representations of interviews are not exhaustive of various discussions within the literature (Bourgeault, Dingwall and de Vries, 2010; Denzin and Lincoln, 2011; Gubrium, Holstein, Marvasti and McKinney, 2012; Hesse-Biber and Leavy, 2011), they highlight some of the ongoing debates relating to the assumptions, practices and outcomes of using interviews within qualitative research. Regardless of the infinite nuances and possibilities for discussing the representations of interviews and interviewing, some fairly 'generic' practical considerations underlie getting ready for and undertaking interviews.

Fundamental considerations

Practical considerations underlie interviews and interviewing, such as deciding on the type of interview and undertaking the interview. These considerations have been described in detail in other texts (Bourgeault, Dingwall and de Vries, 2010; Denzin and Lincoln, 2011; Gubrium, Holstein, Marvasti and McKinney, 2012; Hesse-Biber and Leavy, 2011, Taylor et al., 2006), so they are outlined here, as a means of reviewing some fundamental aspects, which remain pertinent to qualitative projects undertaken at any level of scope and complexity. Rather than go through each and every point, many of which you may have already applied several times, the outline of practical considerations is posed as a checklist of questions for you to assess how you fare as an interviewer.

There may be more fundamental considerations in getting ready to interview and in conducting interviews than reflected in the questions posed as 'Food for thought'. Interview methods and processes have technical and epistemological intricacies, many of which require attentive consideration. Look beyond simple checklists and one or two sources, to a wide range of strategies and literature, when you are planning interviews in your qualitative or mixed methods project.

Methodological differences

Added to the considerations already discussed in this chapter, interviews and interviewing differ according to the epistemological assumptions of a specific methodology and to the research design in which they are used. Methodologies may differ within their own general classification, for example, there are many, varied feminisms, ethnographies, narrative inquiry approaches, and so on. Research designs differ according to whether they are wholly qualitative or mixed methods, and to the selection of key or combined processes, for example, inductive and/or participatory, collaborative, and/or whatever, and so on. Therefore, the key features of interviews in qualitative methodologies are that they may be selected and enacted to reflect their respective technical and epistemological considerations, but the interview collection and analysis methods and processes are not necessarily prescriptive, exclusive, directive or homogenous.

To exemplify the use of interviews within methodological diversity, this section outlines some differences in convergent, ethnographic, feminist, focus group, life story, mixed methods design, narrative and postmodern trends. This book is devoted to the in-depth description of qualitative methodologies, methods and processes, as are other texts (Bourgeault, Dingwall and de Vries, 2010; Denzin and Lincoln, 2011; Gubrium, Holstein, Marvasti and McKinney, 2012; Hesse-Biber and Leavy, 2011), so in the interests of brevity and comprehensiveness, Table 12.1 provides a comparison of key qualitative methodologies, in relation to their features and possible interview type, methods, processes and analytic strategies, and some useful references for further reading.

The analytic strategies are not strictly prescribed for managing interview data, but researchers tend to reflect the assumptions of their chosen methodology when analysing interviews as transcribed text (Charmaz and Belgrave, 2012; DeVault and Gross, 2012; Nikander, 2012; Riessman, 2012). For example, grounded theory projects using interview data will use grounded theory analysis methods, unless they are really a non-specific type of qualitative research masquerading as grounded theory. Also, some non-specific qualitative projects in search of a structured analysis method use a grounded theory approach to deal with multitudinous data (Charmaz and Belgrave, 2012).

The decision to use a specific methodologically-informed analytic method may be based on a considered, well-articulated rationale, or it may turn out to be loosely applied in a 'hit and miss' fashion. For example, projects claiming to be phenomenological may use semi-structured, relatively deep interviews, but their analytic strategies for interview data turn out to be 'stock standard' approaches, not able to deliver deep illuminative insights into phenomena. Similarly, projects deigning to be ethnographic may use some forms of observation coupled with interviews, but their interview analytic strategies cannot deliver deep descriptions or critiques of cultural groups and their ways of being. If you look for these projects you will find them.

Keeping with the example of grounded theory, the analytic strategies also vary according to the type of grounded theory used, so researchers desiring to maintain a high degree of methodological congruency will use specific methods reflecting the key ideas within a specific type of grounded theory. For example, Charmaz and Belgrave (2012) describe an analytic strategy based on constructivist grounded theory principles, whereas a Glaserian or Strauss and Corbin interview analytic strategy will differ in some respects (refer to Chapter 2 of this book for a comparison).

Another major consideration of interview analysis is the means by which to manage the voluminous data, whether it will be analysed by manual or some form of computer-assisted means. Practicalities of expense, time and effort win out over arguments for detailed manual searches for nuances in interview text, when participant numbers rise and the transcribed data grow exponentially. Qualitative data analysis (QDA) software is useful and indeed necessary in large health and social research projects, and contemporary software systems are becoming increasingly fine-tuned to detect the nuances of various methodological principles (Seale and Rivas, 2012). However, qualitative researchers need to consider QDA carefully, so that qualitative analysis strategies do not become 'the norm'. In the postmodern era when arguments for methodological congruency may be criticized for 'old school' thinking, it is easier for qualitative researchers to become seduced by the logic of 'more data equals better data'. When the mantra becomes 'more interviews result in more interview data to strengthen the rigour of a project', we will have lost sight of the particulars which make philosophies what they are. For example, the phenomenological quest to illuminate a phenomenon does not rely on more data, but on a closer, deeper exploration of what is at hand (refer to Chapter 5 of this book). Therefore, increased numbers of interviews may not be necessary, and manual analytic techniques will be preferable for projects where the epistemological assumptions reflect the ideas that objective truths are suspect, and that inter-subjective meaning is derived from relative, dynamic, partial and contextually interpreted sources.

In summary, decisions about interviews and interviewing are no longer simple or straightforward. Qualitative researchers now have to struggle with technical and epistemological issues, which go well beyond following a comprehensive checklist, to prepare for and undertake interviews, and then find the best means of analysing them. Gubrium et al. (2012) summarize the situation succinctly, when they explain that a 'more reflexive appreciation of knowledge production in general, not just interview knowledge, has prompted a reassessment of the procedures of empirical inquiry, including the interview' (p. 27). The main message to derive from this section is that there is no main message when it comes to interview collection and analysis. Qualitative researchers need to remain mindful of the vast array of possibilities when embarking on projects which feature interviews as knowledge generating sources. To reflect the methodological assumptions of a particular approach, qualitative researchers need to plan and enact careful methods and processes for including interviews in their projects. Otherwise, they may be simply using interviews as an unconsidered means to an end, which may have been reached a lot easier by a well-chosen survey or questionnaire.

Chapter summary

Interviews serve as effective information collecting and knowledge generating methods across the whole range of qualitative research methodologies, consequently, a wide range of sources provide advice on gathering and analysing interview data, much of which 'dives in at different places'. In order to contextualize various descriptions of qualitative interviews and interviewing, this chapter began with some fundamental ideas, such as the types of interviews, according to their different degrees of structure, depth, approximation and sensitivity.

Traditional structural classifications include structured, semi-structured and unstructured, but structural distinctions do not dictate that an interview 'belongs' to a specific qualitative or mixed methods approach. Extending the metaphor of an ocean of knowledge made accessible through qualitative interviews, I suggested that there are three possible types of interview based on depth: 1) overview interviews, consistent with the shallows; 2) intermediate interviews, with the depth of reefs and shoals; and 3) in-depth interviews, with the potential of the deep ocean. In a general sense, the deeper an interview goes into participants' experiential accounts, the deeper insights it reveals about a lived phenomenon.

Approximation refers to the proximity of the interviewer to the interviewee, depending on the size and scope of projects. Therefore, this chapter also described interviews conducted in close approximation face to face, and by distance, by various technological means. Qualitative interviews can be differentiated from relatively low to extremely high sensitivity, so interviews were discussed, in relation to the sensitivity of the research focus, the nature of the participants, and the researcher–participant relationship. Even though researchers may assume that interviews for projects with high sensitivity must be conducted face to face, this is not a solid rule. However, researchers need to be mindful of all the potential ethical risks and be prepared to argue a sound case to human ethics committees for conducting sensitive interviews via distance technologies.

Undertaking interviews with research participants also varies according to the nature of the projects for which they are selected. To demonstrate the methodological versatility of qualitative research interviews, this chapter compared various methodological adaptations in methods and processes for undertaking interviews. Interviews are data collection and knowledge generating methods, which can be used in a variety of qualitative and mixed methods approaches, but they differ according to the methodology for which they are used. In the interests of methodological congruency, researchers decide on the type of interview and the methods and processes to collect and analyse interview data, to best reflect the epistemological assumptions of their chosen methodology.

Key points

- Qualitative researchers are interested in people's individual and collective experiences, so interviews are often used to gather participants' experiential accounts as data.

- Interviews are versatile, serving as effective information collection methods across the whole range of qualitative research methodologies.

- Interviews can be classified according to their structure, depth, interviewer–interviewee approximation, the degree of project and participant sensitivity in interviewing, and specific methodological considerations.

- Decisions about interviews and interviewing are no longer simple or straightforward, because qualitative researchers struggle with technical and epistemological issues, which go well beyond following a comprehensive checklist, to prepare for and undertake interviews, and then find the best means of analysing them.

Critical review questions

1 What are the advantages and disadvantages of collecting interview data?

2 To what extent does interviewing play a part in gathering data for your healthcare profession's key research issues and questions?

References

Benjamin, J. (1988). *The bonds of love: Psychoanalysis, feminism, and the problem of domination.* New York: Pantheon Books.

Birks, M., Chapman, Y., & Francis, K. (2007). Breaching the wall: Interviewing people from other cultures. *Journal of Transcultural Nursing, 18*(2), 150–156.

Bischofberger, I., & Vischer, L.R. (2010). Interviewing sub-Saharan Migrants in Switzerland about HIV/AIDS: Critical reflections on the interview process. *Journal of Transcultural Nursing, 21*(1), 23–28.

Bourgeault, I., Dingwall, R., & de Vries, R. (Eds.) (2010). *The SAGE handbook of qualitative methods in health research.* Thousand Oaks: Sage.

Brinkmann, S. (2007). Could interviews be epistemic? An alternative to qualitative opinion polling. *Qualitative Inquiry, 13*(8), 1116–1138.

Campbell, R., Adams, A.E., Wasco, S.M., Ahrens, C.E., & Sefl, T. (2009). Training interviewers for research on sexual violence: A qualitative study of rape survivors' recommendations for interview practice. *Violence Against Women, 15*(5), 595–617.

Campbell, R., Adams, A.E., Wasco, S.M., Ahrens, C.E., & Sefl, T. (2010). 'What has it been like for you to talk with me today?': The impact of participating in interview research on rape survivors. *Violence Against Women, 16*(1), 60–83.

Charmaz, K., & Belgrave, L.L. (2012). Qualitative interviewing and grounded theory analysis. In Gubrium, J.F., Holstein, J.A., Marvastii, A.B., & McKinney, K.D. (Eds.). *The SAGE handbook of interview research: The complexity of the craft.* 2nd edn. Thousand Oaks: Sage, 347–366.

Creswell, J.W. (2011). Controversies in mixed methods research. In Denzin, N.K., & Lincoln, Y.S. (Eds.). *The SAGE handbook of qualtitive research.* Thousand Oaks: Sage, 269–284.

Denzin, N.K., & Lincoln, Y.S. (Eds.) (2011). *The SAGE handbook of qualtitive research.* Thousand Oaks: Sage.

DeVault, M.L., & Gross, G. (2012). Feminist qualitative interviewing. In Hesse-Biber, S.N. (Ed.). *Handbook of feminist research: Theory and praxis.* 2nd edn. Thousand Oaks: Sage, 206–236.

Driedger, S.M., Gallois, C., Sanders, C.B., Santesso, N. (2006). Interviewing method: Finding common ground in team-based qualitative research using the convergent interviewing method. *Qualitative Health Research, 16*(8), 1145–1157.

Ezzy, D. (2010). Qualitative interviewing as an embodied emotional performance. *Qualitative Inquiry, 16*(3) 163–170.

Genovese, B.J. (2004). Thinking inside the box: The art of telephone interviewing. *Field Methods, 16*(2), 215–226.

Gubrium, J.F., Holstein, J.A., Marvastii, A.B., & McKinney, K.D. (Eds.) (2012). *The SAGE handbook of interview research: The complexity of the craft.* 2nd edn. Thousand Oaks: Sage.

Hamilton, R.J., & Bowers, B.J. (2006). Internet recruitment and e-mail interviews in qualitative studies. *Qualitative Health Research, 16* (6), 821–835.

Harris, R., Kelly, D., Hunt, J.A., Plant, H., Kelley, K., Richardson, A., & Sitzia, J. (2008). Accessing elite nurses for research: Reflections on the theoretical and practical issues of telephone interviewing. *Journal of Research in Nursing, 13*(3), 236–248.

Hesse-Biber, S.N., & Leavy, P. (2011). *The practice of qualitative research* 2nd edn, Thousand Oaks: Sage.

Holt, A. (2010). Using the telephone for narrative interviewing: A research note. *Qualitative Research, 10*(1), 113–121.

Hunt, N., & McHale, S. (2007). A practical guide to the e-mail interview. *Qualitative Health Research, 17*(10), 1415–1421.

James, N., & Busher, H. (2006). Credibility, authenticity and voice: Dilemmas in online interviewing. *Qualitative Research, 6*(3), 403–420.

Lagesen, V.A. (2010). The importance of boundary objects in transcultural interviewing. *European Journal of Women's Studies, 17*(2), 125–142.

McConnell-Henry, T., James, A., Chapman, Y., & Francis, K. (2009). Researching with people you know: Issues in interviewing. *Contemporary Nurse, 34*(1), 2–9.

McCoyd, J.L. M., & Kerson, T.S. (2006). Conducting intensive interviews using email: a serendipitous comparative opportunity. *Qualitative Social Work, 5*(3), 389–406.

Morse, J.M. (2012). The implications of interview type and structure in mixed-methods designs. In Gubrium, J.F., Holstein, J.A., Marvastii, A.B., & McKinney, K.D. (Eds.). *The SAGE handbook of interview research: The complexity of the craft.* 2nd edn. Thousand Oaks: Sage, 193–206.

Nikander, P. (2012). Interviews as discourse data. In Gubrium, J.F., Holstein, J.A., Marvastii, A.B., & McKinney, K.D. (Eds.). *The SAGE handbook of interview research: The complexity of the craft.* 2nd edn. Thousand Oaks: Sage, 397–414.

Olesen, V. (2011). Feminist qualitative research in the millennium's first decade: Developments, challenges, prospects. In Denzin, N.K., & Lincoln, Y.S. (Eds.). *The SAGE handbook of qualitative research,* 4th edn. Thousand Oaks: Sage, 129–146.

Perry, C., Thurston, M., & Green, K. (2004). Involvement and detachment in researching sexuality: Reflections on the process of semistructured interviewing. *Qualitative Health Research, 14*(1), 135–148.

Riessman, C.K. (2012). Analysis of personal narratives. In Gubrium, J.F., Holstein, J.A., Marvastii, A.B., & McKinney, K.D. (Eds.). *The SAGE handbook of interview research: The complexity of the craft.* 2nd edn. Thousand Oaks: Sage, 367–380.

Roulston, K. (2010) Considering quality in qualitative interviewing. *Qualitative Research, 10*(2), 199–228.

Sands, R.J., Bourjolly, R. and Roer-Strier, D. (2007) Crossing cultural barriers in research interviewing. *Qualitative Social Work* 6(3): 353–372.

Seale, C., & Rivas, C. (2012). Using software to analyse qualitative interviews. In Gubrium, J.F., Holstein, J.A., Marvastii, A.B., & McKinney, K.D. (Eds.). *The SAGE handbook of interview research: The complexity of the craft.* 2nd edn. Thousand Oaks: Sage, 427–440.

Tashakkori, A., & Teddlie, C. (1998). *Mixed methodology: Combining qualitative and quantitative approaches.* Thousand Oaks: Sage.

Tashakkori, A., & Teddlie, C. (2010). *Sage Handbook of Mixed Methods in Social & Behavioral Research.* Thousand Oaks: Sage.

Taylor, B., Kermode, S. & Roberts, K. (2006). *Research in nursing and healthcare: Evidence for practice.* Australia: Nelson.

Walby, K. (2010). Interviews as encounters: Issues of sexuality and reflexivity when men interview men about commercial same sex relation. *Qualitative Research, 10*(6), 639–657.

Winchatz, M.R. (2006). Fieldworker or foreigner?: Ethnographic interviewing in nonnative languages. *Field Methods, 18*(1), 83–97.

13

Group work and analysis

Bev Taylor

There is a wide range of groups in health sciences research, which are similar to, and in some cases overlap with therapeutic treatment groups. Therefore, the first task of this chapter is to differentiate between groups and the work they do in the health sciences, before delineating the types of qualitative research group work into methodologically-influenced group work and focus group work. Having made arbitrary distinctions between the two main types of research groups, I then guide you through some possibilities for thinking about methods and processes for undertaking group work and for selecting and applying appropriate analytic strategies.

Types of group work

As is the case for all of the qualitative research methods and processes featured in this book, group work is versatile, because it has many forms and uses. Used in health sciences professions, group work in research can become blurred with group work for therapeutic reasons, and in some cases, groups can be used simultaneously for both purposes. For example, group work can be used solely for therapeutic purposes, such as in psychoanalysis or narrative therapy, and the same therapeutic purposes can be adapted into research designs for detailed analyses (Lorentzen, 2006; White and Epston, 1990).

While accepting that some research groups can also have therapeutic intentions, research group work in this chapter will be defined as two or more people meeting together with the expressed purpose of assisting in the fulfilment of research aims and objectives, integral to a research plan approved formally by a human ethics committee as a valid project. Another point to make while 'drawing a line in the sand' in setting up this discussion of research group work, is that while all research groups have a focus, they are not all focus groups per se. Therefore, in this chapter I differentiate between group work methods and processes reflecting the epistemological assumptions of particular methodologies and focus group work that happens when people come together in a declared focus group to concentrate their attention on specified research interests.

Methodologically-influenced group work

Although there has been a recent trend towards considering all group work under a 'catch-all' of focus groups, I argue here that there are differences between group work done within a specific methodological approach, and the generic data collection and analysis activities that happen within focus groups. In the sense I use it within this chapter, methodologically influenced group work refers to group methods and processes used in qualitative research projects, which reflect the particular epistemological assumptions of that approach. Methodologically-influenced group work happens over time as group members meet regularly, developing their own group dynamics as they pursue a research plan based on the epistemological assumptions of a philosophical approach underlying the group work methods and processes. To all intents and purposes, any researcher working within a particular qualitative methodology, or combinations of qualitative or mixed methods methodologies, may choose to include a group or various groups for participants to work together in the research plan at various stages and phases, to assist in fulfilling specific research aims and objectives. However, in my opinion, the 'stand out' qualitative methodologies with the greatest success in research group work are action research (McNiff and Whitehead, 2006; Reason and Bradbury, 2006), critical ethnography (Denzin and Lincoln, 2011; Madison, 2011) and the feminisms (Hesse-Biber and Piatelli, 2012; Olesen, 2011).

My intention in suggesting two main types of research group work is to simplify and 'fine-tune' the discussion. However, as we have seen so often, attempts to typify various aspects of qualitative research into convenient groupings fail as soon as we locate an exception to the rule. For example, Bradbury-Jones, Sambrook and Irvine (2009) used focus groups in a phenomenological project. Phenomenology intends to illuminate things of interest, usually from the perspective of the experiencing individual. Bradbury-Jones et al.'s (2009) approach suggests that phenomenological interests can be illuminated by focus group work, immediately questioning my working definitions for both methodologically-informed group work and focus group work. Bradbury-Jones et al. (2009) acknowledge the criticism that the individual's unique existential perspectives illuminated through phenomenology have not been seen traditionally as suiting focus group work approaches, but they argue that 'individual lived experience can be preserved within a group context' (p. 663). They further contend that 'group interviews in phenomenology are actually beneficial because they stimulate discussion and open up new perspectives' (p. 663).

I need to respond to Bradbury-Jones et al. (2009) on two levels. Firstly, focus groups have their place in bringing people together to explore a common research focus, but the practicalities of ease, such as the convenience of everyone in the same location and reduced time and costs for data collection and analysis, need to be weighed against the project's specific methodological assumptions and the chances of focus groups achieving the project's aims and objectives, while remaining 'faithful' to key epistemological assumptions.

Secondly, unravelling the intricacies of phenomenological methods is best left to a seasoned philosopher, given that there is a spirited ongoing debate about the misapplications of phenomenology in health sciences research (Crotty, 1996; Norlyk and Harder, 2010). However, if we can agree that the primary intention in phenomenology is to create a spontaneous pre-reflexive telling of experience, who can say that participation in a focus group does not affect that essentialized response? For that matter, is it actually possible *at all* in a formal research project, whether garnered in one-to-one interviews or in group discussion dynamics, to *do* phenomenology? In other words, getting to the things themselves through phenomenological reduction (epoché) may be ultimately abstract and elusive, regardless of the methods we use to harness and reveal them. However, my present view is that the further we move away from the individual's account in a one-to-one in-depth interview in phenomenological research, the more we favour convenience over methodological fidelity, and the less chance we have of getting pre-reflexively to the things themselves.

Food for thought

In these postmodern times, we are living with increasing trends towards knowledge abstractions. In a practical sense, this means that qualitative researchers are witnessing blurred boundaries in methodological thought and the breakdown of typologies. For example, the philosophy of phenomenology, which underlies the epistemological assumptions of phenomenological projects, has the potential of being merged into a generic descriptive approach, thereby losing its key philosophical features. When a methodology loses its philosophical distinctions, particular methods and processes we might select and use to generate and validate that type of knowledge also lose their distinctive nature and purposes. Are we at risk of losing the methodological 'tints' in the fabric of qualitative knowledge we are producing in postmodern times? Is the convenient selection of methods at risk of replacing, even obliterating, methodological distinctions in qualitative research?

Notwithstanding the various exceptions to my categorizations of group work in this chapter, I will persist with the two distinctive types of group work in qualitative research. Action research, critical ethnography and feminisms often feature highly participatory, collaborative methodologically-influenced group work. Each of these methodologies seek to unearth and represent as problematic, complex knowledge and power issues within human interactions, institutions and organizations at various levels of intensity, complexity and influence. In healthcare research, these methodologies often ask critical questions about the status quo, specifically, how, why and by whom it is being maintained within a wide range of public political arenas. Within these methodologies, when contentious issues are identified collaboratively, research group members work together to systematically expose vested interests and power plays, with the intention of generating alternative, transformative action possibilities.

Focus group work

In this chapter I make the point that while all research groups have a focus, they are not all focus groups as such. Therefore, focus group work in qualitative research happens when people come together conveniently, in a declared focus group, to concentrate their attention on specified research interests. The group may meet once or a few times, but there is no intention to develop group dynamics through collaborative processes, rather the focus is on responding directly and succinctly to the previously identified research interest. The group processes are not necessarily in tune with a particular methodology, and the main interest is in canvassing as many participants' perspectives as possible in as few meetings as possible. The coming together to form a research focus group may be face to face or by technological means, for example, in cyberspace as an online focus group (e.g., Kenny, 2005), or by email (e.g., Kralik, Price, Warren and Koch, 2006).

Keeping to the types of group work as methodologically-influenced and as focus group work, this chapter discusses undertaking and analysing group work within each category. Although other possibilities exist, the methodologically-influenced group work I discuss in this chapter are methods and processes qualitative researchers may choose to select and apply within action research. This chapter also describes a range of focus group strategies researchers may enlist in their qualitative and mixed methods projects.

Methodologically-influenced group work

Although there are many qualitative methodologies for which group work methods and processes can be used, methodologies with collaborative, participatory intentions tend to be exemplary of when group work 'works best', such as action research, critical ethnography and feminisms. Any understanding of methodologically-influenced group work must be underpinned by a thorough understanding of the particular methodology's key ideas. For example, critical ethnography is described in detail in Chapter 4 of this book and in other influential research texts (Denzin and Lincoln, 2011; Madison, 2011). Critical ethnography is a reflexive research process, which reveals 'the complex micro politics of social relationships in the situation and the researcher's position within those politics' (Wellard and Street, 1999, p. 133).

Feminisms are described in detail in Chapter 8 of this book and in other influential publications (Hesse-Biber, 2012; Olesen, 2011). Feminisms recognize the existence of multiple contemporary feminisms; so they identify a feminist methodology for a project and provide an epistemological justification for using a particular feminist approach (i.e., gender issues matter), and the research foci for which it would be most useful (e.g., an area of research interest relating to women's work), before putting the methodology into action congruently.

Hereafter, as an example of methodologically-influenced group work, action research will be described as a 'stand out' methodology, to exemplify how particular epistemological assumptions have been integrated into group work methods and processes. Action research is described in detail in Chapter 9 of this book and in other influential research texts (McNiff and Whitehead, 2006; Reason and Bradbury, 2006). Action research usually involves the stages of a research group working collectively in planning, acting, observing and reflecting in progressive cycles of action. An action plan is usually generated and further acting, observing and reflecting are undertaken systematically, until an action plan is applied which best works towards solving identified research and practice problems (Dick 1995; Stringer 1996). Sometimes the action research phases are named differently, but they are essentially a set of interconnected problem solving steps in cyclical form, which keep on repeating until the action research aims and objectives have been addressed.

The precise structure of an action research project is open to interpretation, so the details of the research plan can vary from being projected as a series of meetings with participants as co-researchers (Rowley and Taylor, 2011; Taylor, 2001; Taylor et al. 2002) to using action research as a unifying methodology for a mixed methods project (Jinks and Chalder, 2007), with various creative iterations in between. In this evidence-based era, action research fits well with a mixed methods design, because it can include any type of data collection method to gather information during the progressive planning, acting, observing and reflecting cycles. For example, Jinks and Chalder (2007) used action research to analyse the roles of a group of mental health consultant nurses, in order to 'enable a group of mental health consultant nurses in the UK to map the scope and dimensions of their roles' (p. 1323). The study used

> action research as a form of self-reflective enquiry … Initial data were generated through use of four focus group discussions, which were held with a group of consultant nurses employed predominately at a mental health National Health Service Trust. Five structured confirmatory questionnaires developed from the focus group data were also administered … Analysis of the focus group data gave five themes, 71 categories and 271 items that were used to inform development of the questionnaires. Responses to the questionnaire showed that 61% (n = 166) of the items had non-consensus responses. It was found there was most consensus relating to leadership theme with 63% (n = 19) items having consensus responses. Least agreement was found in the education theme where there was <15% (n = 5) agreement to individual items. The study demonstrated complexity and variety in how the consultant nurses' roles in the UK are being developed.
>
> (Jinks and Chalder, 2007, p. 1323)

When researchers read project reports of methodologically-influenced group work in refereed journal articles, various restrictions such as word limits and journal stylistic considerations often mean that it is difficult to get a real sense of just what to do and how to do it when using group work as part of a qualitative research plan. For this reason, I am presenting here in some detail a distillation of my experience from projects in which I have been involved, so I can share some of the 'insider thinking' behind the somewhat 'sanitized' journal reports of the projects (Rowley and Taylor, 2011; Taylor, 2001; Taylor, Bulmer, Hill, Luxford, McFarlane and Stirling, 2002; Taylor, Edwards, Holroyd, Unwin and Rowley, 2005).

In an action research project conducted in Australia, Rowley and Taylor (2011) focused on improving the end-of-life care to residents with a non-malignant disease, who were dying in residential aged care facilities. I acted in the role of PhD supervisor for this project, guiding Jo Rowley, a PhD candidate and an experienced Registered Nurse, through an action research and reflection approach. Given that the publication was the overview of the entire project, the journal article (Rowley and Taylor, 2011) could not hope to capture what the group work within the meetings was actually like for the facilitator and how she adapted constantly to departures from what she thought might be expected group work processes. Even with the benefit of more words, the PhD thesis (Rowley, 2010) was unable to capture the full description of the thoughts and feelings Jo had as she worked her way through weeks of meetings with the nurses.

Jo had been involved in an action research project previously (Taylor et al., 2005), but she had not facilitated an action research group herself, and she was also facing the various challenges of undertaking her PhD part-time, while remaining in a busy managerial and research position at a local hospital. After ethical clearance, Jo recruited participants to two groups, each being within a different aged care facility within the local region. Although the numbers were the same in each group (n = 8), from the first meeting, the groups took on their own identity and group dynamics and the participants generated different practice foci. Even though Jo used the action research and reflection method with which she was familiar, many unforeseen challenges came up within the groups, requiring her to 'think on her feet'.

During the time Jo spent 'in the field' attending the facilities weekly for one hour over a four-month period, we stayed in weekly contact via a one-hour PhD supervisory session telephone call. During these calls, I often acted as a critical friend helping Jo to work reflectively through the group work issues in retrospect. No issues became overwhelming, but Jo still felt the impact of them as they occurred. For example, during one meeting a senior person arrived at the door and demanded the participants attend to work matters, even though the project requirements had been approved previously by the management personnel of the aged care facility. Another issue within the group work was that some participants used harsh, inappropriate language to describe some aspects of their practice stories. In this instance, Jo and I talked through how she might be able to challenge the language within the group process, while still allowing participants to feel they could speak openly and honestly.

As qualitative researchers, even though we attempt to disclose the details and account for the 'messiness' of our group work methods and processes, the published reports of our projects often cannot capture the whole of the experience. Sometimes, we may even choose to avoid trying to relay the intricacies of the group work processes, because of the twists and turns they take and the overburden of wordy details. Research methods seldom go to plan and this is particularly so in methodologically-influenced group work, when participants meet regularly, sometimes for many months, developing their own group dynamics. In the end, in methodologically-influenced group work all we really have to fall back on in assessing the 'worthiness' of our group work processes, is the extent to which the activation of the planned group work activities reflects the key ideas of the methodology by which they were informed.

In action research, the key ideas which guide the group work methods and processes can often be traced to the discipline of education (Kemmis and McTaggart, 1988) and the transformative intentions of critical theory, and Habermas's (1972, 1973) three different forms of knowledge-constitutive interests adapted to three forms of action research: technical, practical and emancipatory. Technical action research aims to improve techniques and procedures by having practitioners work collaboratively to test the applicability of results generated elsewhere. Practical action research aims to improve existing practices and to develop new ones by taking deliberate strategic action. Emancipatory action research involves a group of practitioners taking responsibility for freeing themselves from the constraints of their practice through understanding and transforming the political, social and economic conditions that keep them from doing their work as they would ideally choose.

The key intentions of group work in action research are to create the group dynamics through systematic phases of planning, acting, observing and reflecting in progressive cycles, until an action plan is activated with the potential of bringing about changes and improved conditions in the research interest. Central to this cyclical method are participatory, collaborative processes, which require group work in which each member cooperates and participates actively. To be successful the group work in action research projects involves the researcher and participants sharing the workload and responsibilities of the research project and assisting one another to create a co-researcher process. To do this well, each member needs to feel valued as an important, equal member of the group, free to share in discussions and decisions openly and honestly.

I worked with nurses in their clinical settings (Taylor 2001; Taylor et al. 2002, 2005) and we generated an approach to group work in action research, which you may find useful. As for any research, the preliminary steps are to firstly locate the healthcare professionals to form a research group of two or more people, who are ready to make a commitment to the research group. The participants need to know 'up front' that they need to commit to working together through their work issues, and to meet regularly, reflect on their work and share their thoughts with the group. Next, the co-researchers decide on a venue and a regular meeting day and time. The venue must allow for privacy, so co-researchers can speak openly and confidentially. The meeting day and time is negotiated by the healthcare professionals involved. If there is not one already in existence, a brief research proposal is written as a guide for the group, as well as for any other interested audiences, such as a funding body or an ethics committee. (The proposal and ethics approval process is the first consideration if you are going as a researcher into a venue to enlist support for a research project.)

The group work in action research continues with getting the project underway and deciding on who facilitates meetings. Decide if you will have one facilitator for every meeting, or if you will use a 'rotating chair' system, in which everyone takes a turn at guiding the agenda of the regular meetings. You may decide to keep minutes of meetings as a successive account of the research process and for information that can be included in the research report for dissemination.

The first few meetings are crucial in setting the tone for the group work. Very early in the life of the action research group, it is important to discuss the group processes openly, and to get a shared understanding of the key ideas and intentions in an action research methodology. The participants talk about what they want from the group in terms of how they will work together. For example, they may say that they want to be able to speak openly, with trust and confidentiality, and that nothing discussed in the group will be open to public discussion and so on. So that everyone understands the fundamental ideas in action research, the methodology is discussed and participants may be directed towards readings and any other useful resources to increase their understanding of some basic ideas in action research and how they relate to researching their work experiences.

Reflection is an important component of action research, so I usually guide group members through an initial reflective task. Learning to reflect effectively gives participants in the research group confidence in writing or recording their reflections and sharing them in the group. A simple reflective task is to think of someone or something in their childhood from whom/which they learned their 'rules for living' (values), and to then reflect on how these values have been integrated into their adulthood, contributing to how they now live and work. When each participant shares his or her responses, it is important that the other co-researchers listen attentively and non-judgementally. This may be the first trusting contribution co-researchers make to the group, so it is important to respect and honour the responses for the insights they give into the personal-professional life of the participant.

In the next part of the action research group work, members begin to reflect on their present or past practice stories, to identify a common theme ('thematic concern', in action research language) through which to work collaboratively. The group take as many meetings as they need to work through the first part of the process, because it is important that participants share at least two practice stories with the group. The aim of the research group work is to locate issues of common interest to participants, in order to raise awareness and change practice through action research and reflective processes. After the group has worked together for a while, through discussion, disagreement and consensus, they decide on issues that are common to everyone (thematic concerns) and use an action research approach to work through them.

When each participant shares her or his practice stories, it is again important that the other co-researchers listen attentively and non-judgementally. It is not usually a part of healthcare culture to speak openly about practice stories that did not go well, so encourage participants to be careful to honour the stories, allowing the storyteller to find his or her own insights. Co-researching participants may act as critical friends by asking questions for a fuller description, or to encourage a wider exploration of the issue, but they should not offer easy solutions, because it is best to avoid early foreclosures on action possibilities.

Locating the thematic concern is part of the group work analysis process. I find it useful to keep summary notes of each story shared within the group and I have devised a method for analysing the contents. I find it useful to construct a grid with four columns, including 1) story summary, 2) the issue(s), 3) the healthcare professional's feelings about the issue(s), and 4) how the issue(s) came about. The second column is most useful in locating the issues to find some thematic concerns common to each participant. For example, the analysis may show that participants have issues relating to relationships, such as with other healthcare professionals, patients, relatives and so on. The third column identifies the emotions and feelings participants experience in day-to-day practice, which are foundational to perceptions of their practice. The fourth column locates the various sources of participants' work issues, which affect the ways in which they negotiate their practice conditions. The group spends some time discussing the analysis of the stories, with particular interest in the practice issues that are identified. Collectively, they then see if there are any issues that come up consistently in the stories, to decide on an issue to research together using an action research approach. If there are several thematic concerns and enough participants in the group to work on them effectively, it may be possible to work on many issues at the same time.

In this form of action research, the next task of group work is to generate the action plan and begin the action research cycles. This phase of the research lasts as long as it takes for the group to reach satisfactory outcomes. The group is now at the point where they are ready to 'do' action research. The main phases of action research are: Plan, Act, Observe, Reflect (PAOR). Participants begin with a thematic concern (common to enough of them to matter) and move through a series of cycles of PAOR until they feel that the issue is addressed in whatever way they envisaged.

The group work for the planning phase of action research is generally as follows:

- The group projects a plan in relation to the thematic concern.

- The plan must be flexible to allow for unforeseen effects and constraints.

- The action prescribed by the plan must take account of the social risks involved and recognize the material and political constraints in the situation.

- The plan allows participants to go beyond their present constraints to empower them to act more effectively in the situation.

- The group plans by collaborating openly and honestly with one another and by analysing and improving their understanding of the situation.

A practical way for creating an action plan is to construct a grid with three columns, including 1) the thematic concern, 2) the source(s) of the thematic concern, and 3) what can be done about it. The second column is useful in locating the sources of the thematic concerns, because they are the work aspects that need some adjustment. For example, if a source of the thematic concern is due to economic constraints, a strategy for the action plan may involve inviting a person 'holding the purse strings' to meet with the group to discuss the concern. If the source of a concern is cultural, in its broadest sense of the way people relate to one another, the focus will be on interpersonal relationships, and a strategy may be to observe interpersonal interactions at work in order to examine, and work towards changing, the cultural foundations of these relationships.

When the group is discussing the strategies for the action plan, keep in mind the basic principles listed previously. It is very important to maximize the potential for the success of the action plan by making the strategies within it reasonable for managing the risks and ensuring the best possible outcomes. The action plan is instituted in the work settings and the results of the changed approach to the thematic concern are noted, through continued PAOR. The action plan undergoes revision until it achieves positive changes in successfully managing the identified thematic concern in practice.

The group work for the acting phase is:

- The group makes a critically informed, careful and thoughtful variation to practice by putting their plan into action.

- As the strategies in the action plan may be potentially risky, participants need to be flexible and open to change in the light of the real-time situation.

- Acting may involve material, social and political struggle towards improvement and negotiation, and compromise may be necessary.

- Participants may need to be content with modest gains that gradually get bigger based on previous gains (in other words, they may not always be able to 'fix things' the first time).

The group work for observing is what makes the project action research, because:

- It involves documenting the effects of critically-informed action.

- Participants use their powers of observation and stay responsive, open-eyed and open-minded to see how the plan of action is working.

- Participants record their observations in their journal or by whatever additional means they decide.

- Participants observe the action, the effects of the action (intended and unintended), the circumstances and constraints of the action, and any other issues that may arise.

Reflecting in action research group work:

- Recalls action as it has been recorded in the observation, but it is active in making sense of processes, problems, issues and constraints that may manifest in the strategic action.

- Is aided by group discussion in research meetings so participants can reconstruct the meaning of the social situation and revise the plan if necessary.

- Asks participants to evaluate the effects and the issues and to suggest ways of proceeding.

- Allows reconnaissance for further action research cycles as necessary. Participants keep using the action plan in daily practice until they know they have achieved their aims (plans) relating to the specific issues they raised.

In action research, the group work continues through the finalizing phases of the project, such as in working together on writing a research report and disseminating the findings. If participants in the group have not had previous professional publication and presentation experience, they need to ask for help of people who have, and invite them to assist the group in the final stage. Alternatively, the group can choose to learn the processes needed by working together through information for contributors supplied by journals and conference committees, ensuring a fair division of labour in preparing and presenting the information, for which they are duly acknowledged.

Summary

Methodologically-influenced group work reflects the key ideas of the underlying philosophy. For example, action research, critical ethnography and feminist projects often feature highly participatory, collaborative methodologically-influenced group work, because they are essentially collective, transformative philosophies. Group work in these methodologies seeks to expose and challenge problematic knowledge and power issues within human interactions, institutions and organizations and ask critical questions about the status quo, specifically, how, why and by whom it is being maintained.

In this section I described in detail the group work methods and processes I use when I facilitate action research projects. My reason for sharing my own research strategies was to disclose an 'insider's view' of the inner dynamics of a project. While other methodologically-influenced group work may be planned and undertaken quite differently, my intention in featuring action research group processes in this section was to exemplify the careful consideration that is applied to ensuring that group work reflects the key assumptions of a particular qualitative methodology.

Focus group work

Focus group work is gaining popularity in qualitative and mixed methods research, because it brings together many people to generate and collect data in a group interview and discussion format, thereby having practical and substantive advantages over one-to-one data collection methods and processes. Focus groups are not new, having their genesis in a variety of different fields in the 1940s and 1950s, but most notably in organizational and market research. In their early days, focus groups were mainly geared towards bringing a group of people (usually as consumers) into one place to seek their views on a particular organizational innovation, or product and marketing pitch. Applied to human research interests, focus groups have been used in various disciplines, such as education and the health sciences, for group interview purposes (Hesse-Biber and Leavy, 2011).

Initially, focus groups in research projects were used mainly for their practical advantages, such as reducing project costs and minimizing the time and effort to collect and analyse data. Considerable effort has been invested over the last six decades or so by researchers in developing focus group methods and processes, so that they have moved beyond opinion polling, to data collection and analysis methods, and ultimately to knowledge generation and validation events. As I mentioned previously, some researchers use focus groups within specific methodologies (Bradbury-Jones et al., 2009), and for some researchers, research group work means focus groups.

There are many varieties of focus groups, which differ according to the structure, depth and scope of research intentions. Some authors focus on the practical aspects of setting up and running focus groups (Barbour, 2010; Hesse-Biber and Leavy, 2011; Morgan, 2012), and others also look into the epistemological possibilities within the focus group dynamics (Kamberelis and Dimitriadis, 2011; Morgan, 2012). In the postmodern research era, focus group work is being 'troubled' in the form of a performative turn that reimagines 'qualitative inquiry … as asking and dwelling in new questions that are not necessarily answerable in finalizable ways' (Kamberelis and Dimitriadis, 2011, p. 547). Essentially, postmodern perspectives situate 'focus group work within a performative idiom', within the construct of multifunctionality, which is used to 'explain complexity and contingency within many different disciplines' (Kamberelis and Dimitriadis, 2011, p. 545).

Given that contemporary focus groups range from practical to performative, for them to be of any use to you as a qualitative researcher in the health sciences, it is important to have a grasp on their various methods and processes. For example, the proliferation of many different research focus groups, while advantageous in many practical ways, has led authors to caution researchers to avoid using focus groups opportunistically (Barbour, 2010), to differentiate focus group interviews from in-depth interviews (Hesse-Biber and Leavy, 2011), to take care in co-constructing meaning (Morgan, 2012), and to consider the 'contingent articulations of pedagogy, politics, and inquiry' in focus groups (Kamberelis and Dimitriadis, 2011, p. 545).

Barbour (2010) takes a practical approach to the use of focus groups as a method of collecting data which is 'efficient and amenable to a broad range of topics'. However, she cautions that 'the attractiveness of the method masks some of its subtleties and can lead to its lazy and uncritical use' (p. 327). In Barbour's (2010) view, focus groups are inappropriate when they are based on opportunistic reasons, unrealistic expectations, a poor match of moderator to group, a lack of methodological positioning, and inadequate analysis procedures. The effect of the focus group moderator is a paramount consideration to Barbour, who points out that a moderator's skills are far more refined than those required in effective interpersonal communication, because thorough planning and in-the-moment creativity and responses are needed to conduct research focus groups well.

Much of the advice offered by Barbour (2010) in her chapter on focus groups relates to when to use focus groups, how to recruit participants and deal with ethical issues, sampling and group composition issues. She also covers practical considerations about the focus group venue, whether to audiotape discussions, how to moderate using topic guides and other stimulus material, and challenges in analysing focus group data, but she is silent on the actual group work processes within the focus groups. Group work is not just what participants and moderators do, but how they do it. For example, group process questions are: How do participants perceive their roles within the group and get to know each other? What 'rules' of conduct operate within the group? How do participants discuss issues and decide on what matters to them? How are the research requirements (aims, objectives, data management, insights, results dissemination) negotiated within the group?

Hesse-Biber and Leavy (2011) turn their attention to focus group interviews, in which 'multiple participants are interviewed together, making the focus group distinct from one-on-one methods of interview' (p. 163). They differentiate between in-depth interviews and focus group interviews based on group influences on interaction and conversation. Hesse-Biber and Leavy (2011) point out that in focus group interviews 'participants, even if they hold similar views, attitudes, and life experiences, are not merely responding to questions posed by a researcher but they are also responding to each other and the group dynamics as a whole' (p. 166). Even with repeat focus groups, different conversations are likely to occur. Therefore, focus group interviews are actually discussions moderated by group effects; they are not the considered, relatively uninterrupted view of an individual as he or she responds to an in-depth interview prompt or guide.

Hesse-Biber and Leavy (2011) acknowledge the role of the researcher as moderator in focus groups, in influencing 'the flow of the conversation and therefore the group dynamic and manner of the group narrative' (p. 181). They emphasize the practical strategy of the moderator planning and posing the opening question, to give the group focus and to be the stimulus for group discussion. The next consideration is the role of the moderator in structuring and controlling the group interview, so that there is sufficient standardization and flow. They make the point that in marketing research and in some projects using structured quantitative methods, the moderator needs to maintain a high degree of standardization and control, but this is not so or necessary in social science approaches. In the health sciences, where projects may be qualitative or mixed methods research, focus groups tend to use less structure and control, to allow the free exchange of ideas and experiences.

Morgan (2012) has been writing about focus groups for some time (Morgan, 1997, 1998, 2002), mainly about practical considerations for setting up, facilitating and analysing focus group work. His recent interest lies in social interaction on focus groups, viewed and interpreted mainly through a symbolic interactionist perspective (Morgan, 2010, 2012). Morgan's (2012) recent work explores the co-construction of meaning through social interaction in focus groups. Morgan (2012) differentiates between content-oriented and conversation-oriented research. Content-oriented research focus groups 'use a more directed style of moderating to elicit useful information on their topic of interest' (p. 163). Conversation-oriented researchers 'typically use a less structured style that lets them hear how participants set their own agenda' (p. 163). Morgan's (2012) distinctions of moderator style fit well with Hesse-Biber and Leavy's (2011) discussion about structure and control. By sharing and comparing, focus group participants move between conversations and creating the content, thereby fulfilling the dual purposes of social interaction while accomplishing research aims.

In the later part of focus groups, Morgan (2012) observes that organizing and conceptualizing takes place through a process of co-constructing meaning. He uses a symbolic interactionist interpretation to label as *social objects* the organizing and conceptualizing that happens in focus groups, because they emerge in the course of the focus group conversations. The co-construction of social objects occurs as 'participants expand on a research topic and consolidate their discussion through the more abstract processes of organizing and conceptualizing' (Morgan, 2012, p. 171). He suggests that procedures that promote focus group organizing and conceptualizing processes include using variations in group interviewing techniques, using concept mapping, and in undertaking repeated interviews.

Kamberelis and Dimitriadis (2011) leave the practical aspects of focus groups to other writers and centre their attention on the pedagogical, political and inquiry aspects of focus groups. They explain that the 'pedagogic function basically involves collective engagement designed to promote dialogue and to achieve higher levels of understanding of issues critical to the group's interests and/or the transformation of conditions of its existence' (p. 547). The political function is 'to transform the conditions of existence of the stakeholders' through activism and consciousness-raising activities (p. 547). The third function of focus groups, inquiry, is to 'generate rich, nuanced, and even contradictory accounts of how people ascribe meaning to and interpret their lived experience, with an eye toward how these accounts might be used to affect social policy and social change' (Kamberelis and Dimitriadis, 2011, p. 546). Kamberelis and Dimitriadis (2011) make the point that 'the boundaries between inquiry, pedagogy and politics within focus groups are porous' (p. 547).

My reading of Kamberelis and Dimitriadis (2011) is that they are basically putting forward a case for methodologically-influenced group work, which they position within the generic category of focus groups. The examples they use of pedagogy, politics, and inquiry fall into democratizing, transformative philosophies introduced by critical social scientists and expanded by later post-structuralist and postmodern epistemological trends. I read their work as a call to investigate group work beyond its practical advantages of relatively convenient group data collection and analysis, to a deeper analysis of the group work processes as instructive in teaching and learning, personal and institutional power analyses, and research inquiry with epistemological possibilities.

There is no consensus about the best methods of analysing focus group work, however, grounded theory methods provide some structure and rigour (Barbour, 2010) and concept mapping (Hesse-Biber and Leavy, 2011; Morgan, 2012) assists in the process. For information on grounded theory analysis, please refer to Chapter 2 of this book. Concept mapping is a stimulus strategy for the analysis process, which

> requests participants to organize the content from their prior discussion ... This approach typically relies on a two-part question, where the participants begin by either generating a list of concepts or using a predetermined list, with the goal of creating a 'map' (actually a structured diagram) that shows the relationships among the concepts. The second part of the question asks participants to step back from their map and talk about how they chose to create it the way they did – that is, why they organised the concepts into this set of relationships.
>
> (Morgan, 2012, p. 173)

A simple guideline to keep in mind when thinking about analysing focus group work outcomes is that the type of analysis depends on the type of focus group data. If focus groups are used as group interview sessions, it will be reasonable to analyse audiotaped transcripts for themes and subthemes. If focus groups are used for narrative inquiry, some form of narrative analysis will be advisable (see Chapter 14 of this book). As is the case in all qualitative research, the pre-planned methods and processes, as outlined in the research proposal, will lead to the best way of dealing with the data that emerge from focus groups. The actual analysis procedures may happen within the group work as a collective activity, or the data may be analysed by the researcher(s) remote from the focus group venue, by manual or software analysis means, with little or no input from the focus group members.

Chapter summary

As there is a wide range of groups in health sciences research, sometimes overlapping with therapeutic treatment groups, the first task of this chapter was to differentiate between groups and the work they do in the health sciences. I defined research group work in this chapter as two or more people meeting together with the expressed purpose of assisting in the fulfilment of research aims and objectives, integral to a research plan approved formally by a human ethics committee as a valid project. I also made the point that while all research groups have a focus, they are not all focus groups per se. Therefore, in this chapter I differentiated between methodologically-influenced group work methods and processes reflecting the epistemological assumptions of particular methodologies and focus group work that happens when people come together in a declared focus group to concentrate their attention on specified research interests.

Methodologically-influenced group work, for example, in action research, critical ethnography and feminist projects, often feature highly participatory, collaborative methodologically-influenced group work, because they are essentially collective, transformative philosophies. Group work in these methodologies seeks to expose and challenge problematic knowledge and power issues within human interactions, institutions and organizations and ask critical questions about the status quo, specifically, how, why and by whom it is being maintained. I described in detail the group work methods and processes I use when I facilitate action research projects, to exemplify the careful consideration that ensures that group work reflects the key assumptions of a particular qualitative methodology.

The final part of this chapter explored focus group work, which brings together many people to generate and collect data in a group interview and discussion format, thereby having practical and substantive advantages over one-to-one data collection methods and processes. I explained that initially focus groups in research projects were used mainly for their practical advantages, but considerable effort has been invested over the last six decades or so to move focus groups beyond opinion polling, to data collection and analysis methods, and ultimately to knowledge generation and validation events.

I reviewed some ideas from a variety of focus groups, in relation to the practical aspects of setting up and running focus groups (Barbour, 2010; Hesse-Biber and Leavy, 2011; Morgan, 2012), and the epistemological possibilities within the focus group dynamics (Kamberelis and Dimitriadis, 2011; Morgan, 2012). The methods of focus group data analysis vary, but the present trend is toward adopting structured grounded theory analysis approaches and concept mapping.

If you are thinking of using group work in a qualitative or mixed methods project, my advice to you is to firstly write a full and detailed research proposal, with clear aims and objectives. I suggest that you decide which type of research group work you are doing and why, which will give you the answer to whether you are undertaking methodologically-influenced group work, or whether you are running a focus group for specific group work purposes. The project may be seated in a qualitative methodology, or it may be a broad qualitative and/or mixed methods approach with no particular methodological orientation. The research aims, objectives and questions, plus the practicalities of the project's timelines and costs, will direct you towards the nature of the group work you need to include in your research plan. The group work methods and processes you then apply will be likely to serve the research interests well and increase the likelihood that the participants will be engaged actively and effectively in the group work.

Key points

- Research group work is defined as two or more people meeting together with the expressed purpose of assisting in the fulfilment of research aims and objectives, integral to a research plan approved formally by a human ethics committee as a valid project.

- While all research groups have a focus, they are not all focus groups per se.

- Methodologically-influenced group work happens over time as group members meet regularly, developing their own group dynamics as they pursue a research plan based on the epistemological assumptions of a philosophical approach underlying the group work methods and processes.

- Although there are many qualitative methodologies for which group work methods and processes can be used, methodologies with collaborative, participatory intentions tend to be exemplary of when group work 'works best', such as action research, critical ethnography and feminisms.

- Focus group work in qualitative research happens when people come together conveniently, in a declared focus group, to concentrate their attention on specified research interests in a group interview and discussion format, thereby having practical and substantive advantages over one-to-one data collection methods and processes.

- Considerable effort has been invested to develop focus group methods and processes, so that they have moved beyond opinion polling, to data collection and analysis methods, and ultimately to knowledge generation and validation events.

- A simple guideline to keep in mind when thinking about analysing methodologically-influenced group work or focus group work outcomes is that the type of analysis depends on the type of collected group data.

Critical review questions

1 What are the advantages and disadvantages of collecting group data?

2 To what extent does group work play a part in gathering data for your healthcare profession's key research issues and questions?

References

Barbour, R. (2010). Focus groups. In Bourgeault, I., Dingwall, R., & De Vries, R. (Eds.). *The SAGE handbook of qualitative methods in health research*. Thousand Oaks: Sage, 327–352.

Bradbury-Jones, C., Sambrook, S., & Irvine, F. (2009). The phenomenological focus group: An oxymoron? *Journal of Advanced Nursing* 65(3), 663–671.

Crotty, M. (1996). *Phenomenology and nursing research*. Melbourne: Churchill Livingstone.

Denzin, N.K., & Lincoln, Y.S. (Eds.) (2011). *The SAGE handbook of qualitative research*, 4th edn. Thousand Oaks: Sage.

Dick, R. (1995). A beginner's guide to action research. *ARCS Newsletter, 1*(1), 5–9.

Habermas, J. (1972). *Knowledge and human interests*, London: Heinemann.

Habermas, J. (1973). *Theory and practice*, London: Heinemann.

Hesse-Biber, S.N. (2012). *The handbook of feminist research: Theory and praxis* 2nd edn. Thousand Oaks: Sage.

Hesse-Biber, S.N., & Leavy, P. (2011). Focus group interviews. In Hesse-Biber, S.N., & Leavy, P. (2011). *The practice of qualitative research*. 2nd edn. Thousand Oaks: Sage, 163–192.

Hesse-Biber, S.N., & Piatelli, D. (2012). The feminist practice of holistic reflexivity. In Hesse-Biber, S.N. *The handbook of feminist research: Theory and praxis* 2nd edn. Thousand Oaks: Sage, 557–582.

Jinks, A.M., & Chalder, G. (2007). Consensus and diversity: An action research study designed to analyse the roles of a group of mental health consultant nurses. *Journal of Clinical Nursing, 16*, 1323–1332.

Kamberelis, G., & Dimitriadis, G. (2011). Focus groups: Contingent articulations of pedagogy, politics, and inquiry. In Denzin, N.K., & Lincoln, Y.S.. *The SAGE handbook of qualitative research*. Thousand Oaks: Sage, 545–561.

Kemmis, S., & McTaggart, R. (Eds.) (1988). *The action research planner*, 3rd edn. Geelong, Australia: Deakin University Press.

Kenny, A.J. (2005). Interaction in cyberspace: An online focus group. *Journal of Advanced Nursing, 49*(4), 414–422.

Kralik, D., Price, K., Warren, J., & Koch, T. (2006). Issues in data generation using email group conversations for nursing research. *Journal of Advanced Nursing, 53*(2), 213–220.

Lorentzen, S. (2006). Analysis special section: Contemporary challenges for research in groups. *Group Analysis, 39*, 321.

Madison, D.S. (2011). *Critical ethnography: Method, ethics, and performance*. Thousand Oaks: Sage.

McNiff, J., & Whitehead, J. (2006). *All you need to know about action research*. London: Sage.

Morgan, D.L. (1997). *Focus groups as qualitative research*. 2nd edn. Thousand Oaks: Sage.

Morgan, D.L. (1998). *The focus group guidebook*. Thousand Oaks: Sage.

Morgan, D.L. (2002). Focus group interviewing. In Gubrium, J., & Holstein, J. (Eds.) *Handbook of interview research*, Thousand Oaks: Sage, pp. 141–160.

Morgan, D.L. (2010). Reconsidering the role of interaction in analyzing and reporting focus groups. *Qualitative Health Research, 20,* 718–722.

Morgan, D.L. (2012). Focus groups and interaction. In Gubrium, J.F., Holstein, J.A., Marvasti, A.B., & McKinney, K.D. (Eds.). *The Sage handbook of interview research: The complexity of the craft,* 2nd edn. Thousand Oaks: Sage, 161–176.

Norlyk, A., & Harder, I. (2010). What makes a phenomenological study phenomenological? An analysis of peer-reviewed empirical nursing studies. *Qualitative Health Research, 20*(3), 420–431.

Olesen, V. (2011). Feminist qualitative research in the millennium's first decade: Developments, challenges, prospects. In Denzin, N.K., & Lincoln, Y.S. (Eds.). *The SAGE handbook of qualitative research,* 4th edn. Thousand Oaks: Sage, pp. 129–146.

Reason, P., & Bradbury, H. (2006). *Handbook of action research.* London: Sage.

Rowley, J. (2010). Dying in a rural residential aged care facility: An action research and reflection project to improve end-of-life care to residents with a non-malignant disease. *Unpublished PhD Thesis,* Southern Cross University, Lismore, Australia.

Rowley, J., & Taylor, B. (2011). Dying in a rural residential aged care facility: An action research and reflection project to improve end-of-life care to residents with a non-malignant disease. *International Journal of Nursing Practice, 17,* 591–598.

Stringer, E. (1996). *Action research: A handbook for practitioners.* Thousand Oaks: Sage.

Taylor, B.J. (2001). Identifying and transforming dysfunctional nurse–nurse relationships through reflective practice and action research. *International Journal of Nursing Practice, 7*(6), 406–413.

Taylor, B.J., Bulmer, B., Hill, L., Luxford, C., McFarlane, J., & Stirling, K. (2002). Exploring idealism in palliative nursing care through reflective practice and action research. *International Journal of Palliative Nursing, 8*(7), 324–330.

Taylor, B.J., Edwards, P., Holroyd, B., Unwin, A., & Rowley, J. (2005). Assertiveness in nursing practice: An action research and reflection project, *Contemporary Nurse,* 20(2), 324–347.

Wellard, S. & Street, A.F. (1999). Family issues in home-based care. *International Journal of Nursing Practice, 5,* 132–136.

White, M. and Epston, D. (1990) *Narrative means to therapeutic ends.* New York: W.W. Norton.

Narrative analysis

Bev Taylor

Narrative analysis is inextricably interwoven into the fabric of narrative inquiry, making it a highly diversified qualitative research methodology (see Chapter 6 of this book). Narrative analysis began in the social sciences, as a systematic means of literary critique through investigating the imagery of metaphor and the flow and impact of stories. Since the emergence of qualitative research approaches as valid epistemological choices for researching human experiences, narrative inquiry and analysis have been considered appropriate methods and processes for researching the human condition. The popularity of narrative inquiry and analysis has led to an ever increasing array of qualitative research approaches, which claim to use narratives and storytelling in their projects.

Due to the versatility of narrative approaches in qualitative research, it is almost impossible to typify the existing and emerging methods and processes of narrative analysis. Narrative analysis is a vast, densely overgrown jungle of epistemological possibilities. If we could hover over it high up from a bird's eye point of view, we could choose to drop down into the terrain of narrative analysis from myriad starting points and explore the detail by many pathways from multiple perspectives. To clear a path through the jungle of narrative research possibilities, in Chapter 6 I suggested narrative inquiry spins around a three-pronged axis of 1) the importance of the stories, depicting people's lived experiences (Bell, 2009; Riessman, 2008); 2) the storytellers, and how they narrate their experiences, constructing meaning for themselves and their audiences (Chase, 2010; Hole, 2007) and 3) the listeners, focusing on the reflexive interplay between the narrative practices and environments (Gubrium and Holstein, 2009), and in sometimes finding deeper meaning by aligning themselves experientially within participants' stories (Myerhoff, 1979; Behar, 2007).

Rather than get lost in the jungle of narrative analysis by creating other possible storylines, for the sake of simplicity and continuity, in this chapter I will continue to traverse the broader pathway of the three-pronged axis of narrative inquiry and analysis I took in Chapter 6. The story, the storyteller and the listener are important in narrative inquiry and analysis, because they encompass narrated life experiences as forms of discourse, from which we can learn about human knowledge and existence (Chase, 2011). Data collection and analysis methods chosen for narrative inquiry projects are subsumed within various approaches to inquiring into people's narratives, and they are chosen to suit the particular emphases on the story, the storyteller and the listener. Therefore, there is a wide variety of potential choices available to researchers for describing people's lived experiences, the ways storytellers narrate their experiences, the construction of meaning, the reflexive interplay between the narrative practices and environments, and the ways researchers find deeper meaning in participants' stories.

Narratives are integral to human communication, and they qualify as research when researchers take interest in collecting, analysing and interpreting contextualized life events as ontological experiences (Bamberg, 2007; Clandinin, 2007; Denzin and Lincoln, 2011; Gubrium and Holstein, 2009; Knowles and Cole, 2008; Lindsay, 2011; Riessman, 2008); politicized experience and action (Hall, 2011); and highly relativistic, personalized accounts of 'truth' (McAllister, 2001).

When they are collected, how will the stories be analysed? How will the overall quality of the project be ascertained? In this chapter, I describe these questions relating to narrative analysis by elaborating on selected examples of narrative research undertaken in the health sciences, from the perspectives of the stories, the storytellers and the listeners. The narrative research projects highlighted in this chapter are not described fully; for detailed descriptions please refer to the original articles. My intention here is to overview the projects, to set a context for focusing mainly on the methods and processes they used to analyse the data.

Stories: Health and illness narratives

In narrative inquiry, beginning with the story, or series of stories, choices need to be made about what stories will be collected, with what focus, for what purposes, by what means. In the health sciences, stories convey research participants' experiences, often presented as health and illness narratives. For example, publications report health and illness narratives in palliative care (Bingley, Thomas, Brown, Reeve and Payne, 2008), mental health (Lewis, 2006), family health (Lindenmeyer, Griffiths, Green, Thompson and Tsouroufli, 2008) and cancer care (Sinding and Wiernikowski, 2008). There is no prescriptive approach to narrative analysis methods and the means of judging a project's trustworthiness also vary.

For example, UK researchers Lindenmeyer et al. (2008) interviewed midlife women about their family history and their perceived risk of disease. The researchers were interested in 'how personal experience translates into a sense of vulnerability' (p. 277). The researchers became interested in the research focus when participants being interviewed about their experiences of HRT, mammography and bone densitometry began to talk spontaneously about their present and future health concerns in relation to close family members. The women's discussion of their perceived health risks and family history prompted the researchers to undertake a secondary analysis of the interview data. The women's focus on family history became evident when

Of 98 women (who) were interviewed, 61 mentioned their mothers' health, often together with that of other close relatives, while another eight did not talk about mothers but mentioned fathers, siblings, or both, giving a total of 69 women in this analysis. Of the 29 participants who did not mention family members and were therefore excluded from this analysis, seven were Pakistani women interviewed through an interpreter, a situation that may not be conducive to storytelling. On other socio-economic dimensions, there were no major differences between those included or excluded from this analysis, except there were more graduates among the women included (pp. 278–279).

As is so often the case with research journal articles, there is very little mention of the narrative analysis methods. In this case, the statement was that 'the interviews were entered into NVivo software for ease of data retrieval, and any mention of health in relation to family members was coded' (Lindenmeyer et al., 2008, p. 279). There is no mention of strategies applied to ensure the project's trustworthiness.

Uncertainty about the future was a major emergent theme. Women lived with uncertainty because they were worried about the future, in relation to a specific condition and uncertainty about their genetic links. Even though they expressed certainty about increased risk or inevitable decline, some participants also expressed optimism about the future and they cited disconfirming cases in which genetic characteristics had not been passed down. The researchers discussed these themes in terms of resemblance and kinship, because in their narrative accounts women shared perceptions of likeness, of being 'unlike', and of 'becoming like', other family members.

Lindenmeyer et al. (2008, p. 275) concluded that 'perceptions of vulnerability to illness are strongly influenced by the salience given to personal experience of illness in the family … (and) this salience is created through autobiographical narrative, both as individual life story *and* collectively shaped family history'. They assert that 'both types of narrative provide a sense of continuity in an uncertain world' (p. 277).

In this narrative research, the transcribed semi-structured interview data were managed by software analysis. The data were gathered as autobiographical accounts and the women were apparently at ease telling their experiential stories, because the researchers found more in the participants' responses than they expected originally. The NVivo analysis strategy was necessary, practical and useful, given the number of in-depth interviews and the richness of the data. The transcribed words and sentences were organized within the NVivo software into themes (although the article also refers to codes and categories). The emergent themes provided deeper insights into how these women perceived their illness risks and their family history, so this project is an example of how narrative analysis can use software analysis successfully.

Canadian researchers Sinding and Wiernikowski (2008) explored older women's cancer narratives and challenged the idea of chronic illness as disruption to consider it as 'normal hardship'. This qualitative study referred to as the '70+ women and cancer study' was part of the Intersecting Vulnerabilities research programme, which is 'a series of linked studies focused on the cancer experiences of older women, women living on low incomes, Aboriginal women with women diagnosed with cancer in their 70s or 80s' (Sinding and Wiernikowski, 2008, p. 393). Each study within the research programme uses participatory research to engage researchers and participants actively as collaborators in the research methods and processes. After a comprehensive recruitment and sampling strategy, the participants' demographic data specific to age and cancer diagnosis were

> of the 15 women interviewed, six were between 70 and 74 years old, four between 75 and 79 and five 80 or older ... of the 10 women diagnosed with breast cancer, six had lumpectomies and four had mastectomies; six also had radiation and one had chemotherapy. Of the five diagnosed with gynaecological cancer, four had surgery and one also had radiation; one declined all treatment. Most (10) were within one year of diagnosis, four were between one and two years and one was between two and three years from diagnosis.
>
> (Sinding and Wiernikowski, 2008, p. 395)

Two audiotaped semi-structured interviews averaging 1.5 hours were conducted with each participant. Notably, 'the three interviewers (two of whom are cancer survivors, and all three in their late 60s or early 70s) were drawn from the Project Team' (p. 395). The interview guide focused on participants experiences of how they found out about their diagnosis and how they felt about their subsequent healthcare experiences.

Possibly reflecting the open-minded (and hearted) participatory nature of the project, the researchers provided a succinct description of the narrative analysis procedures they used, which are best relayed in their own words:

> In keeping with our participatory approach, each interview transcript was reviewed by all Project Team members. At team meetings (usually half a day, approximately every two months), we shared our reflections on what was striking, puzzling, unexpected or moving about the narratives. Drawing from detailed minutes taken at these meetings, CS developed a coding framework and coded the transcripts using the qualitative software program NVivo ... Both naturally and by design, the Project Team's analysis employed key grounded theory methods ... (such as) constant comparison within and between accounts, and attention to the conditions under which phenomena arise and the consequences associated with the phenomena. As each interviewer presented an interview she had done, members of the team recalled aspects of other participants' narratives, quite naturally noting similarities and differences among them.
>
> (Sinding and Wiernikowski, 2008, p. 396)

The researchers explained that as the collaborative analysis processes continued they started to see that participants were telling them that cancer was not 'an especially "big deal" in their lives' (Sinding and Wiernikowski, 2008, p. 396). They located many sentences in which 'not' appeared and even though 'the link between the construction of cancer as unproblematic and (their) overall research question was not immediately clear' the researchers began to see how 'other health or social problems seemed to overshadow cancer' for some participants (p. 396). The researchers explained that for study participants

> the disruption cancer occasioned often receded in significance in relation to historical, current or anticipated health and social problems (their own or those of significant others), or was mitigated by resources drawn from long and often difficult histories. These findings lend support to the notion that long, hard lives render any one chronic illness relatively non-disruptive. However, it was not only in contexts of struggle that cancer was described as unproblematic. Cancer was sometimes represented this way in the context of lives assessed as sufficiently long and marked by certain satisfactions … As well, contexts of old age and struggle occasionally had the opposite effect, rendering cancer especially disruptive.
>
> (Sinding and Wiernikowski, 2008, p. 397)

In the article the researchers discuss the debates reflecting chronic disease as 'biological disruption' and as 'normal hardship'. They note that for these research participants, the fact that their cancer experiences as older women tended to be mainly perceived as normal hardship, explains why the women tended not to dwell on their diagnosis. The researchers make a very good point, which comes directly from their attention to the participants' cancer stories and from recent literature, that for 'people who are old, already living with illness, and/or socially marginalized, (another) chronic illness is often not experienced as a disruption' (p. 407). However, they point out a fundamental issue, that when marginalized people speak of non-disruption it is easy to overlook 'the social forces that obscure and mute their suffering' (p. 409).

If we look at this research as an example of narrative analysis, we see that the researchers have been influenced to a large extent by their adherence to their participatory, social equality research principles in the way they selected their research methods and processes. In particular, the inclusion as interviewers of older women with cancer experiences themselves points to the researchers' intention to reflect their equity principles within the research processes. The thoughtful selection of these women as interviewers would have optimized the chances that they would be able to 'go with the flow' of the participants' stories, so that their 'what happened next?' prompts could bring out rich, deep participants' accounts of living with cancer. Added to this, their inclusion in the collaborative analysis process ensured that the interviewers were able to feed back their impressions to the analysis group of talking with the particular participants, which I imagine would have assisted the team immensely in unearthing the nuances in the participants' 'no big deal' statements.

The combined analysis procedures for the Sinding and Wiernikowski (2008) project are interesting, because they include group collaboration in identifying themes, grounded theory principles and the use of NVivo. Grounded theory provides a structured analysis method and NVivo tracks participants' ideas and researchers' connections well, so these seem reasonable choices for data analysis. In terms of how they might be suited to narrative analysis, the selection of multiple analysis possibly demonstrates the research team's intentions to 'drill down' into the data for the best possible interpretations. Personally, if I am reading the project design correctly, for 15 participants interviewed twice, I imagine that the team's collective abilities to analyse the data together would have been sufficient. Even though the article is limited in what intricate details of the team process it can convey, it seems to me that this team worked together well and their deep discussions about the directions that data were taking would have been thorough and sufficient, without the addition of grounded theory and NVivo.

Food for thought

Do you think it is possible to 'over-analyse' qualitative data? While triangulation and other methods of ensuring 'rigour' are standard procedures in present-day approaches, given the relativistic, context-dependent knowledge assumptions about qualitative research knowledge, is it possible we are being 'too wary and worried' about qualitative data analysis?

These research projects are just two of so many other examples of how health science researchers have used narrative inquiry and applied various analysis methods to participants' narratives of health and illness. I selected the projects as illustrating narrative analysis from the orientation of the story, as a medium for constructing, analysing and making meaning of health and illness narratives.

Storytellers: Constructing meaning

Another way of looking at narrative analysis is to focus on the storytellers as research participants. Qualitative researchers are often interested in people's private and personal experiences, because they intermesh so often with incompletely or unexplained phenomena. Getting to these private phenomena is often through interviewing methods and processes that enhance participants' in-depth disclosures (see Chapter 12).

I make the point in Chapter 12 that it is possible to consider interviews as connected to sensitivity issues. I argue that qualitative researchers are often interested in deep accounts of participants' lived experiences, so interviews may be classified as sensitive, depending on the research focus, the nature of the participants, and the researcher–participant relationship. These classifications are particularly likely to be of importance in narrative inquiry, because participants are often encouraged to describe their life stories through in-depth interviews.

Sensitive research foci involve projects seeking to explore areas not often disclosed and discussed publicly, which may have ethical and legal implications. *Sensitive research participants* are those people deemed vulnerable, if they fit within definitions and categories pre-determined by various national and global health research committees as having sensitivities according to their: age, such as children and ageing people; condition, such as debilitated and frail people; ethnicity, such as indigenous people and diverse migrant groups; and disadvantage, such as low socio-economic groups, homeless people and minority groups. *Researcher–participant sensitivities* are associated with relatively high ethical risks when intersubjective research processes intentional blur traditional researcher–participant roles in close relationships and highly participatory processes, to lessen or eradicate researcher–participant power imbalances.

If we accept that interview sensitivities are often reflected in researchers' choices of stories and storytellers for narrative inquiry projects, we can possibly also accept that storytellers and their stories require our special consideration. This is not to say that all storytellers involved in narrative inquiry are vulnerable, because narrative researchers in the health sciences can also be interested in participants' stories of health and lifestyle successes. Vulnerable storytellers may be children (Nordyke, Myléus, Ivarsson, Carlsson, Danielsson, Högberg, Karlsson and Emmelin, 2010), victims of sexual violence (Wiklund, Malmgren-Olsson, Bengs and Öhman, 2010), pregnant teenagers (Harlow, 2009), older women with cancer (Sinding and Wiernikowski, 2008), or young men and women with cancer (Hilton, Emslie, Hunt, Chapple and Ziebland, 2009).

In view of narrative researchers' interests in learning from storytellers' lived experiences, caution has been sounded. For example, De Haene, Grietens and Verschueren (2010) 'question narrative inquiry's predominant ethics of benefit when engaging in narrative research on trauma and social suffering'. When they explored the use of a narrative methodology in refugee health, De Haene et al. (2010) identified how narrative trauma research with vulnerable respondents can 'evoke the replay of traumatic experience within the research relationship itself' (p. 1664).

Given the ethical ramifications of conducting narrative research with vulnerable participants, Hall (2011) took an advocacy stance for participants' interests, using a critical feminist standpoint approach when she directed an interdisciplinary team in a large-scale 'constructivist, feminist, narrative study describing the trauma recovery process' (p. 3). Being fully aware of the ethical pitfalls in sensitive research with vulnerable participants, Hall (2011, p. 3) used feminist principles to navigate her way through this narrative study, which was 'focused on success or thriving in women surviving childhood maltreatment'.

The research example I have selected here to highlight participants as storytellers is the project by Nordyke et al. (2010) conducted with 12-year-old children involved in coeliac disease (CD) screening in Sweden. I have chosen it because it is a good example of researching a vulnerable group in relation to their age, but it also exemplifies making meaning out of 'sketchy' data by using thorough narrative analysis methods. After approval from the researchers' university Research Ethics Committee, 15 children's classes were approached during CD screening 'after blood sampling, but prior to learning of the test results' (p. 351). The researchers reported that school nurses and teachers forwarded information letters to the parents as part of the consent process and that consent to participate was given by 271 children, and 240 (89 per cent) of these submitted narratives, with drop-outs mostly due to being absent on the day of narrative writing. Most children wrote their name on the narrative, which along with their unique identification number, (mostly) allowed gender to be ascertained (107 girls, 109 boys, 24 unknown) ... For ethical reasons, families who had declined participation in the screening were not approached again even if the researchers believed that their experiences could have contributed to an understanding of non-participation (Nordyke et al., 2010, p. 352).

The children were also given a letter letting them know the focus of the project, that there were no wrong answers, and that the researchers 'wanted the children to focus their narratives around: (i) their feelings when deciding to participate, (ii) their thoughts and feelings on the day of the blood sampling, (iii) how they felt when waiting for the answer, and (iv) what they think is important to consider for participating children in the future' (p. 353).

The researchers used a form of content analysis to analyse the written narratives. They explained that the analysis began

> with the first (KN) and second (AM) authors reading the transcribed narratives from one class, writing a brief summary of each student's narrative and forming a naive interpretation of the class as a whole. Through this initial step, a flexible frame of reference was developed that guided further analysis. A portion of texts were then coded by KN and AM and these codes, along with potential categories and themes, were discussed with ME to negotiate the interpretation. The narratives were fairly brief and thus were considered as condensed meaning units. The analysis continued by KN labelling all the text with codes. More abstract labels, grouping the content that shared a commonality, were conceptualised into subcategories and categories. Properties and dimensions were added to illustrate the variation, an approach associated with grounded theory.
>
> (Nordyke et al., 2010, p. 353)

After analysis, the overall experience of the screening was captured in the theme 'A Journey towards Confidence', which illustrated 'that, although some children faced fear or anxiety, overall they had or were provided tools allowing them to cope well and experience a journey towards confidence' (p. 353). The categories contributing to the theme were *being involved*, which reflected 'the importance of involvement in receiving information and deciding to participate'; *being a good citizen*, which referred 'to feeling a duty to help and a trust to be treated fairly'; *being able to cope*, which was 'influenced by the children's ability to manage sensations and support received' during screening; and *being able to balance risk*, which illustrated 'that the children were able to balance the risks of screening when they had a realistic understanding of the disease and their vulnerability and had tamed their anxiety' (pp. 353–354). The researchers quite rightly concluded that the 'study increases the understanding of how 12-year-old Swedish children experienced participating in a CD screening and describes conditions important for a positive experience' (p. 357).

Qualitative researchers might well imagine that written narratives, especially those penned by children, may not reveal much about an area of research interest. However, this research demonstrates that a well-planned and facilitated narrative inquiry project with young children can tell us a great deal of how they experience necessary but potentially scary health screening procedures. As health professionals move increasingly towards using primary health screening procedures of all types of diseases for all age groups, we need to know what those procedures are like for the people experiencing them.

Nordyke et al.'s (2010) research is also noteworthy as an example of narrative analysis in that the researchers identified the strategies through which they achieved trustworthiness criteria. They outlined how they used

> interdisciplinary triangulation of researchers and continued peer debriefing sessions aimed at creating creditability. The researchers (had) expertise in CD research, qualitative research, paediatrics and nursing practice. Also, an audit trail was maintained throughout the study by taking field notes, meeting notes and analytical memo notes. To increase validity, the subcategories, categories and, finally, the theme were continuously compared to the narratives to ensure that the results were well grounded in the empirical text. The study's integrity was strengthened by the primary researcher and the principal qualitative researcher not being involved in the planning of the screening.
>
> (Nordyke et al., 2010, p. 353)

In summary, narrative analysis can focus on the storytellers as research participants, because qualitative researchers are often interested in people's private and personal experiences, intermeshed with incompletely or unexplained human phenomena. Interviewing methods and processes that enhance participants' in-depth disclosures are a means of getting to these private phenomena. Because participants are often encouraged to describe their life stories, in-depth interviews may be classified as sensitive, depending on the research focus, the nature of the participants, and the researcher–participant relationship.

Listeners: Reflexive interplay

What is the point of telling a story if there is no-one there to hear it? Listeners are integral to narrative inquiry in attending to narrative practices and environments (Gubrium and Holstein, 2009), and in sometimes finding deeper meaning by aligning themselves experientially within participants' stories (Myerhoff, 1979; Behar, 2007). With this in mind, when narrative researchers plan their projects, they need to ask themselves important questions in relation to their audiences, such as: Who will listen, with what focus, for what purposes, by what means? What is the role of the researcher as listener? To what extent will the listener contribute to the stories? Will the listener add in their own storied experience to the research?

Narrative inquiry is directed to listeners, who may be in various receptive roles, however specified, such as patients, clients and consumers. Listeners are also the researchers, who hear participants' accounts initially and have the responsibility of making sense of and disseminating the participants' messages on to other listeners. In the health sciences, narrative inquiry usually tries to create salient messages for listeners about health and illness, so that listeners have a chance to learn from the storytellers' experiences. It is by listening to the participants' experiential stories that personal, lived knowledge is shared, insights are gained and sometimes lives are changed.

Larkey and Hecht (2010) were interested in the effects of narrative as culture-centric health promotion. They were aware that 'health promotion interventions designed for specific cultural groups often are designed to address cultural values through culturally adapted messages' and that narrative theory has become a central medium for 'expressing and shaping health behaviour'. To this end, they present a *Model of Culture-Centric Narratives in Health Promotion* to test the 'narrative characteristics and psychosocial mediators of behavior change in a broad range of health interventions' (p. 114). The model:

> begins with proposing the salient narrative characteristics considered important in a story to be used in a health promotion message or intervention. These include personally engaging elements of the characters and story as well as more culturally embedded aspects of stories that create cultural resonance. These are seen to influence a set of mediators (i.e., responses to narratives that have been shown to be predictors of attitudinal and, in some cases, behavior change) including identification with the characters and transportation into the story (also called engagement). As individuals experience these responses to a story, the responses may trigger action in real-world contexts, such as discussion, group role modeling, and reinforcement. The combined set of mediators is expected to influence intentions (via attitudes and perception of social norms) about the behaviours being promoted, encouraging change patterned after the identified role models. Thus, we suggest a layered ... view of narrative, both as (a) a medium with characteristics that shape individual attitudes and beliefs, and as (b)

an expression of culture embedded in the telling of stories in group contexts.

(Larkey and Hecht, 2010, p. 121)

The model shows the importance of using culture-centric narratives for health promotion. While this example is not of a research project, the discussion of the model nevertheless highlights the importance of directing message-laden stories to listeners to raise awareness and potentially bring about lifestyle changes. The authors encourage testing the model by a number of quantitative tests for measuring the relationships between variables in the model, which is reasonable, given that their focus is on measuring the usefulness of the model in practice. The stories told within the parameters of the model present a different analysis challenge, because they are experiential stories told in culture-centric ways, so they require qualitative analysis methods.

Berkley-Patton, Goggin, Liston, Bradley-Ewing and Neville (2009) undertook narrative inquiry into *Adapting Effective Narrative-Based HIV-Prevention Interventions to Increase Minorities' Engagement in HIV/AIDS Services*. The researchers identified a need to produce culturally-specific role model stories to assist in improving HIV-prevention strategies for at-risk minorities in the Kansas City metropolitan area. The research aimed to talk with community members and HIV-positive minorities to identify barriers and facilitators related to HIV healthcare engagement. Role model narratives were then developed with a direct focus on the specific needs of the consumer group (who in this case were both storytellers and listeners).

The data collection methods included semi-structured interviews, focus groups and a survey. The semi-structured interviews were conducted with '12 key stakeholders in the HIV/AIDS community (e.g., healthcare providers, community advocates, AIDS service organization (ASO) staff' (p. 202). The focus of the interviews was 'HIV prevention, treatment, and social services provided; demographics of patients/clientele; steps required of patients to access services; funding for services provided; gaps in services; and challenges in providing/seeking their services' (p. 202).

A grounded theory analysis method was used to generate codes and themes from the interview transcriptions. The community stakeholders identified 'several challenges for minorities, particularly African Americans, in accessing HIV-related services'. The researchers 'categorized these challenges under three broad themes related to the continuum of HIV care. These themes and their descriptive aspects (shown in brackets) were (a) HIV screening [HIV testing, linkage to care], (b) HIV medical treatment [maintenance of appointments, patient–provider interactions, comorbidities, funding and system issues], and (c) HIV survivorship [supportive services, stigma] (Berkley-Patton et al., 2009, p. 202).

Berkley-Patton et al. (2009) also conducted focus groups with 18 'HIV positive persons who (a) accessed HIV health services at least twice a year, (b) were on a steady antiretroviral regimen for 9 months or longer, (c) self-reported adherence >90%, (d) had a stable viral load, and (e) had overcome barriers to care' (p. 202). The focus group discussion identified 'barriers, facilitators, motivators and strategies for managing HIV disease and accessing supportive services' (p. 202).

The data from the four focus groups averaging 90 minutes each were also coded using grounded theory analysis. Although it is not mentioned in the article, the focus group discussion must have been audiotaped to provide the transcribed data with which to undertake a grounded theory analysis. Four primary thematic categories related to disease management and engagement in health and ancillary services emerged from the focus group analyses. These themes were:

> (a) maintaining supportive medical care [appointments kept and lab work done on a regular basis; valued patient–provider communication and relationships; informed providers], (b) seeking out HIV information for personal empowerment [gathering HIV information from multiple sources, advocating for self/others], (c) using support systems [supportive people, groups, and strategies], and (d) having a positive outlook on life [dealing with HIV disease-related challenges, hope in living].
>
> (Berkley-Patton et al., 2009, p. 203)

The focus group participants also agreed to complete a survey before each group discussion. The survey questions were on the degree to which barriers and facilitators impacted their disease and the types of HIV ancillary services they had used. The researchers used univariate analyses to report the survey data. The survey data results, combined with the results from the semi-structured interviews and the focus groups' feedback, provided rich data from which to develop role-model narratives of specific relevance to the consumer group. The thematic issues identified in the research were developed into storylines, which illustrated to consumer audiences how to best approach their personal and organizational issues when navigating their way through HIV-related lifestyle and treatment challenges.

When we look at Berkley-Patton et al.'s (2009) project as an example of narrative analysis, we see that it exemplifies the common principle that the type of data analysis chosen is that which best fits the data collection method used. The project is unusual in that it was undertaken to enhance the use of role-model narratives in HIV prevention and treatment. Although the participants may have responded to the various interview and focus group questions in a narrative style, this does not mean that the researchers were seeking rich narratives on which to base the development of their role-model narratives. Even so, given the extreme variability in what constitutes narrative inquiry projects, this project seems a reasonable choice to highlight as an example of how the narrative researchers have undertaken their analyses. In this case, the results relied on storied accounts as told by the community stakeholders and the HIV participants, so in this project the individuals with HIV were at the same time storytellers and potential listeners.

Conclusion

The opportunities for using and developing narrative analysis methods and processes are as wide and deep as narrative inquiry itself. This chapter could not hope to gather in all of the possibilities for narrative analysis and so many other approaches have not been discussed. For example, performative narrative acts out stories on a stage, leaving the interpretations open to the particular audiences (Smith and Sparkes, 2011). Other researchers perform a narrative analysis of extant research literature on a given focus (Vallido, Wilkes, Carter and Jackson, 2010), while others co-create narratives (Antelius, 2009). All of the existing approaches to narrative inquiry and those yet to be imagined employ analysis methods and processes (or choose to leave stories open, neither analysed nor interpreted). Whatever the choices now or in the future, the field of narrative inquiry is wide open, meaning the responses of narrative analyses are wide open also.

Due to the versatility of narrative approaches in qualitative research, it is almost impossible to typify the existing and emerging methods and processes of narrative analysis. To clear a path through the jungle of narrative research possibilities, I suggested an approach to narrative analysis around a three-pronged axis of: the importance of the stories, depicting people's lived experiences; the storytellers, and how they narrate their experiences, constructing meaning for themselves and their audiences; and the listeners, focusing on the reflexive interplay between the narrative practices and environments, and in sometimes finding deeper meaning by aligning themselves experientially within participants' stories. The story, the storyteller and the listener are important in narrative inquiry and analysis, because they encompass narrated life experiences as forms of discourse, from which we can learn about human knowledge and existence. In the health sciences our learning is about how to understand and enhance people's experiences of health and wellbeing and to journey with them meaningfully through their illness trajectories.

Key points

- As a highly diversified qualitative research methodology, narrative analysis is inextricably interwoven into the fabric of narrative inquiry.

- Due to the versatility of narrative approaches in qualitative research, it is a complex undertaking to typify the existing and emerging methods and processes of narrative analysis.

- The story, the storyteller and the listener are important in narrative inquiry and analysis, because they encompass narrated life experiences as forms of discourse, from which we can learn about human knowledge and existence.

- In the health sciences, researchers value participants' life stories, so they use narrative inquiry and applied various analysis methods to explore participants' narratives of health and illness and to offer insights to health professionals and consumers as listeners.

Critical review questions

1 What are the advantages and disadvantages of collecting narrative data?

2 To what extent does narrative research play a part in your healthcare profession's key research issues and questions?

References

Antelius, E. (2009). Whose body is it anyway? Verbalization, embodiment, and the creation of narratives. *Health: An Interdisciplinary Journal for the Social Study of Health, Illness and Medicine, 13*(3), 361–379.

Bamberg, M. (Ed.) (2007). *Narrative-state of the art.* Philadelphia: John Benjamins.

Behar, R. (2007). *An island called home: Returning to Jewish Cuba.* New Brunswick, NJ: Rutgers University Press.

Bell, S.E. (2009). *DES daughters: Embodied knowledge and the transformation of women's health politics.* Philadelphia, Temple University Press.

Berkley-Patton, J., Goggin, K., Liston, R., Bradley-Ewing, A., & Neville, S. (2009). Adapting effective narrative-based HIV-prevention interventions to increase minorities' engagement in HIV/AIDS services. *Health Communication, 24,* 199–209.

Bingley, A.F., Thomas, C., Brown, J., Reeve, J., & Payne, S. (2008). Developing narrative research in supportive and palliative care: The focus on illness narratives. *Palliative Medicine, 22,* 653–658.

Chase, S.E. (2010). *Learning to speak, learning to listen: How diversity works on campus.* Ithaca, NY: Cornell University Press.

Chase, S.E. (2011). Narrative inquiry: Still a field in the making. In Denzin, N.K., & Lincoln, Y.S. (Eds.). *The SAGE handbook of qualitative research,* 4th edn. Thousand Oaks: Sage, 421–434.

Clandinin, D.J. (2007). *Handbook of narrative inquiry: Mapping a methodology.* Thousand Oaks: Sage.

De Haene, L., Grietens, H., & Verschueren, K. (2010). Holding harm: Narrative methods in mental health research on refugee trauma. *Qualitative Health Research, 20*(12), 1664–1676.

Denzin, N.K., & Lincoln, Y.S. (2011). *The SAGE handbook of qualitative research.* 4th edn. Thousand Oaks: Sage.

Gubrium, J.F., & Holstein, J.A. (2009). *Analyzing narrative reality.* Thousand Oaks: Sage.

Hall, J. (2011). Narrative methods in a study of trauma recovery. *Qualitative Health Research, 21*(1), 3–13.

Harlow, E. (2009). Eliciting narratives of teenage pregnancy in the UK: Reflexively exploring some of the methodological challenges. *Qualitative Social Work, 8*(2), 211–228.

Hilton, S., Emslie, S., Hunt, K., Chapple, A., & Ziebland, S. (2009). Disclosing a cancer diagnosis to friends and family: A gendered analysis of young men's and women's experiences. *Qualitative Health Research, 19*(6), 744–754.

Hole, R. (2007). Narratives of identity: A poststructural analysis of three deaf women's stories. *Narrative Inquiry, 17,* 259–278.

Knowles, J.G., & Cole, A.L. (Eds.) (2008). *Handbook of the arts in qualitative research: Perspectives, methodologies, examples, and issues.* Thousand Oaks: Sage.

Larkey, L.K., & Hecht, M. (2010). A model of effects of narrative as culture-centric health promotion. *Journal of Health Communication, 15,* 114–135.

Lewis, B. (2006) Listening to Chekhov: Narrative approaches to depression. *Literature and Medicine* 25(1), 46–71.

Lindenmeyer, A., Griffiths, F., Green, E., Thompson, D., & Tsouroufli, M. (2008). Family health narratives: Midlife women's concepts of vulnerability to illness. *Health*, 12, 275–293.

Lindsay, G.M. (2011). Patterns of inquiry: Curriculum as life experience. *Nursing Science Quarterly, 24*(3), 237–244.

McAllister, M.M. (2001). In harm's way: A postmodern narrative inquiry. *Journal of Psychiatric and Mental Health Nursing, 8*, 391–397.

Myerhoff, B. (1979). *Number our days: Culture and community among elderly Jews in an American ghetto.* New York: Meridian.

Nordyke, K., Myléus, A., Ivarsson, A., Carlsson, A., Danielsson, L., Högberg, L., Karlsson, E., & Emmelin, M. (2010). How do children experience participating in a coeliac disease screening? A qualitative study based on children's written narratives. *Scandinavian Journal of Public Health, 38*, 351–358.

Riessman, C.K. (2008). *Narrative methods for the human sciences.* Thousand Oaks: Sage.

Sinding, C., & Wiernikowski, J. (2008). Disruption foreclosed: Older women's cancer narratives. *Health: An Interdisciplinary Journal for the Social Study of Health, Illness and Medicine, 12*(3), 389–411.

Smith, B., & Sparkes, A. (2011). Exploring multiple responses to a chaos narrative. *Health, 15*(1), 38–53.

Vallido, T., Wilkes, L., Carter, B., & Jackson, D. (2010). Mothering disrupted by illness: A narrative synthesis of qualitative research. *Journal of Advanced Nursing 66*(7), 1435–1445.

Wiklund, M., Malmgren-Olsson, E-B., Bengs, C., & Öhman, A. (2010). 'He messed me up': Swedish adolescent girls' experiences of gender-related partner violence and its consequences over time. *Violence Against Women, 16*(2), 207–232.

15

Discourse analysis

Karen Francis

Discourse analysis (DA) is the intimate study of talk and text (Traynor, 2006; van Dijk, 2012). As a research methodology it is used to interpret, understand and in some cases to critique the function of talk, communication or text. The elements of discourse that are of interest include the style of the communication, the underlying social structures that permit or limit the communication or text and the message that is being delivered that is inclusive of both the overt and covert. As with other research methodologies there are various forms of discourse analysis (Lupton, 2004). DA that are interpretive only focus on how language, text is created and used while critical DA approach advocates assume that discursive practices provide for a power base that legitimates the speaker/ authors' (of the talk/text) authenticity and therefore validates primacy. Being heard and thus having power is time and context specific; that is, it is relational to social influences and dominant ideologies at the time the talk is generated (Rudge, Holmes, and Perron, 2011). The critical DA theorists assert that there is a political intent of discourse embedded in the constructions each speaker has of who they are and their ideological beliefs that inform their understandings, which can be revealed through a DA process (Cheek and Rudge, 1997; Gillett, 2012; Mulligan, Elliot, and Schuster-Wallace, 2012; Rudge et al., 2011).

The versatility of discourse analysis

Through language people communicate and investigate the world, learning about the social traditions and practices that define the behaviours of individuals, groups and cultures (Gillett, 2012). There is no single discourse analysis methodology, however all approaches, irrespective of where they are located on the interpretivist–critical interpretivist continuum (see Figure 15.1), allow researchers to describe and/or critique talk, communication, discourse, dialogue or text (Lupton, 2004). As such, DA enables researchers to explain relationships and can also be used to uncover

> ... the operation of power exercised by investigating how concepts and linguistic categories are developed and used at the institutional and societal level.
>
> (Traynor, 2006, p. 71)

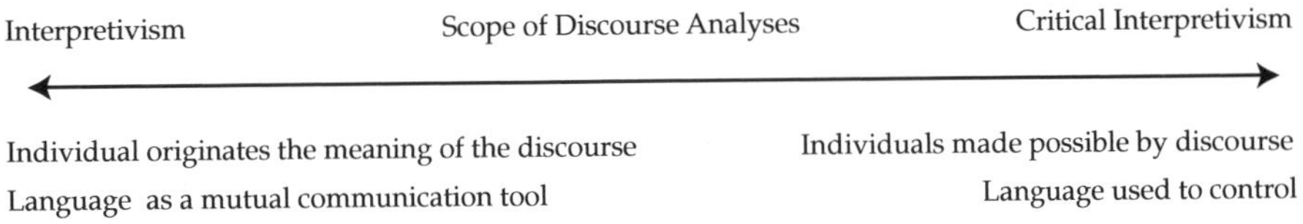

Figure 15.1 The scope of discourse analyses (based on Traynor, 2006)

DA studies generally access data that already exists, which is often cited as a strength although some authors have argued that it is a weakness, stating it was not produced for the purposes of research (Crowe, 2005; Matusov and von Duyke, 2012; Perakyla, 2008).

Types of discourse analysis

As previously highlighted, there are many forms of discourse analysis that most authors argue are reflective of the theoretical positions accepted by the researchers (Perakyla, 2008). These positions, suggests Traynor (2006, p. 65), range from a belief that individuals are free thinking and that they have autonomous control over language which they use to articulate their thoughts, to a belief that individuals are a product of the social structures of the society in which they live. This ideology maintains that each individual's capacity for autonomous thought and action is limited by opportunities that arise at specific points in time when ideologies change (Alvesson and Karreman, 2000; Traynor, 2006).

In attempting to explain the various DA approaches, Traynor (2006) used three different theorists' work to clarify subtle variations in philosophical thinking that influence the style of DA approaches. Firstly, he asserted that the interpretivist DA approaches view language as a mutually shared tool that allows for common understanding, while the critical DA proponents view it as method to enforce social, political and philosophical beliefs on individuals, groups and societies. The next method he offered is focused on how language is used and analysed. Interpretivist DA approaches see language as person initiated and it is used to communicate with others. This approach accepts that the initiator of the message is central, while the polar opposite approach views language as a mechanism to control how humans interpret and exist in their worlds. The final method he proposed is a four-category classification based on the work of Taylor (2001). Traynor's conceptualization of these classifications is described below:

- *'Identifying code': language properties and linguistics.* The DA researcher focuses on the properties of language; what is said and understood by others. This approach aligns with the philosophical positioning of the interpretivist paradigm. It provides for superficial consideration of the influence of the context only.

- *'Use and interaction': conversation analysis.* DA researchers are interested in language as an interaction tool. Proponents of this approach accept that talk is constrained by socially determined conversational practices.

- *'Interpretive repertoires': studies of occupation.* Similar to the previous categories, DA researchers aligning with this approach are fascinated by the relationship of language as a tool for communicating which they understand to be socially contextualized and constrained. This category adds a new dimension, the analysis of how individuals behave and engage through language with and in occupational groups (Rudge et al., 2011).

- *'Social discursive practices': studies of discourse and power.* DA approaches that fall within this category examine how discursive practices reflect societal and individual values and beliefs (Traynor, 2006, 64–65). Critical DA approaches are included in this grouping. Critical DA holds that language or discourse constructs, illustrates and defines reality. The analysis of discourse using this approach locates why, who and for what purposes the text or dialogue exists, and why it has pre-eminence (Mulligan et al., 2012; Perakyla, 2008; Traynor, 2006). Foucault's 'the Clinic' illustrated how medical dominance evolved as disciplinary knowledge was established through the creation of a new language (discursive practice) for medical personnel and excluded others. Discourse as argued by Foucault is used to affirm and maintain power, and therefore to create opportunity for domination of others (Gillett, 2012; Graham, 2005; McIntyre, Francis, and Chapman, 2012; Traynor, 2006).

Figure 15.1 illustrates the scope of discourse analysis approaches that range from being purely interpretivist in nature to aligning with the critical interpretivist positions as previously described.

Traynor (2006) summarized the variation in DA approaches on the basis of theoretical orientation. He qualified his arguments, however, stating that some DA researchers combine elements from a number of different approaches along the DA continuum to meet specific research needs. It is our contention that such practices lead to the evolution of methodology.

Undertaking a discourse analysis

Generating data

Researchers contemplating undertaking a study using DA decide on what theoretical approach will be appropriate for their study. The framing of the research question/s informs this stage of the research process. Traynor's (2006) work and that of the authors he referenced (Taylor, 2001; Alvesson and Karreman, 2000) provides a useful guide to assist researchers to understand the array of approaches to DA and their points of difference. Once this decision is finalized, isolating the text that will constitute the data is finalized. The text or talk that is the sample may be government or organizational reports, commentaries in the media, scholarly writings or personal communications to name just a few. Researchers next decide how large the sample will be (the number of texts) and how the data will be accessed (Lupton, 2004). McIntyre et al. (2012) utilized a critical DA methodology to investigate how key stakeholders who they grouped as Government, maternity healthcare professionals, public press and consumers, used discursive power to influence the direction of maternity care reform. The data accessed for their study were submissions from stakeholders to the Australian National Review of Maternity Services website and also media articles published in *The Australian*, a national newspaper. The latter data were limited to a three-year period (2008–2011) subsequent to the release of the government report on maternity services that addressed maternity issues.

Data analysis

The method adopted for analysis of the data is informed by the theoretical approach. Researchers interested in understanding language as a communication method, interrogate the data for what information, messages, are conveyed. Lupton (2004) offered that counting the number of times identified information appears in text is one way to identify overt or superficial messages. This deductive approach of analysing data does not take into consideration the socio-cultural influences that may have influenced the production of the text (van Dijk, 2012). Researchers using an approach that is more aligned to the critical interpretivist end of the continuum as described by Traynor (2006), employ more qualitative data analysis methods and probe the data for understanding of why and for what purpose the discourse exists. Lupton (2004) contended that researchers at this end of the continuum ask the data questions that include:

- How are things said?
- What is the underlying meaning of what is said?

If a critical DA methodology is adopted the text is further scrutinized by asking more probing questions that Lupton (2004) suggests allow for deconstruction of the text. The type of questions that are used include:

- Why are certain words, phrases and images used?
- What are the deeper, covert meanings and assumptions imbued in the text?
- Whose interests are being served by the text?
- What sorts of moral and political judgements are being expressed in the text?
- How are social groups represented and what implications does this have for society? (Lupton, 2004, p. 489)
- What is the basis for the speaker/s' legitimacy and who has given them power to speak?

Fairclough (2003) provides a useful approach to guide critical DA that is useful for health researchers. His approach 'links textual and sociological processes' (Traynor, 2006) allowing for issues of power, resistance and identity to be recognized (Rudge et al., 2011). McIntyre et al. (2012, p. 5) utilized Fairclough's method which they stated involves three phases of targeted questioning of the text. The three phases involved review of the text from different perspectives that included:

- Sociocultural influences
- Discourse practices
- Textual analysis.

Sociocultural influences are identified by uncovering unspoken and unstated assumptions embedded in the text that legitimate the speaker's authority to have a voice. *Discourse practice* analysis encompasses discovering why the text was produced, how it has been distributed and who is using the text. *Textual analysis* refers to the construction of the text, the language and style used to convey meaning (McIntyre, Francis, and Chapman, 2011).

A number of authors have advocated developing templates that allow for data to be categorized or sorted. Each text document is read and then reread. The researcher distinguishes the styles adopted for each individual text and through this process heightens their awareness ensuring that they are able to expose the overt messages. As the researcher becomes more familiar with the text a secondary analysis is undertaken that results in the exposure of assumed knowledge and covert messages within the text/s. This process is achieved by asking the text questions as described previously; deconstructing the data from which a reconstruction or analysis is realized. Using a template that provides a framework for doing and reporting on the process of analysis coupled with journaling thoughts that have informed decision making is advocated as the decision making process can be tracked and provides a decision pathway thus supporting arguments for how rigour was maintained. There are no rules governing the development of an analysis template. Prior (2011) described concept mapping or concept clustering as a useful system for sorting data and identifying relationships.

Once the data is mapped, visual interrogation with reference to the research questions and the particular DA approach used can assist researchers to detect overt and covert messages. Next, relationships can be located and pursued as further insights lead to isolating reasons for why the text exists. Another method proposed to manage data analysis is to use the 'highlight and comment' tools on a word processing program such as Microsoft Word. Text is read and segments of text highlighted that are of significance to the researcher. Comments can be inserted tagging the data segment as important. These tags can aid the researcher to further theorize about the data. These data segments may be used as evidence supporting arguments of social influences, discursive practices and as examples of how language has been used (Prior, 2011).

McIntyre et al. (2012) developed a table that was used to categorize sorted data that reflected Fairclough's three-stage analysis process; these were: key stakeholder, text source, presentation, and discourse. They argued that by revealing the selected texts for inclusion in their study and ensuring equal representation of the discourses for all stakeholder groups included in the study they had controlled for researcher bias (McIntyre et al., 2012).

Data analysis is a complex and exhaustive process that requires intimacy with the data. Knowing the data, reflecting on it with continual reference to the tenets that underpin the DA approach used is fundamental to completing the project. Once the researcher is convinced that the data has been analysed thoroughly, findings generated are compared with the literature. Points of consistency are described and difference explicated. Finally, the contribution that the DA makes is emphasized.

Limitations

DA is a qualitative research methodology that many authors have commented can lead to a biased analysis of the data (Matusov and von Duyke, 2012). Data used for DA studies has not been generated for research purposes, which some commentators have claimed is a weakness of the methodology (Matusov and von Duyke, 2012; Perakyla, 2008). Other antagonists of this methodology have stated that DA is an etic research endeavour and therefore it fails to provide the insider, emic perspective (Perakyla, 2008). Finally, results of DA studies are not generalizable, however like all qualitative methodologies the findings of DA research inform understanding.

Chapter summary

This chapter has provided an overview of the diversity of DA methodologies. The process for completing a research investigation using a DA approach has been described.

Key points

- As a research methodology, discourse analysis is used to interpret, understand and in some cases to critique the function of talk, communication or text.

- Discourse analysis is an interpretative qualitative research methodology that allows researchers to describe and/or critique talk, communication, discourse, dialogue or text.

- There are many forms of discourse analysis that most authors argue are reflective of the theoretical positions accepted by the researchers.

- The method adopted for analysis of the data is informed by the theoretical approach, for example, researchers interested in understanding language as a communication method interrogate the data for what information, messages are conveyed.

Critical review questions

1 Discuss the range of DA approaches, identifying the theoretical tenets that underpin them.

2 Locate a contemporary health issue that has been described in the public press and undertake a critical DA of the text. Identify what is being said, who is saying it, for what purposes and who has given them the authority to speak. Discuss the implications of this analysis for healthcare professionals and the broader community.

References

Alvesson, M., & Karreman, D. (2000). Varieties of discourse: On the study of organisations through discourse analysis. *Human Relations, 53*(9), 1125–1149.

Cheek, J., & Rudge, T. (1997). The rhetoric of healthcare? Foucault, healthcare practices and the docile body – 1990's style. In O'Farrell (Ed.), *Foucault the legacy* (1st edn). Brisbane: Queensland University of Technology.

Crowe, M. (2005). Discourse analysis: towards an understanding of its place in nursing. *Journal of Advanced Nursing, 51*(1), 55–63.

Fairclough, N. (2003). *Analyzing Discourse: Textual Analysis for Social Research.* London: Routledge.

Gillett, K. (2012). A crtitical discourse analysis of British national newspapers representations of the academic level of nurse education: too clever for our own good. *Nursing Inquiry, 19*(4), 297–307.

Graham, L.J. (2005). *Discourse analysis and the critical use of Foucault.* Paper presented at the Australian Association for Research in Education Sydney. eprints.qut.edu.au/2689/1/2689.pdf.

Lupton, D. (2004). Discourse analysis. In V. Minichiello, G. Sullivan, K. Greenwood & R. Axford (Eds.), *Research Methods for Nursing and Health Science* (2nd edn, pp. 483–497). Frenchs Forest, NSW: Pearson Education Australia.

Matusov, E., & von Duyke, K. (2012). Broader outside social discourses, embodiment, and technism in James Cresswell's critique of discourse analysis methodology. *Discourse & Society, 23*(5), 609–618. doi: 10.1177/0957926512455883.

McIntyre, M., Francis, K., & Chapman, Y. (2011). Shaping public opinion on the issue of childbirth; a critical analysis of articles published in an Australian newspaper. *BMC Pregnancy and Childbirth, 11.*

McIntyre, M., Francis, K., & Chapman, Y. (2012). Critical discourse analysis: Understanding change in maternity services. *International Journal of Nursing Practice, 18*(1), 36–43.

Mulligan, K., Elliot, S.J., & Schuster-Wallace, C.J. (2012). Global publc health policy transfer and dengue fever in Putrajaya, Malaysia: a critical discourse analysis. *Critical Public Health 22*(4), 407–418.

Perakyla, A. (2008). Analyzing talk and text. In N.K. Denzin & Y.S. Lincoln (Eds.), *Collecting and Interpreting Qualitative Materials.* (3rd edn, pp. 351–374). Los Angeles: Sage.

Prior, L. (2011). Using documents in Social Research. In D. Silverman (Ed.), *Qualitative Research* (pp. 93–110). Los Angeles: Sage.

Rudge, T., Holmes, D., & Perron, A. (2011). The rise of practice development with/in reformed bureaucracy: discourse, power and the government of nursing. *Journal of Nursing Management, 19*, 837–844.

Taylor, S. (2001). Locating and conducting discourse analytic research. In S. Taylor & S. Yates (Eds), *A guide for Analysis.* London: Sage/Open University Press.

Traynor, M. (2006). Discourse analysis: theoretical and historical overview and review of papers in the *Journal of Advanced Nursing* 1996–2004. *Journal of Advanced Nursing 54*(1), 62–72.

van Dijk, T.A. (2012). A note on epistemics and discourse analysis. *British Journal of Social Psychology, 51*(3), 478–485. doi: 10.1111/j.2044-8309.2011.02044.x.

16

Creative forms of qualitative data collection and analysis

Bev Taylor

Anything we do in the name of seeking qualitative research data and making sense of it is in some way creative, because it requires us to dig into our imaginations to create the methods and processes most likely to unearth fresh, new insights into what it means to be human. Some forms of enquiry and analysis, however, are just that little bit more creative, because they step outside the boundaries of what have now, to some extent, they become conventional practices. For example, once upon a time unstructured, conversational interviewing was considered creative, because it dared to transgress the structural rules that standardized how we accessed participants' experiential accounts. Now, in the light of many decades of experience, qualitative researchers are at ease with free-flowing interviewing styles and participants enjoy deeper connections to the research process as collaborators and co-researchers. As qualitative researchers move further away from needing to constantly defend their practices against the yardstick of the scientific research method, and relax into the postmodern freedoms of relativism, abstraction and multiple representations of knowledge, contemporary, creative data collection and analysis methods and processes have emerged, and will keep on emerging.

This chapter discusses creativity and how this fits with human research, especially in the health sciences. Even though creative research approaches spill over into one another, to exemplify the possibilities, the methods and processes of art works, autobiographies, performance and photography are discussed.

Creativity in research

The doors are wide open for creativity in qualitative research, inviting researchers to step through to epistemological and ontological realms of multiple, tentative representations, interpretations, relativities and abstractions. Since the advent of qualitative research at the turn of the 20th century, paradigmatic shifts have taken qualitative researchers further and further away from the black and white certain and objective assumptions of positivism, to the brightly coloured tentative and subjective knowledge possibilities beyond postmodernism. The creative research influences have been felt not only in the social and human sciences, but also in the earth sciences, such as geography.

We might reasonably expect to see creativity in research in the social sciences, such as the arts, because they are by their very nature creative. However, while this implicit creativity has been foundational to their ontological roots, the arts have struggled to be seen as legitimate knowledge- and research-based disciplines. Even though the arts of music, dance, painting, sculpture, literature, drama and others are established social media for upturning firmly held conventions about human existence, until the critiques of positivism they were seen 'as largely emotive rather than primarily informative' (Eisner, 2008, p. 3). While other social sciences such as psychology and sociology gained their epistemological credibility by adopting positivistic assumptions and methods, the content and form of the arts on the whole have not been conducive to quantification and the strict controls of the scientific method. In this contemporary era, however, the arts are not only established as valid epistemological sources, they also offer methods and processes for gathering knowledge in all areas of qualitative research (Knowles and Cole, 2008).

We might be less likely to expect to see creativity in the earth sciences, but the discipline of qualitative geography has slipped out of the constraints of objective space and place inquiry, to embrace the full range of creative, methodologically-based research possibilities. DeLyser, Herbert, Aitken, Crang and McDowell (2010) explain how the transition occurred from quantitative to qualitative research:

> Aligned, for the most part, with a putatively positivistic science, quantitative geography forged forward, carried on waves of technological advances (in statistical methods and computational capability), constructing and employing large data sets in the pursuit of generalizable knowledge, until, for a time in the mid-twentieth century, a quantitative-inspired paradigm became dominant in the discipline ... Amid this fervour for numerical sophistication and explanation, qualitative human geographers, traditionally mute on the subject of methods and methodology, initially offered little response. By the 1970s, however, humanist, feminist and some radical geographers argued for a qualitative *human* geography that recognized and validated human experience, and they led campaigns for the recognition of qualitative work as valid and valuable (p. 5).

Although it has experienced some ongoing criticism, mainly casting it in poor light against quantitative research assumptions and methods, human geographers have continued to progress their human perspectives of space and place. For example, in their *Handbook of Qualitative Geography*, DeLyser et al. (2010) feature writers describing various creative encounters and collaborations. In Part Two of the book, chapters feature: Ethnography and Participant Observation (Watson and Till, 2010); Autoethnography as

Sensibility (Butz, 2010); Interviewing: Fear and Liking in the Field (McDowell, 2010); Life History Interviewing (Jackson and Russell, 2010); Focus Groups as Collaborative Research Performances (Bosco and Herman, 2010); Visual Methods and Methodologies (Crang, 2010); and Performative, Non-Representational, and Affect Based Research: Seven Injunctions (Dewsbury, 2010). Not only are these approaches groundbreaking and highly creative for qualitative geographers, they are also instructive for researchers open to creativity in all fields, including the health sciences.

Creative approaches in qualitative research spill over into each other, so that it is difficult and somewhat unnecessary to try to extract one from the other. The mixing and merging of creative research approaches is evident in the next section, which addresses creativity in a sequential manner, even though creative methods and processes in research projects are often experienced as being in no particular sequence, non-delineated and utterly interconnected.

Undertaking and analysing creative forms of qualitative data collection

Creative expressions seldom exist alone. Music goes well with dance, dance favours lighting, costumes and backgrounds, writing loves characters who attract readers, who listen to music as they read, and so on. So it is with qualitative research, where creative approaches tend to prefer company. In qualitative research, creative data forms often combine to enliven one another, adding to the depth and richness of the accounts and the interpretations of the meanings. For example, in the ethnographies the methods go beyond the traditional options of participant observation and interviewing to the creative possibilities of performance ethnography (Alexander, 2008) and critical ethnography as street performance (Madison, 2008), both of which interpret performance through drama, dance, music and so on.

Creativity in research tends to break free from methodological boundaries, to embrace and play with a wide range of philosophical and practice assumptions. Keeping to the example of performance ethnography, its creative approaches are

> both interdisciplinary and polydisciplinary: interdisciplinary because it relies on and forges connections between a variety of fields – communication and theater studies, for example, or music and folklore. It is polydisciplinary because so many areas claim and contribute to it: anthropology, communication, dance, ethnomusicology, folklore, performance studies, theater studies ... Performance ethnography is inter- and polydisciplinary because performance itself demands it.
>
> (Hamera, 2011, p. 317)

Although many creative research approaches are emerging all the time, in this chapter I have selected art works, autobiography, performance and photography to highlight as possibilities for qualitative data collection and analysis.

Art works

Pablo Picasso is purported to have claimed: 'I never made a painting as a work of art, it's all research' (McNiff and Whitehead, 2008, p. 29). Art is both the focus of art-based research and it is also a means of data collection, analysis and interpretation. McNiff and Whitehead (2008, p. 29) makes the distinction between art-based research and the use of art as data when he explains that art-based 'research can be defined as the systematic use of the artistic process, the actual making of artistic expressions in all of the different forms of the arts, as a primary way of understanding and examining experience by both researchers and the people that [sic] they involve in their studies'. This means that doing arts as action is the focus of arts-based research, whether it is in creating a painting, choreographing a dance, or composing a piece of music. Whatever the art form, art-based researchers show

> a willingness to start the work with questions and a willingness to design methods in response to the particular situation, as contrasted to the more general contemporary tendency within the human sciences to fit the question into a fixed research method. The art-based researcher extends to the creation of the process of inquiry.
>
> (McNiff and Whitehead, 2008, pp. 33–34)

Finley (2008, p. 71) identifies a transformative purpose in arts-based research, when she claims, as a 'form of performance pedagogy, arts-based inquiry can be used to advance a subversive political agenda that addresses issues of social inequity. Such work exposes oppression, targets sites of resistance, and outlines possibilities for transformative praxis'. In contrast, arts-informed researchers are not artists per se, neither do they necessarily hold transformative agendas, but drawing on their

> artistic sensibilities, relationship to the arts, and respect for ways in which artists of all genres have throughout history, tackled society's pressing socio-political concerns and confronted public audiences with their messages, (they) turned (their) attention to the relationship between art and research and the possibilities inherent in infusing processes and representational forms of art into social science inquiry ... by dabbling with two and three-dimensional art, performance, and fiction mainly for the purposes of representation ... (and by exploring) media of poetry, literary prose, playwriting, visual arts, dance, and music as alternative approaches to knowledge representation and advancement.
>
> (Cole and Knowles, 2008, p. 58)

It is possible to integrate the arts into health science research as both art-based research and arts-informed research. The arts-based artist as researcher opens up to locating and exploring phenomena through artistic media, while arts-informed researchers and co-researchers explore deeper meanings of lived experiences as project participants assisted by various artistic strategies. For example, Clover (2011) undertook a feminist arts-based participatory approach with homeless/street-involved women in Victoria, Canada. The creative research methods used were 'group interviews and the creation of collective and individual artworks to explore their personal and political realities and share these with a larger audience' (Clover, 2011, p. 19). Over an 18-month period, two feminist university researchers, two facilitators and two artists made themselves available to approximately 20 homeless/street-involved women, who came to the project voluntarily. The women made a commitment

> a) to work with diverse mediums and professional artists … ; b) to meet at least twice a week and; c) to mount at least one exhibition. (They) then brainstormed the elements of the actual study agreeing the questions would uncover the changes (or not) the arts were making in their lives and the impact of the art-making. (They) also agreed (they) would ask the audience about their impressions at the exhibitions. The women were adamant also that everyone – the researchers and facilitators – participate in the art-making.
>
> (Clover, 2011, p. 16)

The women's artworks gave them a medium through which to find their own voices about the meaning they made of their homeless and street living experiences. The individual art works created included 'masks, poetry, collages, paintings, bead work, miniature mosaics, and a dress designed from old plastic bags … Collective works were a quilt, a mural, a life-size marionette, a collage, a decoupage on wood, and a tile mosaic featuring a phoenix taking flight' (Clover, 2011, p. 16). The benefits of the project were that the women learned to trust one another and how to build community through empathic sharing. They also experienced and developed aesthetic identity and personal and collective empowerment. However, Clover (2011, p. 16) indicated that 'tensions and challenges emerged around art as education versus therapy, individual and collective works, the role and place of men, and mental health and the police, two things ever present in the lives of these women'. Therefore, this project was not only about using art works as creative research methods for exploring participants' lived experiences, it was also about letting a participatory process evolve within the project itself.

Food for thought

Imagine a research project you have done or contemplated previously. If you have neither example, choose a qualitative (essentially 'standard') project you have read. Now re-vision it to include art works and a participatory process. How does the revised research plan differ in content and potential complexity from your original plan? What are the likely advantages and disadvantages of incorporating art works into a qualitative research plan?

Across a wide range of disciplines, health science researchers are using art works in qualitative research projects. In psychology, the arts are research strategies for knowing self (Higgs, 2008). The arts provide agencies for critical imagination in social work (Chambon, 2008). In nursing, art forms such as drawings, paintings, narrative videos and drama are transformative research strategies, which inspire a deeper exploration of illness and wellness mediated through nursing care (Bergum and Godkin, 2008). Health policy researchers are using theatre as a creative knowledge generation and validation modality (Nisker, 2008) and arts-informed inquiry is being used in disability studies (Ignagni and Church, 2008).

In summary, whether art works are used in art-based research or arts-informed research, or in merged identities of both, art forms have the creative potential to enrich and deepen participants' and researchers' epistemological and ontological understandings of human experiences. In the health sciences, art works assist participants to find their voices and share actively in research projects, while they uncover their personal and collective insights into the phenomena being explored. Researchers have the potential to explore new research topographies and stretch the boundaries of methods and processes they use in undertaking research, while creating and validating new insights into research questions about human experiences.

Autobiographies

The creative research possibilities of autobiography arbitrarily included and described in this section are reflective topical autobiography (RTA) and performative autoethnography. These approaches are creative, and they confidently answer the questions: How can a study of self be acceptable as research? Is *that* real research?

Reflective topical autobiography (RTA)

Two of the most interesting PhD projects I have supervized using RTA were undertaken by candidates with very different backgrounds, interests and life stories (Myers, 2008; Zammit, 2008). Estelle Myers' PhD came about because of her boundless energy and lifelong pursuit of good causes. Carmen Zammit's PhD came about because she was dying and wanted to give a first person account of the experience. Both women were passionate about reflecting on their life experiences, with abundantly rich stories to tell, and deeply personal messages to impart.

Autobiographies provide personal, partial, context-bound knowledge from which other people can benefit. According to Richardson (2003), autobiographical research is not only a way of knowing, it is also a process of discovery. Reflective topical autobiography is a focused autobiographical method that can be used by researchers to retrace the events of their lives and the sense they have made of them through reflection. Johnstone (1999, p. 24) suggested to nurses that this form of historical research 'is an important research method in its own right, and one which promises to make a substantive contribution to the overall project of advancing nursing inquiry and knowledge'. Although Johnstone was keen to encourage nurses to see the worth of RTA, this creative qualitative research approach can be used by all researchers who want to make a knowledge contribution to any human-centred discipline.

Johnstone (1999, p. 25) encouraged the 're-visioning of an original topical self-life story', which 'leaves open to the self-researcher the opportunity to return at will to his or her life story again to re-read, re-vision and re-tell the story in the light of the new insights, understandings and interpretations of meaning acquired through ongoing lived experience'. In this sense, RTA is positioned in the interpretive paradigm, integrating storytelling with history, and it also resonates well with postmodern epistemological assumptions, that knowledge is personal, contextual, partial and transitory. When used as a research approach RTA does not deign to render a 'true account of the self (as some researchers subscribing to the tenets of positivistic research expect...), but to render an account of the lived experience of self that advances shareable understanding of common human experiences' (Johnstone, 1999, p. 25).

Estelle (Myers, 2008) sorted through a lifetime of personal archives to locate topical aspects of her life. The research aim of her RTA was 'to reflect on and recount (her) own life stories and the life lessons learned, in order to identify patterns, trends and insights from (her) life to offer these insights to others' (p. 7). The thesis began with personal reflections on her childhood and young adulthood, connecting these experiences to her later major initiatives in freeing cetacea, championing water births, mediating for world peace and growing spiritually herself. The RTA is laid out systematically as a PhD thesis with all the usual academic inclusions, such as a literature review, ethics clearance considerations and a methodology chapter. Estelle also substantiated her personal growth and action claims with photographs, reflective writing, newspapers excerpts and a DVD. The combination of these methods not only made for enjoyable reading, it also provided a comprehensive, validated account of topical aspects of Estelle's life, which are instructive for others with whom they resonate.

Carmen (Zammit, 2008) wanted to describe her experience of dying and to describe the impact on family, friends and others. Her RTA objectives were to give an account of dying to help her own genetic family and to 'reach those interested parties who would benefit from this information and knowledge, particularly those who were diagnosed with a life-threatening illness' (Zammit, 2008, p. 3). Carmen's PhD was awarded posthumously and websites have been created: http://carmenhealingjourney.com/about.htm and http://carmenhealingjourney.com/.

As an accomplished artist, Carmen chose to her portray her RTA through images and stories, the lived experience of which she then interpreted for herself and for others. For example, in the thesis document (Zammit, 2008, pp. 103–105) the image: *Living Horror* (Figure 16.1) is depicted and described thus:

Living Horror

This image comes to mind when I recall my demeanour, when I was critically ill and expecting to die. At that time, I was thin, and unable to eat. I was aware of the fact that I had metastatic cancer that had now spread throughout my body (represented by the red spots in the drawing). The largest tumours – on my thigh, lower back and shoulder – created lumps that could be seen and felt through my skin. The doctors' efforts now seemed futile. There was no relief, no escaping this reality. In this image, the female figure represents me at this time. My demeanour is one of utter terror and horror. I am bound by rope to convey the paralysis I felt, and I was unable to move, unable to escape. Any movement at that time was excruciatingly painful, so I lay quite still. In spite of the morphine I was taking, I was conscious of my circumstances – that I was critically ill, that Western medicine was ineffective at this point, that I was about to die at any time, and in a horrible, dreadful manner. There had already been some close calls, and finally there would be the bullet that was aimed to kill. I would die the victim in life's macabre game of Russian Roulette.

As I reflect on this illustration, I notice some features that reveal truths that were not drawn consciously. For instance, neither my hands nor feet are drawn. The omission of hands indicates to me the powerlessness I felt at the time; I felt unable to do anything at all about my situation. The omission of legs and feet describes my actual inability to move, to stand

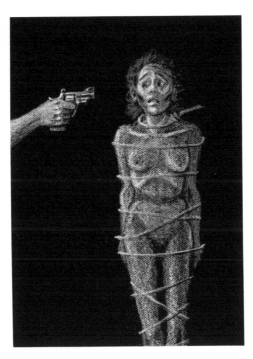

Figure 16.1 Living Horror

and to walk. I interpret the image of the gun pointing at my head as imminent and sure death. I also see it as a metaphor for the need to bring to an end my conditioned inclination to relate to my life and the world predominantly 'from my head', that is, from my thought-processes and intellect alone. There is no figure attached to the gun pointing at my head. In my mind, the figure is definitely masculine. It represents the aggressive, destructive and exploitative aspects of patriarchy.

This, for me, was ultimately a transformative and life enhancing event. I allowed myself to experience fully the feelings I had at the time – I was paralysed with fear, threatened with the real danger of losing my life, feeling extreme pain and futility. From this immersion, I noticed a sense of familiarity – I had experienced these feelings before. They were there in my childhood. I was shocked by my sudden discovery, that in spite of all my determined lifelong efforts, I had never truly transcended my childhood legacy. I had never really found the true peace of mind I had so longed for. My whole life had been one of struggle, full of effort to overcome my difficulties. At that point of realization, I experienced profound and heart-felt compassion for myself, for the hardships I had endured, for the never-realised goal I had set for myself. I had believed wrongly that peace was something I would achieve in the future (after much hard work), however, as such, it remained in the future. This was a profound insight, one not understood merely by the intellect. It was an insight that I experienced with my whole being. I finally, profoundly, completely, understood.

This insight led to my consciously choosing a different way of being in the world. My previous focus on 'doing' things (to overcome my difficulties) was clearly mistaken. My state of 'being' was now paramount – a truth I had neglected unknowingly all my life, until then. Even during this very difficult and (seemingly) very late stage of my life when all seemed hopeless and futile, when I was racked with pain believing that I would not survive, I decided to live my life – however much longer it was to be – in the way I had always wanted to live it. I had believed previously that I had to struggle hard to overcome my difficulties that I had to earn peace of mind and freedom from suffering. Everything in my culture seemed to support this delusion. I saw finally my life's mistake clearly. I finally understood deeply – when I believed it was too late – an adage of profound wisdom and compassion: *'There is no way to peace – peace is the way'* (A.J. Muste).

In summary, an RTA is an account of self, written in the first person, as personal experiences of potential interest and insights for others. As an academic thesis an RTA is usually recorded as text (for the ease of examiners), but it is possible to imagine an RTA using DVD and online technologies. The creative data sources for an RTA can be anything at all, such as: DVD recordings of talk, music, songs, dance, dramatization, art works and so on; photographs; written or spoken text, verses and poetry; newspaper clippings;

and so on. The media chosen will be those that best relate the self story. The 'data' analyses and interpretations are made by the reflecting researcher, who then leaves the RTA 'laid open' for multiple interpretations from readers.

Performative autoethnography

Sometimes the epistemological assumptions about the research worth of autobiographies merge into knowledge assumptions about the value of ethnography and performance studies, and the result is performative autoethnography. The autobiography is valid as a personal, local narrative of self and the ethnographic component is the account of the socio-political and cultural experience of living in a time and place. The performative aspect is in the artistry of the words, which bring together the personal narrative of experience of events and phenomena in such a way as to refresh and deepen history from written accounts of first person participation.

Spry (2011) defined performative autoethnography in ever enlarging word circles to encapsulate autobiography as critical ethnography within performance studies. Spry (2011) layers the meaning of performative autoethnography thus:

> Performative auto ethnography is a critically reflexive methodology resulting in a narrative of the researcher's engagement with others in particular sociocultural contexts. Performative autoethnography views the personal as inherently political, focuses on bodies in context as co-performative agents in interpreting knowledge, and holds aesthetic crafting of research as an ethical imperative of representation (p. 498).

> The process of performative autoethnography starts with a body, in a place, and in a time (p. 500).

> Embodied knowledge is the research home, the methodological toolbox, the 'breadth' of the performative ethnographer (p. 502).

> Making writing perform. Making the story answerable to its own sociocultural emergence, to its own performance, to its own life as art and back again ... Performative autoethnographic writing is about the continual questioning, the naming and renaming and unnaming of experience through craft, through heart, through the fluent body (p. 509).

Spry's (2011) writing exemplifies the methodology, as she moves softly and deeply between definitions and the philosophies into and through her own experiences of grief and loss. When I began reading Spry's (2011) words, I had a fleeting, almost anxious feeling, that I might not get the gist of her meaning. Then, like the unravelling of awareness that comes with gentle coaxing, I followed her words into an experience of performative autoethnography and sensed not only the meaning of the methodology, but also a deeper insight into her lived grief. The performative aspect of performative autoethnography comes from performance studies, which rests on exploring knowing as embodied experience. My reading of this creative methodology is that, essentially, the performance of embodied sociocultural and inherently political personal experience in performative autoethnography is through the creative performance of words and sentences in text, by discussing, philosophizing, critiquing, questioning, disclosing and poeticizing, to present a deeply reflected lived phenomenon.

In summary, experiences of living are set in time against social and cultural backdrops, and because they involve the person in context, they are intensely political. Postmodern assumptions about the partiality of knowledge and the value of personal narratives give health science researchers opportunities to explore their own experiences as performative autoethnographies. Writing is performance. We are writers of our personal histories. Researchers and participants are the same, as writers of their own experiences. Performative autoethnography provides a creative qualitative research option for accounting for lived history.

Performance

Performance of human situations and experiences can be incorporated into teaching (Denzin, 2003) and research (Denzin and Lincoln, 2011) as either a pedagogical or inquiry strategy. Performances may be enacted as drama, dance, music, art installations and so on, separately or in any possible combination, because performance is wide open to presentation, representation and interpretation. Qualitative research projects use performance as the focus of inquiry or to represent possible interpretations. While performance has boundless applications in qualitative research projects, its application is most visible within the ethnographies.

Hamera (2011) distinguishes between ethnography and performance ethnography in this way:

> Where traditional ethnography asks, 'How and why do my research interlocutors express what they do?' performance ethnography takes a more layered and critical approach, examining expression *about* the site as well as *within* it. It demands explicit attention to the politics of representing that expression, not just to conventions of accurately recording and interpreting it. Performance ethnography lifts up the 'graph', the always already taken-for-grantedness of writing … this is far more complex than an imagined dichotomy between text and performance (p. 320).

Hamera (2011) explores performance, ethnography, performativity and aesthetics as four of many possible 'elastic' keywords within performance ethnography, to highlight the freedom to play with the ideas. However, even though 'there are no prescriptions for operationalizing performance ethnography' she suggests that 'a set of key questions for performance ethnographers raised throughout the research process reminds us of our aesthetic, ethical, and intellectual responsibilities' (p. 322). Essentially, the main key questions are:

How does performance merge in my research site?

Where is my performance located in time and place, and how do these times and places intersect with history, with other places, other institutions?

When I use 'performance' and reflect on my own assumptions underlying this use, which scholarly conversations am I participating in, however implicitly?

How do I conceptualize the act of research itself as a performance, beyond the simple ideas of demonstrating 'competent execution': the techno bureaucratic definition of the term?

How and where does my research make meaningful interventions?

(Hamera, 2011, p. 323)

Performance is creative in its application to qualitative research of all types, such as in exploring and critiquing culture (Alexander, 2008) and in critical ethnography as street performance (Madison, 2008). Performance within research inquiry has also been explored and applied within the health sciences (Denzin, 2002; Gray, Sinding and Fitch, 2001; Kontos and Naglie, 2006; Smith and Gallo, 2007; Washington and Moxley, 2008). For example, Washington and Moxley (2008, p. 155) brought 'together in close correspondence social science, the humanities, and the helping professions' when they used performance in a narrative approach to assist 'older homeless African American women get and stay out of homelessness in the city of Detroit, Michigan, USA'. The research was part of an ongoing Leaving Homelessness Intervention Research Project (LHIRP) through which women told their individual stories of experiencing homelessness. Washington and Moxley (2008, p. 155) describe how, through

performance (such as gospel singing) undertaken by homeless and formerly homeless women, audiences experience the stories behind the data, which illuminate in first person detail the tragic toll this social issue takes in health and well-being, the strengths and virtues of the women, and the strategies that they see as useful in the successful resolution of homelessness.

In summary, performance in research inquiry is creative and highly versatile, but that does not mean it is applied thoughtlessly for added interest, or taken up haphazardly as entertainment. Performance adds depth and scope to qualitative projects if it is incorporated thoughtfully, with key questions in mind, to ensure that it is applied aesthetically, ethically, and intellectually. Performance contributes to qualitative research inquiry when it plays an important part in constituting research capable of generating and validating new and adapted forms of knowledge in areas of research interests.

Photography

Still photographs as individual images, or set into rapid sequence in film and DVDs, are becoming increasingly acceptable as valid, creative means of collecting and interpreting qualitative research information (Downing and Tenney, 2008; Frohmann, 2005; Iedema, Long, Forsyth and Bonsan, 2006; Knowles and Cole, 2008; Lorenz, 2011). In particular, photovoice has become popular in health sciences research (Castleden, Garvin, First Nation, 2008; Drew, Duncan and Sawyer, 2010; Findholt, Michael and Davis, 2010; Goodhart, Hsu, Baek, Coleman, Maresca and Miller, 2006; Martin, Garcia and Leipert, 2010; Novek, Morris-Oswald and Menec, 2012).

Photovoice is 'a participatory action research methodology that involves the use of photography and enables people to document, reflect upon, and communicate community needs to policymakers for the purpose of promoting social change' (Findholt et al., 2010, p. 186). The use of photography gives research participants a voice in the project. The basic process is for participants to take photographs representing their perceptions on a research interest and to share their thoughts in research group discussions. As the photographic images are representations, they do not assume a given 'truth', therefore, they rely on the person taking the photograph to share their perceptions and interpretations, and in so doing, find voice and also possibly gain deeper insights into the research focus.

Photographs have been used in qualitative research for some time, especially as a creative method to augment observation and interviewing in ethnographic research (Magilvy, Congdon, Nelson and Craig, 1992). Photographs have also been used in research with a range of participants to depict their experiences. For example, Frohmann (2005, p. 1396) used 'participant-generated photographs and photo-elicitation interviews as methods for exploring with women, in support group settings, the meanings of violence in their lives and their approaches to creating safer spaces'. In a project with patients, Lapum, Ruttonsha, Church, Yau and Matthews (2011) created a large installation of poetry and photography 'to research, interpret and exhibit patients' narratives of open heart surgery in "The 7,024th Patient" project – an arts-informed, narrative study' (p. 100). In both projects, the photographs provided deeper insights into participants' experiences than what may have been conveyed by words alone.

Given that photographs as images are representations of possible realities with many potential interpretations, their use 'comes with a warning' to qualitative researchers, in general and health science researchers, in particular. For example, the intentions and interpretations of the person taking the photograph as a research participant may be different from the person analysing and interpreting the image as a researcher. Increasingly, research participants are being given disposable cameras and invited to take images of anything representing their perceptions of a research area (Castleden, Garvin, and First Nation, 2008; Drew, Duncan and Sawyer, 2010; Findholt, Michael and Davis, 2010; Goodhart, Hsu, Baek, Coleman, Maresca and Miller, 2006;

Martin, Garcia and Leipert, 2010; Novek, Morris-Oswald and Menec, 2012). In this regard, when Lorenz (2011) revisited photographs taken previously by brain-injured research participants, she checked her original analytic perceptions with participants. In a process of careful conversation with participants who had taken the photographs, she gained fresh insights into 'the limits of researcher empathy and analysis' (p. 259). What researchers see in participant's photographs is coloured is by their own experiences, so even well-intentioned interpretations may be well off the mark. The lesson learned here is that the research participants' interpretations are what they are, and the best researchers can do is to provide the research conditions in which these insights can be teased out carefully and described as fully as possible.

In all human research, participants' rights for privacy and confidentiality must be protected. Researchers in the health sciences recognize the need for these rights on a professional and ethical level, because patients' diagnoses and treatments are confidential, closely guarded information. In health science research the use of photographic images, whether in still photographs or rapid sequence frame films and DVDs, have the potential of identifying patients and the places and people connected to their care. Also, if a person consents to be identified in any form of photographic image, the direct presentation of their identity is potentially long lasting as research data. If their image has been captured on DVD, along with spoken words about how they perceived and responded to research questions posed in that moment in time, they may change their perceptions and responses over time. Unsurprisingly, given these issues, ethical considerations are paramount in relation to using photographic images in qualitative research.

Even though Tenney and MacCubbin (2008) were directing their ideas towards social science researchers and video vision, their advice on ethical matters is sound for health science researchers seeking to use photographic images in any form in their projects. They summarize the main points in using photographic images in research as:

Ensure that your research is well designed;
    Create a consent form that facilitates informed consent with informed choice for potential participants;
    Demonstrate that you can identify when someone is giving true informed consent and that you have the ability to facilitate optimal conditions to meet the processes for obtaining informed consent ...;
    Create a separate consent and release process for your use of video (and photographs) in the form of an agreement between you and the people you are working with;
    Define how you will meet the standards set forth in the Nuremberg Code (1947), Declaration of Helsinki (1964) and the Belmont Report (1979);
    Create and give the IRB (or any specific ethics committee) replications of the video (photographic) techniques that you intend to employ by writing scripts and having actors perform scenarios (if appropriate);

Ensure that members of the (specific ethics committee) keep abreast of cutting edge (visual) technologies – such as video; and

Triangulate the principle of *Respect for Persons* from the Belmont Report (1979) to facilitate ethical research.

(Tenney and MacCubbin, 2008, pp. 16–17)

In summary, photographic images have been used in qualitative research for some time, and with developing technologies and increasing tendencies towards creative methods in qualitative research, they are likely to be used far into the future. However, photographic images need to be used carefully, after a full analysis of the risks and benefits to research participants. Also, even though the use of photographic images may deepen and enrich research data, care needs to be taken to ensure that participants are active in dialoguing with researchers about their interpretations, insights and implications from photographic data, so that researchers do not unwittingly impose their own context-bound perceptions on the data.

Chapter summary

In this chapter, I discussed creativity and how this fits with human research, especially in the health sciences. Creative research approaches are seldom contained to one modality or tradition, and this is evident in the proliferation of creative qualitative research approaches that borrow their artistic and epistemological ideas from many disciplines. Although there are many other extant and developing examples, in this chapter I described some creative research methods and processes relating to art works, autobiographies, performance and photography.

Key points

- As qualitative researchers move further away from needing to constantly defend their practices against the yardstick of the scientific research method, and relax into the postmodern freedoms of relativism, abstraction and multiple representations of knowledge, contemporary, creative data collection and analysis methods and processes have emerged, and will keep on emerging.

- In this contemporary era, the arts are not only established as valid epistemological sources, they also offer methods and processes for gathering knowledge in all areas of qualitative research.

- In qualitative research, creative data forms often combine to enliven one another, adding to the depth and richness of the accounts and the interpretations of the meanings.

- It is possible to integrate the arts into health science research as both art-based research and arts-informed research.

- The arts-based artist as researcher opens up to locating and exploring phenomena through artistic media, while arts-informed researchers and co-researchers explore deeper meanings of lived experiences as project participants assisted by various artistic strategies.

- Reflective topical autobiography is a focused autobiographical method that can be used by researchers to retrace the events of their lives and the sense they have made of them through reflection.

- The performance of embodied sociocultural and inherently political personal experience in performative autoethnography is through the creative performance of words and sentences in text, by discussing, philosophizing, critiquing, questioning, disclosing and poeticizing, to present a deeply reflected lived phenomenon.

- Performance adds depth and scope to qualitative projects if it is incorporated thoughtfully, with key questions in mind, to ensure that it is applied aesthetically, ethically, and intellectually.

- Photographic images have been used in qualitative research for some time, and with developing technologies and increasing tendencies towards creative methods in qualitative research, they are likely to be used far into the future.

- Photographic images need to be used carefully, after a full analysis of the risks and benefits to research participants, and care needs to be taken to ensure that participants are active in dialoguing with researchers about their interpretations, insights and implications from photographic data.

Critical review questions

1 What are the advantages and disadvantages of collecting creative forms of data?

2 To what extent does creativity play a part in gathering data for your healthcare profession's key research issues and questions?

References

Alexander, B.K. (2008). Performance ethnography: The reenacting and inciting of culture. In Denzin, N.K., & Lincoln, Y.S. (Eds.) *Strategies for qualitative inquiry.* Thousand Oaks: Sage, 75–118.

Belmont Report (1979). *The Belmont Report: Ethical principles and guidelines for the protection of human subjects of research.* Retrieved September 7, 2012 from hhs.gov/ohrp/humansubjects/guidance/belmont.html.

Bergum, V., & Godkin, D. (2008). In Knowles, J.G., & Cole, A.L. (2008). *Handbook of the arts in qualitative research: Perspectives, methodologies, examples, and issues.* Thousand Oaks: Sage, 603–612.

Bosco, F.J. and Herman, T.H. (2010) Focus Groups as Collaborative Research Performances. In D. DeLyser, S. Herbert, S. Aitken, M. Crang and L. McDowell (eds) *The SAGE Handbook of Qualitative Geography*, New York: Sage.

Butz, D. (2010). Autoethnography as Sensibility. In D. DeLyser, S. Herbert, S. Aitken, M. Crang and L. McDowell (eds) *The SAGE Handbook of Qualitative Geography*, New York: Sage.

Castleden, H., Garvin, T., & First Nation, H. (2008). Modifying photovoice for community-based participatory indigenous research. *Social Science & Medicine, 66*, 1393–1405.

Chambon, A. (2008). Social work and the arts: Critical imagination. In Knowles, J.G., & Cole, A.L. (2008). *Handbook of the arts in qualitative research: Perspectives, methodologies, examples, and issues*. Thousand Oaks: Sage, 591–602.

Clover, D. (2011). Successes and challenges of feminist arts-based participatory methodologies with homeless/street-involved women in Victoria. *Action Research, 9*(1), 12–26.

Cole, A.L., & Knowles, J.G. (2008). Arts-Informed Research. In Knowles, J.G., & Cole, A.L. (2008). *Handbook of the arts in qualitative research: Perspectives, methodologies, examples, and issues*. Thousand Oaks: Sage, 55–70.

Crang, M. (2010). Visual methods and methodologies. In D. DeLyser, S. Herbert, S. Aitken, M. Crang and L. McDowell (eds) *The SAGE Handbook of Qualitative Geography*, New York: Sage.

Declaration of Helsinki (1964) The World Medical Association, Helsinki, Finland. Retrieved September 7, 2012 from http://aix-scientifics.com/en/_helsinki1964.html.

DeLyser, D., Herbert, S., Aitken, S., Crang, M., and McDowell, L. (eds) (2010) *Handbook of qualitative geography*. London: SAGE.

Denzin, N.K. (2002). Social work in the seventh moment. *Qualitative Social Work, 1*(1), 25–38.

Denzin, N.K. (2003). *Performance ethnography: Critical pedagogy and the politics of culture*. Thousand Oaks: Sage.

Denzin, N.K., & Lincoln, Y.S. (Eds.) (2011). *The SAGE handbook of qualitative research* 4th edn. Thousand Oaks: Sage.

Dewsbury, J.D. (2010). Performative, non-representational, and affect based research: seven injunctions. In D. DeLyser, S. Herbert, S. Aitken, M. Crang and L. McDowell (eds) *The SAGE Handbook of Qualitative Geography*, New York: Sage.

Downing, M.J. & Tenney, L.J. (2008). *Video vision: Changing the culture of social science research*. Newcastle on Tyne: Cambridge Publishers.

Drew, S.E., Duncan, R.E., & Sawyer, S.M. (2010). Visual storytelling: A beneficial but challenging method for health research with young people. *Qualitative Health Research, 20*(12), 1677–1688.

Eisner, E. (2008). Art and knowledge. In Knowles, J.G., & Cole, A.L. (2008). *Handbook of the arts in qualitative research: Perspectives, methodologies, examples, and issues*. Thousand Oaks: Sage, 3–12.

Findholt, N.E., Michael, Y.L., & Davis, M.M. (2010). Photovoice engages rural youth in childhood obesity prevention. *Public Health Nursing, 28*(2), 186–192.

Finley, S. (2008). Arts-based research. In Knowles, J.G., & Cole, A.L. (2008). *Handbook of the arts in qualitative research: Perspectives, methodologies, examples, and issues*. Thousand Oaks: Sage, 71–81.

Frohmann, L. (2005). The framing safety project: Photographs and narratives by battered women. *Violence Against Women, 11*(11), 1396–1419.

Goodhart, F.W., Hsu, J., Baek, J.H., Coleman, A.L., Maresca, F.M., & Miller, M.B. (2006). A view through a different lens: Photovoice as a tool for student advocacy. *Journal of American College Health, 55*, 53–56.

Gray, R.E., Sinding, C., & Fitch, M.I. (2001). Navigating the social context of metastatic breast cancer: Reflections on a project linking research to drama. *Health, 5*(2), 233–248.

Hamera, J.A. (2011) Performance ethnography. In D Soyini Madison (ed.) *Critical ethnography: Method, ethics and performance*. Los Angeles: Sage.

Higgs, G.E. (2008). Psychology: Knowing the self through arts. In Knowles, J.G., & Cole, A.L. (2008). *Handbook of the arts in qualitative research: Perspectives, methodologies, examples, and issues*. Thousand Oaks: Sage, 545–556.

Iedema, R., Long, D., Forsyth, R., & Bonsan, L.B. (2006). Visibilising clinical work: Video ethnography in the contemporary hospital. *Health Sociology Review, 15*(2), 156–168.

Ignagni, E., & Church, K. (2008). Disability studies and the ties and tensions with arts-informed inquiry: One more reason to look away? In Knowles, J.G., & Cole, A.L. (2008). *Handbook of the arts in qualitative research: Perspectives, methodologies, examples, and issues*. Thousand Oaks: Sage, 625–638.

Jackson, P., & Russell, P. (2010). Life history interviewing. In D. DeLyser, S. Herbert, S. Aitken, M. Crang and L. McDowell (eds) *The SAGE Handbook of Qualitative Geography*, New York: Sage.

Johnstone, M.J. (1999) Reflective topical autobiography: an under utilised interpretive research method in nursing. *Collegian* 6(1), 24–29.

Knowles, J.G., & Cole, A.L. (2008). *Handbook of the arts in qualitative research: Perspectives, methodologies, examples, and issues*. Thousand Oaks: Sage.

Kontos, P.C., & Naglie, G. (2006). Expressions of personhood in Alzheimer's: moving from ethnographic text to performing ethnography. *Qualitative Research, 6*(3), 301–317.

Lapum, J., Ruttonsha, P., Church, K., Yau, T., & Matthews, D.A. (2011). Employing the arts in research as an analytical tool and dissemination method: Interpreting experience through the aesthetic. *Qualitative Inquiry, 18*(1) 100–115.

Lorenz, L.S. (2011). A way into empathy: A 'case' of photo-elicitation in illness research. *Health, 15*(3), 259–275.

Madison, D.S. (2008). Critical ethnography as street performance: Reflections of home, race, murder, and justice. In Denzin, N.K., & Lincoln, Y.S. (Eds.) *Strategies for qualitative inquiry*. Thousand Oaks: Sage, 243–256.

Magilvy, J.K., Congdon, J.G., Nelson, J.P., & Craig, C. (1992). Visions of rural aging: Use of photographic method in gerontological research. *The Gerontologist, 32*(2), 253–257.

Martin, N., Garcia, A.C., & Leipert, B. (2010). Photovoice and its potential use in nutrition and dietetic research. *Canadian Journal of Dietetic Practice and Research, 71*(2), 93–97.

McDowell, L. (2010). Interviewing: Fear and liking in the field. In D. DeLyser, S. Herbert, S. Aitken, M. Crang and L. McDowell (eds) *The SAGE Handbook of Qualitative Geography*, New York: Sage.

McNiff, J. & Whitehead, J. (2008) Demonstrating quality in action research for social accountability. In S. Noffke and B. Somekh (eds) *The SAGE Handbook of Educational Action Research*. London, Sage.

Myers, E. (2008). Midwife to Gaia, birthing global consciousness: A reflective topical autobiography. Unpublished PhD Thesis, Southern Cross University, Lismore, NSW, Australia.

Nisker, J. (2008). Health-policy research and the possibilities of theater. In Knowles, J.G., & Cole, A.L. (2008). *Handbook of the arts in qualitative research: Perspectives, methodologies, examples, and issues*. Thousand Oaks: Sage, 613–624.

Novek, S., Morris-Oswald, T., & Menec, V. (2012). Using photovoice with older adults: Some methodological strengths and issues. *Ageing & Society, 32*, 451–470.

Nuremberg Code (1947) In Mitscherlich, A. & Mielke, F. (1949) *Doctors of infamy: The story of the Nazi medical crimes*. New York: Schuman, xxiii–xxv. Retrieved September 7, 2012 from http://www.cirp.org/library/ethics/nuremberg.

Richardson, L. (2003). Writing: A method of inquiry. In Denzin, N.K., & Lincoln, Y.S. (Eds.) (2003). *Collecting and interpreting qualitative materials,* 2nd edn. Thousand Oaks: Sage, 499–541.

Smith, C.A., & Gallo, A.M. (2007). Applications of performance ethnography in nursing. *Qualitative Health Research* 17(4), 521–528.

Spry, T. (2011). Performative autoethnography: Critical embodiments and possibilities. In Denzin, N.K., & Lincoln, Y.S. (Eds.) (2011). *The SAGE handbook of qualitative research* 4th edn. Thousand Oaks: Sage, 497–511.

Tenney, L.J., & MacCubbin, P. (2008). When no one was watching: Human subjects protections and videotaping (take one). In Downing, M.J., & Tenney, L.J. (Eds.) Video vision: Changing the culture of social science research. Newcastle Upon Tyne, UK: Cambridge Scholars Publishing, 14–79.

Washington, O.G.M. & Moxley, D.P. (2008). From narrative to exhibit in illuminating the lived experience of homelessness among older African American women. *USA Journal of Health Psychology*, 13(2), 154–165

Watson, A., & Till, K.E. (2010). Ethnography and participant observation. In D. DeLyser, S. Herbert, S. Aitken, M. Crang and L. McDowell (eds) *The SAGE Handbook of Qualitative Geography*, New York: Sage.

Zammit, C. (2008). The experience of dying: A reflective topical autobiography. Unpublished PhD Thesis, Southern Cross University, Lismore, NSW, Australia.

17

Uptake of qualitative research in health sciences

Karen Francis

This chapter discusses the uptake of qualitative research in health sciences. Health professionals are encouraged, indeed expected, to base practice on evidence. Traditionally, incontestable outcomes of research such as the randomized clinical trial were viewed as the most reliable forms of evidence to inform practice. While the evidence arising from studies of this nature was useful, many aspects of healthcare service delivery did not lend themselves to these types of investigations. To accommodate the humanism of healthcare, evidence is drawn from both quantitative and qualitative studies and is informing healthcare service delivery. Combining studies and performing meta-analysis of the data achieve strengthening of the evidence provided by small-scale quantitative and qualitative studies. Nonetheless all rigorous research studies have the potential to inform practice and therefore health outcomes.

Interdisciplinary collaboration in health sciences research

As the 21st century dawned a new discourse started to infiltrate the world of research, interdisciplinary practice, and collaborative interprofessional/ interdisciplinary/transdisciplinary research. Major funding bodies in Australia changed their instructions to researchers promoting projects submitted by collaborative, interdisciplinary and international teams. There was a relaxation of the focus on large-scale intervention style quantitative studies to ones that embraced more holistic investigations of health concerns and incorporated both physiological and social causation of ill health. In short, there has been a move from the dominance of the biomedical research agenda to one that at least recognizes that health outcomes will only be achieved when the totality of what makes us human is understood and included in research endeavours.

Practice development

Engaging in reflective practice to promote best practice has been a commonly discussed expectation of health professions for many decades. In recent years nursing internationally has adopted a research-inspired approach to reviewing, renewing and promoting best practice: practice development (NSW Nursing and Midwifery Office, 2012). Practice development (PD)

> is a continuous process of developing person-centred cultures. It is enabled by facilitators who authentically engage with individuals and teams to blend personal qualities and creative imagination with practice skills and practice wisdom. The learning that occurs brings about transformation of individual and team practices. This is sustained by embedding both processes and outcomes in corporate strategy.
>
> (Manley, McCormack and Wilson 2008, p. 9
> cited by NSW Nursing and Midwifery Office, 2012)

A discourse analysis of PD was undertaken that demonstrated that this methodology has become synonymous with quality improvement (Rudge, Holmes, and Perron, 2011) and as such is accepted and advocated by healthcare organizations wanting to improve the efficiency and effectiveness of healthcare (NSW Nursing and Midwifery Office, 2012). Teams of healthcare professionals who have utilized PD methodology have been empowered to appraise and refine their practice. Practice development is similar to action research methodology in that it is action orientated and involves groups of people who interact collaboratively to achieve a common goal and objectives.

There are numerous examples of research projects that have adopted a PD framework to address a problem that is inclusive of supporting those involved to refine their skills and knowledge for a common outcome. Dempsey (2008) reported that reducing the incidence of falls in acute care and residential aged care environments is an effective method for limiting risk to patients and residents (aged care). She led a practice development project to promote improved falls risk management procedures. PD techniques were employed to support a group of nurses assess current practice, review the contemporary literature and construct a falls risk chart to guide practice that was more useful than the instrument previously used in the context in which the project occurred (Dempsey, 2008). Managing continence in residential aged care was the focus of another project that utilized practice development methodology to augment cultural change that embraced person-centred and evidenced-based clinical practice (Parlora and McCormack, 2012). These exemplars support the contention that PD does support the quality care agenda and also highlights the importance of supporting teams to capitalize on their expertise and to utilize evidence to underpin change. Healthcare professionals contribute to the generation of evidence as well as the translation of research in their practice. The context in which practice occurs has a direct impact on the usefulness of research evidence. Research that is produced in controlled environments using state-of-the-art technologies managed by experienced experts is not always transferrable. Healthcare professionals who work in human, fiscal and resource-poor contexts need to modify practice recommendations to meet their specific needs. New generations of healthcare professionals have research and clinical decision making skills that facilitate reflexive, innovative and evidence informed practice.

Qualitative research translation

Best practice guidelines are advocated as the gold standard for guiding practice delivery. Based on empirical evidence, best practice guidelines are summaries of current research (Nagy, Mills, Waters, and Birks, 2010). The Joanna Briggs Institute (JBI) and the Cochrane Collaboration are two international entities that generate evidence reports and practice guidelines for healthcare professionals. The JBI evolved initially to support best practice for nursing, midwifery and allied health (Joanna Briggs Institute, 2012b) while the Cochrane Collaboration was originally established to produce systematic reviews of research to support medical practice that was primarily focused on interventions (Volmink, Siegfried, Roberston, and Metin Gulmezoglu, 2004). The Cochrane Collaboration adopted a process for ranking research that gave primacy to the randomized clinical trial and dismissed as poor, any research that used small samples and methodologies that could not produce statistically significant irrevocable results (Joanna Briggs Institute, 2012a). The JBI recognized that much of the evidence produced by nursing and midwifery used qualitative research methodologies. To accommodate this research diversity and in recognition of the ontological as well as epistemological nature of nursing and midwifery practice JBI established methods for appraising, synthesizing and developing best practice guidelines that encompass the breath of excellent research (Joanna Briggs Institute, 2012a). JBI states that

> the Institute and its collaborating entities promote and support the synthesis, transfer and utilisation of evidence through identifying feasible, appropriate, meaningful and effective healthcare practices to assist in the improvement of healthcare outcomes globally.
> (Joanna Briggs Institute, 2012b)

The JBI and the Cochrane Collaboration publish systematic reviews that are a meta-syntheses of the available evidence that has been ranked against rigorous inclusion criteria (Cochrane Collaboration, 2012; Joanna Briggs Institute, 2012b). From these data evidence summaries and best practice guidelines are produced for the use of healthcare professionals.

Future directions

Healthcare is dynamic. Each day new research is generated and new technologies developed that revolutionize how healthcare professionals practise, and how consumers experience the healthcare system. The development of Medical Radiation Imaging (MRI) (Online, 2012) and the isolation of a vaccine to prevent cervical cancers (Cancer Council Australia, 2012) are among the new technologies that have impacted on healthcare professionals who have adjusted their diagnostic and therapeutic intervention regimes to accommodate them. The impact of such innovations on humanity is hard to estimate. There is agreement internationally however that these and other technologies save lives although the costs of development and ongoing refinement, marketing and training associated with delivering healthcare are significant and must be balanced against individual nations' financial capacity (Francis, Chapman, Hoare, and Birks, 2013). Burgeoning healthcare costs are a phenomenon that the most industrialized nations are attempting to address. Developing nations are struggling with the other challenges that include the provision of basic requirements of adequate food, clean water, shelter, waste disposal systems, clothing and access to education. These nations are reliant on the developed world to support healthcare and other technological advances as they do not have the resource base to fund development and implementation where it is necessary. New biological threats such as Avian and Swine Flu and environmental concerns arising from climate change have impacted on all nations. Increased global collaboration to address world health problems and improve population health was recognized and endorsed in 1978 with the signing of the Alma Ata Declaration, and the subsequent international health declarations that continued to isolate improved health status as their primary directive (Francis et al., 2013). The developed and the developing world are encouraged by the World Health Organization to work collaboratively to achieve 'health for all'. Healthcare professionals are the forefront of this agenda in roles that range from prevention to intervention of ill health. Their effectiveness is reliant on their currency of knowledge and capacity to be reflexive.

Participating in the generation and translation of research for practice is an important role of all contemporary healthcare professionals. Knowledge translation guarantees that the best available evidence is understood and informs clinical and non-clinical decision making. A project to establish best practice guidelines for maintaining skin integrity was undertaken in an acute care hospital. Staff were engaged in a process that utilized qualitative and quantitative research methods to review practice, complete an audit of records to identify the numbers and types of skin integrity breakdown and to establish a quality improvement process (Gardiner et al., 2008). Engaging the end users of research in processes that promote research critique, practice innovation and that result in best practice is the future of healthcare practice and a challenge for all clinicians and those involved in health professionals' education. Informed consumers of research understand the breadth of research traditions and their applicability for making sense of the world and the people who reside within it. Bayes et al. (2008) completed a study of women's experiences of labour and birth at a Western Australian Women's Hospital (Bayes, Fenwick, and Hauck, 2008). The data collection was accomplished using a questionnaire instrument that included quantitative and qualitative questions. The qualitative questions asked women to share their experiences of the phenomenon of labour and birthing. These data were analysed using a recursive and integrative thematic approach. The researchers concluded that women experienced varying levels of fear and argued that healthcare professionals, midwives, doctors and nurses can limit anxiety if they provide information, are empathetic and support women's choices. Research conducted to improve mental health service provision by community nurses and general medical practitioners incorporated a mixed method approach (Annells et al., 2011). A systematic review of the literature provided direction for the construction of a clinical pathway to enhance early identification of mental health concerns among a targeted population, war veterans, and prompt appropriate intervention. Nurses and general practitioners were involved in the research as experts providing advice and as participants reviewing and commenting on the efficacy of the developed clinical pathway. These two research studies demonstrate the importance of research for healthcare professions, consumers and health outcomes.

Incorporating research into practice, irrespective of the setting, is an expectation of employers and consumers. Appreciation of research for the contribution and the science that underpins it is an important criteria for evaluating and accepting evidence.

Chapter summary

This chapter has described the impact of research on healthcare and the implications for practice. Practice development as one methodology supporting the translation of research to practice and as a research generation technique has been described. The development of evidence-based practice guidelines that are inclusive of qualitative as well as quantitative research was highlighted as affirmation of changed views regarding quality research. Healthcare must be underpinned by quality research that provides for investigation of the human condition irrespective of research bias, context or the healthcare professionals providing the service.

Key points

- In the 21st century interdisciplinary practice, collaborative research, interprofessional/interdisciplinary/transdisciplinary research have caused a move from the dominance of the biomedical research agenda to one that at least recognizes that health outcomes will only be achieved when the totality of what makes us human is understood and included in research endeavours.

- Teams of healthcare professionals who have utilized PD methodology have been empowered to appraise and refine their practice.

- Best practice guidelines are advocated as the gold standard for guiding practice delivery.

- The JBI and the Cochrane Collaboration publish systematic reviews that are meta-syntheses of the available evidence that has been ranked against rigorous inclusion criteria, from which evidence summaries and best practice guidelines are produced for the use of healthcare professionals.

- Participating in the generation and translation of research for practice is an important role of all contemporary healthcare professionals.

- Incorporating research into practice, irrespective of the setting, is an expectation of employers and consumers.

- Appreciation of research for the contribution and the science that underpins it is an important criterion for evaluating and accepting evidence.

Critical review questions

1 The provision of quality healthcare is an expectation of governments and of consumers. Discuss the methods by which clinicians can contribute to improved healthcare.

2 Discuss the contribution of evidence-based practice guidelines to healthcare.

References

Annells, M., Allen, J., Russell, N., Lang, L., Petrie, E., Clark, E., & Robins, A. (2011). An evaluation of a mental health screening and referral pathway for community nursing care: Nurses's and general practitioners perspectives. *Journal of Clinical Nursing 20*, 214–226.

Bayes, S., Fenwick, J., & Hauck, Y. (2008). A qualitative analysis of women's short accounts of labour and birth in a Western Australian public tertiary hospital. *Journal of Midwifery & Women's Health, 53*(1), 53–61.

Cancer Council Australia. (2012). Cervical cancer vaccine. Retrieved 24 November, 2012, from http://www.cervicalcancervaccine.org.au/.

Cochrane Collaboration. (2012). The Cochrane Collaboration: Working together to provide the best evidence for healthcare. Retrieved 24 November, 2012, from http://www.cochrane.org/.

Dempsey, J. (2008). Practice development in action. *Contemporary Nurse, 29*(2), 123–134.

Francis, K., Chapman, Y., Hoare, K., & Birks, M. (2013). *Community as partner: Theory and practice in Australia and New Zealand.* Sydney: Lippincott, Williams & Wilkins.

Gardiner, L., Lampshire, S., Biggins, A., McMurray, A., Noake, N., van Zyl, M., & Edgar, M. (2008). Evidenced-based best practice in maintaining skin integrity. *Wound Practice & Research, 16*(2), 5–15.

Joanna Briggs Institute. (2012a). Systematc reviews. Retrieved 24 November 2012 from: http://www.joannabriggs.edu.au/Systematic Reviews.

Joanna Briggs Institute. (2012b). Welcome to the Joanna Briggs Institute. Retrieved 24 November 2012, from: http://www.joannabriggs.edu.au/.

Manley, K., McCormack, B. & Wilson, V. (2008). *International practice development in nursing and healthcare.* Oxford: Blackwell.

Nagy, S., Mills, J., Waters, D., & Birks, M. (2010). *Using research in healthcare practice.* Broadway: Wolters Kluwer, Lippincott, Williams & Wilkins.

NSW Nursing and Midwifery Office. (2012). Practice development Retrieved 21 November 2012 from: http://www0.health.nsw.gov.au/nursing/practice_development.asp.

Online, N.S.W.H. (2012). Impact of emerging new treatments and technologies on healthcare, e.g. cost and access, benefits of early detection. Retrieved 24 November 2012, from: http://hsc.csu.edu.au/pdhpe/core1/focus/focus1_4/4009/1-3-1/health_pri1_3_1_5.htm.

Parlora, R., & McCormack, B. (2012). Blending critical realist and emacipatory practice development methodologies: Making critical realism work in nursing research. *Nursing Inquiry, 19*(4), 308–321.

Rudge, T., Holmes, D., & Perron, A. (2011). The rise of practice development with/in reformed bureaucracy: Discourse, power and the governent of nursing. *Journal of Nursing Management, 19*, 837–844.

Volmink, J., Siegfried, N., Roberston, K., & Metin Gulmezoglu, A. (2004). Research synthesis and dissemination as a bridge to knowledge management: The Cochrane Collaboration. *Bulletin of the World Health Organization, 82*, 778–783.

Index

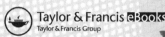